CLINICAL ADVANCES IN PHYSICAL MEDICINE AND REHABILITATION

Frederic J. Kottke, M.D., Ph.D.
Esther Alicia Amate, M.D.
Editors

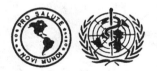

Scientific Publication No. 533

PAN AMERICAN HEALTH ORGANIZATION
Pan American Sanitary Bureau, Regional Office of the
WORLD HEALTH ORGANIZATION
525 Twenty-third Street, N.W.
Washington, D.C. 20037, U.S.A.

1991

PAHO Library Cataloguing in Publication Data

Kottke, Frederic J.
   Clinical advances in physical medicine and
rehabilitation / [edited by] Frederic J. Kottke ;
Esther Alicia Amate. — Washington, D.C. : PAHO,
1991. — 462 p.
   (Scientific Publication ; 533)

ISBN 92 75 11533 8

I. Amate, Esther Alicia
II. Pan American Health Organization
III. Title
1. PHYSICAL MEDICINE
NLM WB460

IV. (Series)
2. REHABILITATION

ISBN 92 75 11533 8

CONTENTS

CONTRIBUTORS

Norman A. Aliga, M.D.
Rehabilitation Medicine Clinic, S.C., Marianjoy Rehabilitation Center, Wheaton, Illinois, U.S.A.

José J. Arvelo, M.D.
Former Chief Physician, Department of Medical Rehabilitation, Ministry of Health and Social Welfare, Venezuela; Member, WHO Expert Committee on Disability Prevention and Rehabilitation

Paul Bach-y-Rita, M.D.
Professor, Department of Rehabilitation Medicine, University of Wisconsin Medical School, Madison, Wisconsin, U.S.A.

Sheldon Berrol, M.D.
Associate Clinical Professor, Physical Medicine and Rehabilitation, University of California, San Francisco, California, U.S.A.

Ralph Buschbacher, M.D.
Chief Resident, Department of Physical Medicine and Rehabilitation, Medical College of Virginia, Virginia Commonwealth University, Richmond, Virginia, U.S.A.

Jeffrey S. Cameron, M.D.
Rehabilitation Medicine Clinic, S.C., Marianjoy Rehabilitation Center, Wheaton, Illinois, U.S.A.

Sandra S. Cole, Ph.D.
Professor and Director, Sexuality Training Center and Sexuality Evaluation Clinic, Department of Physical Medicine and Rehabilitation, University of Michigan Medical Center, Ann Arbor, Michigan, U.S.A.

Theodore M. Cole, M.D.
Professor and Chairman, Department of Physical Medicine and Rehabilitation, University of Michigan Medical Center, Ann Arbor, Michigan, U.S.A.

John F. Ditunno, Jr., M.D.
Michie Professor of Rehabilitation Medicine and Chairman of the Department, Thomas Jefferson University Hospital, Philadelphia, Pennsylvania, U.S.A.

William H. Donovan, M.D.
Executive Vice President for Medical Affairs, Institute for Rehabilitation and Research, The Texas Medical Center; and Professor, Physical Medicine and Rehabilitation, Baylor College of Medicine, Houston, Texas, U.S.A.

Daniel Dumitru, M.D.
Associate Professor and Deputy Chairman, Department of Rehabilitation Medicine, University of Texas Health Science Center at San Antonio, San Antonio, Texas, U.S.A.

Steven V. Fisher, M.D.
Chief, Department of Physical Medicine and Rehabilitation, Hennepin County Medical Center; and Associate Professor, University of Minnesota Medical School, Minneapolis, Minnesota, U.S.A.

Donald C. Fletcher, M.D.
Assistant Professor, Department of Ophthalmology, University of South Florida, Tampa, Florida, U.S.A.

Murray M. Freed, M.D.
Professor and Chairman, Department of Rehabilitation Medicine, Boston University School of Medicine; and Chief of Service, Department of Rehabilitation Medicine, The University Hospital, Boston, Massachusetts, U.S.A.

Lynn H. Gerber, M.D.
Chief, Department of Rehabilitation Medicine, Clinical Center, National Institutes of Health, Bethesda, Maryland, U.S.A.

Daniel Halpern, M.D.
Clinical Professor, Department of Rehabilitation Medicine, Tufts University-New England Medical Center, Boston, Massachusetts, U.S.A.

Lauro S. Halstead, M.D.
Director, Post Polio Program, National Rehabilitation Hospital; and Clinical Professor, Department of Medicine, Georgetown University Medical School, Washington, D.C., U.S.A.

Richard F. Harvey, M.D.
Rehabilitation Medicine Clinic, S.C., Marianjoy. Rehabilitation Center, Wheaton, Illinois, U.S.A.

Rebecca D. Jackson, M.D.
Department of Physical Medicine and Internal Medicine, The Ohio State University, Columbus, Ohio, U.S.A.

Ernest W. Johnson, M.D.
Professor, Physical Medicine and Rehabilitation, The Ohio State University, Columbus, Ohio, U.S.A.

John C. King, M.D.
Assistant Professor, Department of Rehabilitation Medicine, University of Texas Health Science Center at San Antonio, San Antonio, Texas, U.S.A.

W. Jerry Mysiw, M.D.
Department of Physical Medicine and Internal Medicine, The Ohio State University, Columbus, Ohio, U.S.A.

Stephen F. Noll, M.D.
Consultant in Physical Medicine and Rehabilitation, Mayo Clinic, Rochester, Minnesota, U.S.A.

Richard R. Owen, M.D.
Medical Director, Sister Kenny Institute, Minneapolis, Minnesota, U.S.A.

Livio Paolinelli Monti, M.D.
Professor, Physical Medicine and Rehabilitation Service, Clinical Hospital, University of Chile, Santiago, Chile

Gladys del Peso Droguett
Assistant Professor, Medical Technology, Clinical Hospital, University of Chile, Santiago, Chile

Somayaji Ramamurthy, M.D.
Professor, Department of Anesthesia, University of Texas Health Science Center at San Antonio, San Antonio, Texas, U.S.A.

Elizabeth A. Rivers, O.T.R., R.N.
Part-time Clinical Instructor, University of Minnesota; and Burn Rehabilitation Specialist, Ramsey Medical Center, St. Paul, Minnesota, U.S.A.

Karen Snowden Rucker, M.D.
Associate Professor and Chairman, Department of Physical Medicine and Rehabilitation, Medical College of Virginia, Virginia Commonwealth University, Richmond, Virginia, U.S.A.

Vinod Sahgal, M.D.
Professor, Departments of Neurology and Rehabilitation Medicine, Northwestern University Medical School, Chicago, Illinois, U.S.A.

John E. Sarno, M.D.
Professor, Clinical Rehabilitation Medicine, New York University School of Medicine, New York, New York, U.S.A.

Martha Taylor Sarno, M.D.
Professor, Clinical Rehabilitation Medicine, New York University School of Medicine, New York, New York, U.S.A.

Burton J. Silverstein, Ph.D.
Marianjoy Rehabilitation Center, Wheaton, Illinois, U.S.A.

William E. Staas, Jr., M.D.
President and Medical Director, Magee Rehabilitation Hospital, Philadelphia, Pennsylvania, U.S.A.

Stanley F. Wainapel, M.D., M.P.H.
Associate Professor of Clinical Rehabilitation Medicine, College of Physicians and Surgeons, Columbia University, New York, New York, U.S.A.

Nicolas E. Walsh, M.D.
Professor and Chairman, Department of Rehabilitation Medicine, University of Texas Health Science Center at San Antonio, San Antonio, Texas, U.S.A.

Yeongchi Wu, M.D.
Associate Professor, Department of Rehabilitation Medicine, Northwestern University-McGaw Medical Center; and Director, Amputee Program, Rehabilitation Institute of Chicago, Chicago, Illinois, U.S.A.

FOREWORD

Demographic trends indicate that the population of the Region of the Americas is becoming older and more urban—characteristics which are risk factors in the appearance of impairments and disabilities. The elderly population as a whole tends to suffer a high prevalence of these conditions, but individuals of all ages fall victim to accidents and increasingly to violence, and these causes are giving rise to a growing number of disabilities.

The economic crisis in the countries of Latin America and the Caribbean has disproportionately affected the most unprotected groups. In all the countries the prevalence of disabilities and handicaps is higher in impoverished areas; among children and adolescents, disability rates reach values 10 times higher than in developed countries.

The provision of rehabilitation services is generally insufficient and fragmented. The percentage of general hospitals that offer rehabilitative care is very low, ranging between 4% and 14.5%. Compounding this deficit, the education and training of health personnel only exceptionally includes subject matter related to disability. For example, of the 255 faculties and schools of medicine in Latin America and the Caribbean only 6 offer courses in rehabilitation medicine in their basic curriculum.

The Pan American Health Organization considers improving the health of disabled persons to constitute an important challenge. Since the problems faced by the disabled have social and cultural components, a comprehensive and integrated approach within the overall field of public health needs to be adopted.

This publication is directed both to health professionals who specialize in rehabilitation and to generalists. It serves to bridge the gap between community-based rehabilitation, to which PAHO/WHO has dedicated several publications, and the specialized clinical level. We are confident that this book will contribute to enhanced care through providing up-to-date knowledge regarding treatment of the consequences of injuries and disease, and in so doing will benefit an ever-growing number of people.

Carlyle Guerra de Macedo
Director

PREFACE

This publication responds to the need of health professionals in the countries of the Americas for an update on knowledge of the clinical practice of physiatry. The Pan American Health Organization, through the rehabilitation component of its Health of Adults Program, was cognizant of this need, realizing that, in Latin American countries in particular, disadvantageous currency exchange rates prevent most physiatrists from subscribing to the medical journals in which advances are first presented. As a consequence, the most recent information generally available to these physiatrists is contained in textbooks published before 1982. By providing access to the significant clinical information that has come to light over the past 10 years, this publication will greatly enhance the care offered by the practitioners of physical medicine and rehabilitation in those countries. It is recognized that this book also will be valuable to physiatrists in the United States of America, Canada, and elsewhere, because it summarizes in one volume the best of current practices.

The contents of *Clinical Advances in Physical Medicine and Rehabilitation* reflect the most significant clinical areas of physiatry. Physiatrists with special interest in and knowledge of a specific area were invited to select and discuss the important clinical advances that had been reported since 1980. The attempt was made to describe the techniques and equipment involved in these advances in adequate detail so that the clinician can apply them in practice. The wide range of subjects covered represents the major medical problems evaluated and managed by the physiatrist, including brain injuries and encephalopathies, arthritis, amputations, spinal-cord injuries, decubiti, maintenance during intensive care, rehabilitation and maintenance of the frail elderly, burns, acute and chronic pain, multiple sclerosis, and speech and communication problems. Two chapters deal with the clinical phenomenon frequently referred to as "recurrence of poliomyelitis," in which the deteriorations associated with aging add to the impairment resulting from acute polio. Other chapters focus on the rehabilitation management of developmental disabilities and the potential of the central nervous system to compensate and at least partially restore function. The management of visual impairments is discussed, as are advances in the diagnostic techniques of electrodiagnosis and sensory evoked potentials. Functional electrical stimulation is described in applicable detail. Patients with sports injuries are seen by physiatrists with increasing frequency, and the best of current management is presented here. Because physiatrists are concerned with improving quality of life in all respects, both physical and psychological, a chapter on the management of problems related to sexuality is included. An introductory chapter presents an excellent discussion of the epidemiology of rehabilitation. As a compendium of the information that has appeared over the past 10 years, this volume constitutes a valuable and convenient reference for the physiatrist.

We wish to thank the authors of each of the chapters, who readily responded to our request that they give priority to this effort so that it could be produced in the shortest possible time. The value of this volume will be demonstrated by its usefulness to the daily practice of physiatrists throughout the Americas in their efforts to reduce handicaps and improve the quality of life of patients with disabilities.

Frederic J. Kottke, M.D., Ph.D.
Professor Emeritus
Department of Physical Medicine
  and Rehabilitation
University of Minnesota Medical
  School
Minneapolis, Minnesota

Esther Alicia Amate, M.D.
Regional Adviser on Rehabilitation
Health of Adults Program
Pan American Health Organization
Washington, D.C.

Chapter 1

Epidemiology and Rehabilitation

José J. Arvelo

INTRODUCTION

In today's world, the science of epidemiology is indispensable to the practice of medicine. The relationship of disease to the environment was noted by Hippocrates. In the XVII century Graunt saw value in gathering information on diseases, and Farr systematized this data collection in the XIX century, assigning importance to the frequency and distribution of diseases. On this basis, John Snow formulated and proved a hypothesis regarding the origin of the cholera epidemic of 1853 in London, thus laying the foundations of epidemiology as a science applied to the control of diseases.[6] (It is interesting to note that the word "epidemiology" was first coined in Spain by Villalba in 1802,[10] but that the Epidemiological Society of London was not founded until 1850.) However, only in the last 50 years has epidemiology achieved acceptance as the fundamental basis for diagnosis and control of health damages suffered by populations. Today it is believed that a health program cannot be satisfactory unless it is based on knowledge of the magnitude of the problem it addresses, invests its resources according to real priorities, and reorients its activities as the problem changes.

Epidemiology can be defined as a science concerned with the study of health, diseases, and health services among groups or populations, as opposed to the study of aspects of those phenomena as they affect individuals, cells, or molecular processes.[22] Thus, it is one of the sciences subsumed under the heading of public health, along with administration, biostatistics, sociology, demography, medical care, planning, and others.

Its historical evolution can be divided into three stages: (1) an initial *empirical* stage in which it was almost exclusively concerned with the phenomenon of epidemics; (2) a *scientific* stage that sought to describe and establish causal relationships between diseases and factors affecting the individual; and (3) an *ecological* stage that recognizes the importance of the environment in the production of disease and the need for research on the individual. In the second half of this century, the importance of applying epidemiology to the organization and evaluation of health services was recognized. This development marks the culmination of the *ecological-operative* stage and lays the foundation for a stage of *comprehensive epidemiology*, which will make possible the more efficient use of resources, strongly bolster preventive medicine, and aim to improve environmental hygiene.[8]

In Latin America rehabilitation is currently practiced primarily in large institutions, with an isolated and direct doctor-patient relationship. Epidemiology can become the principal instrument for diverting effort into a collective, comprehensive scheme that operates with a sense of social justice, in which the accessibility of services is not a matter of luck for the privileged population that lives close to them. "With the epidemiological approach, evaluation of health and health care services, as well as their organization and operation, acquires a new dimension which makes possible a systematic view of the health of a population, its social surroundings, the conditioning factors, and the true value of our actions. On a parallel, the delivery of services, the training of human resources; and research appear naturally linked."[15] Nevertheless, especially in rehabilitation, considering the multitude of factors that determine and condition disability, epidemiology must be understood as just one of many tools to be applied, since knowledge will also be needed from other branches of public health and even other professions such as economics, engineering, architecture, and marketing. But the most important activity of epidemiology will continue to be that of clearly identifying the profile of a disability in a population, its variations in response to the actions carried out, the risk factors affecting it, and its vulnerability to prevention. The epidemiology of disability can thus be defined as "the early study of disabling manifestations, of their magnitude, transcendence, and vulnerability in relation to the variables of space, time, persons, and living conditions prior to disability, during its treatment, and afterwards, analyzing its repercussions on individuals, families, and society."[19]

Today, the field of epidemiological practice is divided into four major groups of activities,[5] all of which are perfectly applicable to physical medicine and rehabilitation:

(1) studies of the *health situation* of different population groups, its determinants, and trends;
(2) *epidemiological surveillance* of diseases and other health problems;
(3) *causal and explanatory research* on priority health problems; and
(4) *evaluation* of the impact of the health services and other activities on individuals, the environment, and living conditions, and evaluation of the safety and impact of technology.

Thus, epidemiology is no longer limited to identifying the specific causes of high rates of morbidity and mortality. Rather, it is now the best instrument with which to devise policies; develop structures, plans, and services; evaluate their effects; and, furthermore, evaluate the overall context in which disease phenomena are produced, considering society as their source and as a resource for solving them.[12]

EPIDEMIOLOGICAL STUDIES OF DISABILITY

The International Classification of Impairments, Disabilities, and Handicaps (WHO)

For a long time, the start-up of services and development of rehabilitation programs were based on the assumption that there were enough disabled people to justify them. Throughout the years efforts have been made repeatedly, in both developed and developing countries, to measure the magnitude of the problem of disability. Twenty-seven prevalence studies were conducted in 18 countries[23] between 1961 and 1975; their results varied considerably—between 1% and 24.1%—owing to the diversity of the criteria used to define disability and the different methodologies employed. Based on these and other investigations, the World Health Organization (WHO) established 8% to 10% as the proportion of persons in the world disabled for medical reasons.[23] These figures are conservative if one considers the influence that socioeconomic factors certainly have.[11]

The Statistical Office, Department of International Economic and Social Affairs, United Nations Secretariat, has developed a World Bank of Statistical Information on the disabled, which contains information from more than 55 countries obtained through censuses and surveys conducted since 1975.[18] Three of the countries represented are from Central America, four from the Caribbean, and four from South America.[16] In general, the existing statistics on disability have been produced using different criteria and methodologies, making comparisons difficult. They have some value for allowing a clearer picture of the problem, but have little or no value for planning and developing national or local rehabilitation programs.

A lack of adequate data means that incidences of disease consequences cannot be compared, the effect of social interventions and health services cannot be measured, and basic statistics cannot be collected to enable better planning of prevention at various levels;[27] this is particularly true in the case of disability and rehabilitation.

The lack of a classification system for the statistics plays a prominent role in this confused and uncertain situation. The WHO International Classification of Diseases, even in its currently used ninth revision, only includes the "Supplementary Classification of Factors Influencing Health Status and Contact with the Health Services" (V codes) for classifying disabilities, which has not been used extensively in practice.

Concerned about this gap, WHO has promoted studies since 1971 which culminated in the experimental publication in 1980 of the "International

Classification of Impairments, Disabilities, and Handicaps" (ICIDH).[24] It was later translated into Spanish,[25] making it accessible to the Spanish-speaking countries. In brief, "impairment" is defined as a deviation from the norm in an individual's biomedical status with reference to a body part; "disability" is a deviation from the norm with reference to the functioning of the individual as a whole; and "handicap" denotes deviations that arise as the consequence of the interaction of the individual with his or her physical and social environment.

The impact of this classification is threefold:

(1) It broadly complements the WHO International Classification of Diseases in classifying the consequences of disabling diseases.
(2) It has a conceptual basis, establishing a progression from disease toward impairment, disability, and handicap (Figure 1).
(3) It provides an acceptable taxonomy and nomenclature for beginning to classify consequences of diseases. (However, the reservation must be expressed that the section on handicaps is not a taxonomy or a classification that applies to an individual, but rather depends upon the circumstances in which the disabled person may find himself.)

The appearance of this classification follows several applications and critiques carried out in various countries, as well as many important international meetings[17,26,27,29] that analyzed its value and applicability and from which modifications emerged. Its three basic areas of applicability are the production of statistics on the consequences of diseases, the gathering of relevant statistical data regarding the use of services, and the evaluation of

Figure 1. The relationship of the various etiologies to the progressive dysfunction of impairment, disability, and handicap.

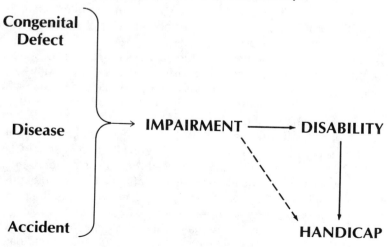

individuals with a view toward improving the grouping and registration of cases.[28]

A fourth area of possible applicability would be that the classification permits comparison of studies of risk factors conducted by different investigators in different circumstances.

In 1981 the Australian Bureau of Statistics[2] conducted a census of the disabled which broadly applied—possibly for the first time—the concepts and definitions of the ICIDH/WHO, although with some changes to adapt them to the characteristics of the census. The questionnaires were administered in three stages: first, to identify people with one or more impairments or disabilities; second, to determine who among them were handicapped; and third, to determine the characteristics and needs of the handicapped. The census found 4.6% of the general population to be disabled but without handicaps and 8.6% to be both disabled and handicapped, for a total of 13.2%. Of all persons with handicaps, 13.2% had severe ones; 24.1% had moderate ones; 20.7% had slight ones; and the severity of the handicap was not specified in 41.9% of the cases.

A survey conducted in Spain in 1986 is the most complete one known to the author in which the ICIDH/WHO was applied.[7] It was performed in a census sample of 75,000 dwellings that housed more than 270,000 people; the sample was representative of the Spanish population. The survey included two phases: detection of persons with disabilities, followed by research on the impairments and handicaps of those people. Diverse variables were analyzed: disabilities, impairments, and handicaps and their characteristics; care received in rehabilitation; economic benefits; and personal (age, sex, etc.), economic, social, and geographic variables. The results were tabulated for the country and the provinces. Overall totals were 14.98% of the general population as disabled and 6.03% with handicaps (Tables 1, 2, and 3).

The author is unaware of any formal study in Latin America in which the ICIDH/WHO was applied to determine the prevalence of disabilities, although some investigations of its value and applicability have been carried out.[4,20]

In light of current experience, the ICIDH/WHO is an indispensable tool for obtaining adequate and comparable statistics on disability and for applying epidemiology to rehabilitation.

APPLICATIONS OF EPIDEMIOLOGY TO REHABILITATION

The development of rehabilitation programs as an integral part of the health services in a country has three fundamental components: integration, intersectoral coordination, and planning.[1] Integration means that health actions should be an indivisible whole with integrated objectives that include rehabilitation, rather than the latter being a "separate" program. This ap-

Table 1. Percentage of persons with impairments, by sex, Spain, 1986.

Impairment	Male	Female	Both sexes
Psychological			
Profound mental retardation	0.13	0.11	0.12
Severe mental retardation	0.24	0.17	0.20
Moderate mental retardation	0.20	0.10	0.15
Mental diseases	0.38	0.55	0.47
Other	0.28	0.18	0.23
Sensory			
Total hearing loss	0.24	0.28	0.26
Hearing loss in one ear	0.83	0.93	0.88
Hearing impairment	1.16	1.28	1.22
Visual loss in both eyes	0.12	0.17	0.15
Visual loss in one eye	0.95	0.87	0.91
Visual impairment	0.83	1.40	1.12
Language impairment	0.34	0.15	0.24
Other	0.46	0.53	0.50
Physical			
Circulatory	1.89	2.54	2.22
Respiratory	1.25	0.64	0.94
Gastrointestinal	0.45	0.47	0.46
Reproductive/urinary	0.17	0.17	0.17
Nervous system	0.27	0.33	0.30
Endocrine/metabolic	0.65	1.03	0.84
Musculoskeletal:			
head and trunk	0.90	1.40	1.16
upper limbs	0.42	0.42	0.42
lower limbs	2.80	4.59	3.72
upper limb deficiencies	0.05	0.01	0.03
lower limb deficiencies	0.09	0.03	0.06
other	0.05	0.10	0.08
Mixed			
Cerebral palsy	0.05	0.05	0.05
Other	0.02	0.02	0.02
Nonspecific	2.12	4.05	3.11
Not recorded	0.01	0.01	0.01
Total with impairments	13.34	16.54	14.98

Source: Encuesta sobre discapacidades, deficiencias y minusvalías, 1986. Instituto Nacional de Estadísticas, España.

proach is particularly important today in light of the priority that should be given to prevention activities and community-based rehabilitation. Coordination must take account of the multisectoral nature of rehabilitation— its medical, educational, labor, and legal aspects, as well as private sector participation. The development of programs and rehabilitation services should be done with acute awareness of the need for linkage within the

Table 2. Percentage of persons with disabilities, by sex, Spain, 1986.

Disability	Male	Female	Both sexes
Vision			
Total blindness	0.13	0.17	0.15
Blind in one eye	0.98	0.91	0.94
Visual disability	0.93	1.58	1.27
Hearing			
Total deafness	0.28	0.33	0.30
Deaf in one ear	0.88	0.99	0.94
Hearing loss	1.25	1.47	1.36
Speech			
Mute	0.11	0.09	0.10
Severe stammering	0.12	0.05	0.08
Incomprehensible speech	0.46	0.21	0.33
Other communication			
Unable to read or write	0.59	0.49	0.54
Unable to make or understand graphic signs	0.44	0.41	0.42
Personal care	1.04	1.25	1.15
Ambulation			
Need wheelchair	0.24	0.33	0.29
Need some help	1.93	1.99	1.96
Climbing stairs	5.29	7.83	6.60
Running	8.53	12.40	10.51
Leaving house	1.35	2.85	2.12
ADL manipulations			
Open or close	0.70	0.90	0.80
Reaching and retrieval	1.60	2.50	2.06
Dependency/endurance			
On some equipment	0.30	0.23	0.26
On strict diet	1.56	1.20	1.78
Balance problems	1.39	2.52	1.97
Environmental	0.69	0.74	0.72
Difficulty identifying/understanding	0.82	0.84	0.83
Difficulty avoiding risks	0.43	0.52	0.48
Disabilities in relationships			
Drug abuse/alcoholism	0.21	0.02	0.11
Aggressiveness	0.20	0.08	0.14
Self-margination	0.55	0.73	0.64
Future disabilities	0.08	0.04	0.06
Total with disabilities	13.34	16.54	14.98

Source: Encuesta sobre discapacidades, deficiencias ỳ minusvalías, 1986. Instituto Nacional de Estadísticas, España.

Table 3. Percentage of persons with handicaps, by sex, Spain, 1986.

Handicap	Male	Female	Both sexes
Orientation	1.05	1.52	1.29
Physical independence	1.44	1.87	1.66
Mobility	1.70	3.22	2.47
Occupation	4.60	4.73	4.67
Social integration	1.65	1.85	1.75
Economic self-sufficiency	2.02	1.50	1.75
Disability without handicap	7.61	10.11	8.89
Not recorded	0.04	0.07	0.06
Total with handicaps	5.69	6.36	6.03

Source: Encuesta sobre discapacidades, deficiencias y minusvalías, 1986. Instituto Nacional de Estadísticas, España.

health sector (with other medical specialties—especially psychiatry, given the importance of mental disabilities) and between sectors (especially with education and labor, and in the formulation of legal provisions that affect the disabled). The need for effective and practical intra- and intersectoral coordination is greatest at the primary level of care.

Health planning means acting to solve a problem through better utilization of resources. Its methodology is essentially the ongoing execution and evaluation of a plan in which the objectives have been specified on the basis of prior diagnosis of the situation; goals must have been established, resources allocated according to priorities, and the results evaluated as to cost-effectiveness of the resources utilized. This is the basic methodology developed in 1962 by the Center for Development Studies of the Central University of Venezuela and technicians from PAHO/WHO (CENDES/PAHO). However, in practice it proved to be relatively rigid and hard to modify in the face of unpredictable social, economic, and political changes. The health-disease-disability process is not the result of purely biological factors. To a significant degree, it is also the product of interactions between the individual patient and his or her familial, social, economic, physical, and environmental setting. In the planning of rehabilitation services, research on conditioning factors external to the patient must be included and, to enable timely decision making, must reveal the interventions needed to produce favorable changes. To this end, classic policy-setting planning is being replaced by new concepts of strategic planning[9] which pose a pragmatic alternative in light of the continuous changes that take place in the external environment and are thus particularly valuable in rehabilitation. Planning includes the phases of diagnosis, programming, execution, and evaluation, which should be a continuous process that parallels execution. Epidemiology can make an important contribution to health planning through application of the epidemiological method and epidemiological research in all phases.

So far, epidemiological knowledge has been scantly applied to rehabilitation, particularly in Latin America and the Caribbean, for two principal reasons: (1) there has been no instrument to allow for the uniform production of comparable statistics (today this difficulty has been, or is being, overcome to a large degree with the ICIDH/WHO); and (2) physical medicine and rehabilitation, particularly with regard to evaluation, etiological diagnosis, and instrumental therapy, has developed as a very clinical specialty, limited to large hospitals or institutions. Rehabilitation programs and services must be rescaled—a task in which epidemiology will have to play an especially important role.

The application of epidemiology to rehabilitation is therefore intimately linked to the use and improvement of the ICIDH/WHO and the reorientation of current physical medicine and rehabilitation programs and services.

It would be difficult to analyze and describe all the possible applications of epidemiology in the field of physical medicine and rehabilitation. This paper merely attempts to point out the most relevant, among which are its usefulness:

- in diagnosing the problem of disability in the population;
- in setting guidelines for the administration of programs and services;
- in evaluating technologies, services, and programs; and
- in research.

Epidemiology in Diagnosing the Problem of Disability in the Population

A national rehabilitation plan cannot be imposed from the top down, that is, from the policy-setting levels to the operational levels. Rather, it must originate in the latter, with the definition of program areas dependent upon multiple criteria including political division, geographic characteristics, social and economic realities, and the existence of health resources. This "sectorization" facilitates application of the concept of equity, understood as equal opportunity for all in access to health services and expressed in the slogan "Health for All by the Year 2000." The strategy for attaining equity starts with the transformation of the national health systems based on development of the local health systems,[13] in which rehabilitation should be included. The necessary first step is to find out the true extent of disability in the local population. It is imperative to know the local situation, since national averages can hide the problems prevalent in some population groups and certain regions.[13]

The only way to discover the facts about disability in different population groups—the various types and their prevalence, their severity, the existing risk factors, and the susceptibility of each group—is through application of the epidemiological method for the following diagnostic purposes:

(1) to identify the frequency, distribution, and grades of severity of different types of disabling consequences of disease in the population;
(2) to identify the subgroups in the population at a higher risk for developing disabilities;
(3) to identify the risk factors susceptible to intervention, not only those within the medical purview but also in the physical and social environment and in the economic context;
(4) to determine the potential impact of the interventions;
(5) to identify the priority groups and areas for treatment; and
(6) to detect the variations that occur in the profile of disability in the population, in both time and space.

Epidemiology in Setting Guidelines for the Administration of Programs and Services

The ultimate goal in health administration is to control the harm caused to the population by an existing health problem or problems. The *control of disabilities* could be defined as the set of actions aimed at preventing, diagnosing, treating, and minimizing disabilities through the use of available techniques that meet standards of equity, cost-effectiveness, efficacy, applicability, and social acceptance. Therefore, a multitude of factors come into play, such as the design of a policy, formulation of a program, structuring of an information system, appropriate allocation of resources, and adequate training of personnel.

Program Design

A rehabilitation policy should be in harmony with the overall objective of health for all by the year 2000 and with the national health policy. It should be based on information produced at the operational levels, set priorities on the basis not only of the type of damages being addressed but also of their distribution among the most marginalized groups, be flexible in the face of change, and respond to biomedical, social, economic, and environmental realities as well as the availability of resources. All these goals will require information in several areas, which can only be made available through the epidemiological method.

Formulation of Plans and Care Programs

In order to improve the disability situation, it is necessary to define objectives and describe a process, which is the program and which gets translated into a document. The consolidation of programs that deal with different types of disability would be the plan. Programming is the second phase of health planning. This activity, like policy design, requires information, but information that is broader in scope as well as more detailed. Provision of epidemiological information is the only way to ensure that plans and programs are well reasoned and demographically sound.

Support for an Epidemiological Surveillance System

Epidemiological surveillance was long understood as a one-way flow of information from the operational level to the central level to aid decision making regarding infectious diseases, usually those for which reporting was compulsory. This simplistic concept has changed substantially in the past few decades to encompass a system with a two-way flow of information that affects policy making, the design and execution of programs, evaluation of the results of interventions, decision making, and guidelines for research projects to study new hypotheses. This broadly conceived epidemiological surveillance system includes three stages within a cycle of continuous evaluation: the gathering of appropriate information on the at-risk population under surveillance; analysis to determine the effects of the interventions conducted; and the response stage, in which new favorable changes are generated. The information-gathering stage is subject to the most obstacles and problems, but the analysis stage is the most difficult because it involves presenting the situation, explaining it, discovering changes that have occurred, and relating them to the interventions conducted.

In order for a system of epidemiological surveillance to be really efficient its structure should be *decentralized by levels*,[21] and the local level, rather than being simply a collector of information, becomes the most important one. It is at this level that valid and timely information is not only gathered but also analyzed and interpreted; the initial decisions should be made and their effects analyzed there. If the local level does not assume these responsibilities, good surveillance cannot be achieved. The regional level consolidates the information received, analyzes it, performs a second evaluation, and makes the decisions corresponding to that level. The national level consolidates the information received from the regions and utilizes it to redefine policies, modify standards, and make comparisons between regions and with other countries. The entire system must give constant feedback to the different levels to facilitate adequate interpretation and timely decision making.

In short, epidemiological surveillance is a permanent process of observation and evaluation of health damages and their severity or relative importance within a population, as well as the interventions carried out to control them. As applied to rehabilitation, the "damage" would be disability in its various forms. There are three basic sources of information:

- the medical and rehabilitation services themselves at all levels, through their record-keeping systems regarding activities performed, their effectiveness, and the population covered;

- household surveys that sample the population to be covered, which must be well designed, representative, uncomplicated, and economical; and
- the community itself through its civic leaders as well as those of cultural, sports, and volunteer organizations, for example.

Community involvement can take many forms. The community can participate in identifying hazards leading to disability so that it can recognize them, avoid them, or minimize them. It can cooperate in the process of diagnosing the magnitude of the disability problem and participate in logistical support actions and activities programmed for its benefit. The community can identify its positive or negative actions in relation to the disabled, participate in the task of reporting new cases of disability or those in need of new interventions, and provide support for the families of disabled persons and their own rehabilitation services.

Current programs and services for physical medicine and rehabilitation, at least in Latin America and the Caribbean, lack epidemiological surveillance systems on disability. This is essentially because of the intrinsic isolation of highly specialized institutional services, the indifference of specialists to the real needs of the population around them, and the ineffectiveness of existing epidemiological surveillance systems.

In conclusion, the following are the basic objectives of a system of epidemiological surveillance on disability:

- keeping up-to-date on the real extent of disability in a given area;
- defining the primary risk factors;
- supplying information to the decision-making process for the purpose of controlling the problem; and
- assessing the effectiveness of the interventions carried out.

Justification for the Allocation of Resources

In Latin America and the Caribbean the health sector is highly dependent on the economic resources provided to it by the State. This situation causes internal competition for the allocation of resources, and the flow of resources is affected by and dependent on such factors as the influence of groups with political, economic, and social power, as well as the real situation of health priorities, apparent demand, and other factors. In order to receive resources, specific health programs must have convincing justifications, which is where epidemiological information is decisive. In the area of rehabilitation, this consideration is particularly important because of the image of rehabilitation as highly specialized and confined to large health institutions, the existence of other priority problems, and the high cost of not only the human resources but the space and equipment required for diagnostic and therapeutic procedures.

Moreover, the image reflects reality. Rehabilitation is in fact offered almost exclusively in terciary health care institutions, without the necessary foundation at the lower levels. While the quality of care is high, coverage is restricted to "privileged groups" to the detriment of the "forgotten groups" that make up the majority of the population. The privileged groups have access to the existing services because they are fortunate enough to live in large cities that have third-level health care institutions and rehabilitation services and also usually have private organizations concerned with disability problems. The members of the privileged groups have political, economic, social, technical, and scientific clout and use it to ensure that the available resources continue to be put at their service. This situation is contrary to equity and may be the greatest challenge that rehabilitation faces today in Latin America, as a medical specialty and as a component of public health programs.

Although they are directed at a general analysis of the health sector, White's concepts[22] are applicable to rehabilitation when he says that in general the knowledge of clinical physicians "is usually based on educational experience that is largely limited to tertiary care hospitals, and there they concentrate on molecular and cellular processes. Many physicians, or the majority of them, especially those who work in academic clinical departments, know very little or nothing about the concepts, methods, and applications of epidemiology. Those are the academic physicians . . . who treat politicians and administrators from around the world, serve as advisors, and exert powerful influence based on their knowledge and the experience they have acquired in teaching hospitals. They are not up-to-date on the majority of the health problems that exist outside of the hospitals where the population lives, works, suffers, and dies. This distorted perspective and experience has caused serious imbalances in the organization of the health services, manpower training, and the establishment of priorities. The net effect is an absurd allocation of resources, unacceptable inequalities in access to health care, and an increase in the cost of care which threatens to bankrupt societies."

This general picture of health care, and specifically rehabilitation, can only change with the gathering of information—which only the epidemiological method can provide—so that resource allocation can be justified and strengthened. Thus, epidemiology is an indispensable instrument in the administration of rehabilitation programs, which need to reorient their resources and obtain new ones so that they may act on priorities while satisfying the need for equity.

Orientation of Training

Personnel in physical medicine and rehabilitation services should have not only a strong academic medical background and specialized training but also a comprehensive, demographic view of disability, to which epidemiology can contribute. This comprehensive, demographic view does not mean the physician is replaced by an epidemiologist. It means rather that the medical specialist should also be able to observe, analyze, and become aware of the true nature of the disability problems in his geographic work area so that he is better equipped to confront them and produce measurable improvements.

The training of human resources in rehabilitation has to become a co-ordinated activity within the common, complementary objectives of the institutions that train these resources and those that employ them. To this end, physical medicine and rehabilitation activities should be carried out within an infrastructure capable of supporting training programs. This means that the services cannot be hidden behind the walls of their institutions, as most of them are now, blind to the realities of disability among the population of their area. On the contrary, they should also take into account the need to gather and analyze statistical information, apply epidemiological knowledge, expand coverage, and evaluate the technologies they use. That is why the isolated training of physiatrists and technicians behind the walls of large health institutions is unacceptable and not even advisable, no matter how academically and scientifically competent the faculty is. In rehabilitation it is necessary to reach a state of integration between the delivery of services, teaching, and research with a demographic perspective. The idea that the problem will be solved simply by training more people must be considered inappropriate. Quantity and quality must go together, with quantity understood as a function of the programs of development and quality based not only on a high degree of scientific excellence but also on a set of attributes such as recognition of the need to stratify rehabilitation into levels of care; the concept of broad coverage of the activities carried out, taking their costs into account; and the ability to develop independent of the specialized commercial apparatus. The training of medical and technical human resources has to be integrated into policy, planning, and the programming of care services. For this reason the bureaus or departments of rehabilitation in the ministries of health and the social security systems have to find lines of common interest with the universities and rehabilitation curricula. In practice, medical-clinical and therapeutic aspects of training have prevailed over the needed epidemiological component. This has produced personnel who are highly qualified to work at the institutional level in various areas of medical rehabilitation, but who do not have training to identify needs or to develop policies or programs for the appropriate services.

The training of personnel in epidemiology, as in administration and planning, should not be done theoretically or abstractly, but instead by integrating important concepts into practice. It is essential that there be a shared commitment on the part of those who train these personnel and those who employ them to develop the necessary infrastructure. The instructional area cannot be indifferent to the delivery of services, nor can the employer be indifferent to the quality of the resources being trained, which it needs. The services have to serve as classrooms not only in the clinical and therapeutic areas but also regarding such topics as administration of the services and evaluation of their activities. This is very important in rehabilitation considered as a component of public health, where such trends as community-based rehabilitation, the structuring of levels of services, compilation of statistics on disease consequences, and recognition of the need to expand coverage are gaining a foothold. These developments cannot continue to be abstract theoretical concepts, but realities to be learned and perpetuated.

In conclusion, the training of medical and technical personnel in rehabilitation must be expanded to include epidemiological practice. The process for accomplishing this would encompass:

- redefining the objectives of instruction so that it covers needs at the different levels;[14]
- ensuring that the content of the curricula also corresponds to demands at the different levels;
- developing the infrastructure of the services needed for teaching;
- continuously evaluating the effectiveness of the training programs, not only in terms of their technical content but also in terms of the capacity they provide for observation, analysis, decision making, and problem solving from both an individual perspective (with patients) and a demographic one (vis-à-vis the problem of disability in a given area); and
- when necessary, modifying the objectives, content, and methodology of the instruction.

In summary, the incorporation of epidemiology into the administration of rehabilitation programs and services would have the following purposes:

- to provide information upon which to base policies and formulate programs;
- to provide information on risks of disability;
- to provide information on the incidence of cases and changes in the profile of disability;
- to reorient the utilization of resources and justify the allocation of new ones according to real priorities, especially with regard to existing services;
- to justify the location of and allocation of resources for new rehabilitation services at all levels of care;
- to guide the changes necessary in the training of personnel; and
- to aid in coordination of different interventions in the fields of medicine (physical and psychiatric), education, and labor.

Epidemiology in the Evaluation of Technologies, Services, and Programs

The evaluation of technologies, services, and programs refers to judging the impact of human and material resources and of technologies on the problem of disability in the population. Knowledge attained through the epidemiological method helps to examine and appraise these parameters in three important ways:

(1) *In terms of resources*: Human and financial resources could be considered the most important ones. In practice, the efficient use of these resources poses many obstacles. It is necessary, particularly in developing countries such as those of Latin America and the Caribbean, to strike a balance between the cost of overcoming a health problem and the results obtained with the interventions. The criteria for using resources must include:

- availability—in other words, the relationship between the existing resources and the needs of the population;
- accessibility—detection and elimination of geographic, organizational, financial, cultural, and functional barriers;
- the projected degree of use of the services by the target population;
- productivity and output—that is, the relationship between the activities carried out, the time available, and the time actually used; and
- quality of the technical and human aspects of the services.

(2) *In terms of the effects of the interventions*: The severity of disability must be evaluated in the individual and the population, for which the ICIDH/WHO is an instrument of irreplaceable value. The following criteria must be applied:

- efficacy—the degree to which interventions resolve problems for the individual and in the population;
- coverage—that is, the proportion of those people who need the services that uses them;
- efficiency—the relationship between the results achieved and the cost of the resources used; and
- effectiveness—the relationship between the efficacy and the coverage attained.

(3) *In terms of technologies*: The available technology influences all areas of medical practice related to disability (prevention, diagnosis, and treatment) and has an impact on efficacy, effectiveness, coverage, cost, etc. Epidemiologic knowledge can help to specify needs and also to determine the distribution of technologies by levels of care, evaluate their efficacy, determine their safety, and analyze their cost.

Technology not only refers to instruments but also drugs and procedures. The use of technology is a complex process of selection, application, adaptation, and innovation in which a multitude of factors come into play. Epidemiological studies can serve to support decision making.

In rehabilitation, much emphasis has been placed on expensive, commercial technologies, without sufficient consideration of whether the costs of those technologies are justified by their effect, or whether the benefits in developing countries are comparable to those attained in the technology's country of origin. A technology whose effectiveness is proven in one place does not necessarily produce acceptably good results in another country where the organization of services, social and economic conditions, cultural acceptance, and training of the personnel who will use it are different. The transfer of rehabilitation technology has been undermined by the tacit acceptance and procurement of equipment before its cost, benefit, effectiveness, or efficiency has been assessed. For this reason the concept of "appropriate technology" has taken hold in the past few years. This term is understood to mean technology that is particularly suited for meeting the needs of individuals or the population, and that has been determined to meet the requirements of the region or local group in terms of efficacy, safety, cost, and cultural compatibility.[3] Therefore, the practice of rehabilitation in developing countries should include the search for technologies appropriate to conditions in those countries. This can mean adapting outside technologies as well as developing other, autochthonous (indigenous) ones. Technologies must be situated at the appropriate level, made accessible, and freed as much as possible from the commercial instrumental technology in which physical medicine and rehabilitation is currently enmeshed. This is fundamental in light of the main challenge confronting rehabilitation: extension of coverage.

In summary, the application of epidemiology to the evaluation of rehabilitation services has the following goals:

- to determine the degree to which the rehabilitation services are available, accessible, and utilized, as well as the productivity and output of resources invested and the quality of the services provided;
- to determine the efficacy, coverage, efficiency, and effectiveness of the interventions carried out; and
- to determine the availability, accessibility, efficacy, cost, and acceptability of technologies at the various levels.

Epidemiology in Research

As in other health programs, research in physical medicine and rehabilitation has been oriented more toward clinical issues than toward the gathering of epidemiological information. However, the latter is essential in enabling us to define the problem to be controlled, adapt the available resources, and identify the results of the interventions. According to Nájera[10] three lines of epidemiological research are needed: (1) research to produce and expand knowledge of the health problems in the community; (2) research to improve effectiveness by identifying inequalities in the application of scientific knowledge; and (3) research to improve efficiency by obtaining better results.

Epidemiological research, therefore, should be inextricably linked to the medical rehabilitation programs in diagnosis of the situation, administration of the services, and their evaluation. Figure 2 illustrates a circle of actions that starts with epidemiological research and then moves to the proposal of strategies to combat disability, testing of strategies in demonstration areas, institution of changes based on the testing, evaluation, and documentation of effects, and the proposal of new research hypotheses.

Physical medicine and rehabilitation as a medical specialty and component of public health programs is supported by a defined body of knowledge. Likewise, epidemiology provides a body of knowledge that has not been sufficiently applied to rehabilitation and that could be expanded considerably through epidemiological research applied to the problem of disability if the countries have the political will to use its results to develop alternatives for intervention and apply them in a continuous process.

Lines of epidemiological research on disability may be grouped as follows:

- definition and quantification of the different types of disability in the population, including frequency and severity;
- identification of the risk factors related to the different types of disability;
- determination of the susceptibility of the priority disabilities to control through available techniques;

Figure 2. Functional linkages between research, programs to control disability, and evaluation of their impact on the population.

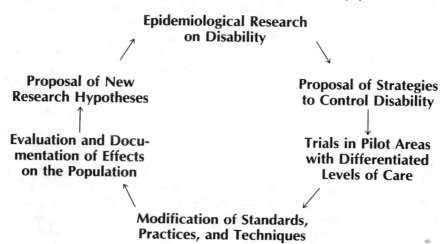

Epidemiological Research on Disability

Proposal of New Research Hypotheses

Proposal of Strategies to Control Disability

Evaluation and Documentation of Effects on the Population

Trials in Pilot Areas with Differentiated Levels of Care

Modification of Standards, Practices, and Techniques

- identification of the local social, economic, and environmental components of disability;
- provision of data to support policies, programs, and allocation of resources;
- evaluation of the interventions over time and geographic area to determine their impact on disability;
- development of theoretical epidemiological models for statistical analysis and simulation.

It is difficult to comprehend that physical medicine and rehabilitation services in Latin America and the Caribbean operate without accurate knowledge about the local disabled population that they were created to serve; they are occupied in large part with problems and situations that are really not their concern and leave unattended the real problems of disability that exist, persist, and grow worse in the surrounding population. The use of epidemiology by rehabilitation specialists and technicians is the best way to change this situation.

CONCLUSION

Epidemiology is no longer confined to the analysis of epidemics. It is a basic health science applicable to the diagnosis of health problems, the modification of interventions, and orientation of research. In the field of physical medicine and rehabilitation, epidemiological knowledge has not been duly applied, particularly in Latin America and the Caribbean. Two fundamental reasons may be the prior lack of a uniform instrument to provide statistics on disability and the predominantly clinical nature of the specialty and services. The appearance of the WHO International Classification of Impairments, Disabilities, and Handicaps is a significant step towards the incorporation of epidemiology into medical rehabilitation programs.

Areas in which epidemiology can be of great value are the diagnosis of the disability situation, administration and evaluation of programs and services, and research. Epidemiological research will be decisively important for the future development of physical medicine and rehabilitation programs.

REFERENCES

1. Arvelo JJ. Rehabilitation in the field of public health and socio-economic development. *Proceedings of the II world congress of rehabilitation international.* Dublin; 1969:377–384.
2. Australian Bureau of Statistics. Handicapped persons—Australia 1981. (ABC catalogue 4343.0).
3. Banta D. Aplicación de la epidemiología en la evaluación de la tecnología médica. *Documentos del seminario sobre usos y perspectivas de la epidemiología.* Buenos Aires: Pan American Health Organization; 1984:199–210. (PNSP 84-47).
4. Bravo-V C. Utilización de la clasificación internacional de deficiencias, discapacidades

y minusvalías en una población seleccionada. [Thesis for the degree of Specialist in Physical Medicine and Rehabilitation]. Santiago, Chile: Instituto de Rehabilitación.

5. XIV Conference of the Latin American and Caribbean Association for Education in Public Health. *Epidemiol Bull [PAHO]*. 1988;9(1):1–8.

6. Hennekens CH, Buring JE. *Epidemiology in medicine*. (Mayrent SL, ed). Boston: Little, Brown; 1987.

7. Instituto Nacional de Estadísticas. Encuesta sobre discapacidades, deficiencias y minusvalías, 1986. Madrid: 1987.

8. Mazzafero VE. Uso de la epidemiología en la planificación de los servicios de salud. *Documentos del seminario sobre usos y perspectivas de la epidemiología*. Buenos Aires: Pan American Health Organization; 1983:37–47. (PNSP 84-47).

9. Motta PR. Planificación estratégica para la monitoría y acción de programas de promoción y protección de la salud del adulto. [Unpublished document].

10. Nájera E. Usos y perspectivas de la epidemiología en la investigación. *Documentos del seminario sobre usos y perspectivas de la epidemiología*. Buenos Aires: Pan American Health Organization; 1983:109–132. (PNSP 84-47).

11. Noble JH. Population and development problems relating to disability prevention and rehabilitation: background paper for meeting of the WHO Expert Committee on Disability Prevention and Rehabilitation, Geneva, 17–23 Feb 1981. [Unpublished document].

12. Pan American Health Organization. Strengthening national capacity in epidemiology. *Epidemiol Bull [PAHO]*. 1985;6(2):1–6.

13. Pan American Health Organization. *Development and strengthening of local health systems in the transformation of national health systems*. Washington, DC: PAHO; 1989.

14. Pan American Health Organization, Health of Adults Program. Niveles de atención en rehabilitación. Washington, DC: 1991. [Working document].

15. Rodríguez H. Discurso inaugural. *Documentos del seminario sobre usos y perspectivas de la epidemiología*. Buenos Aires: Pan American Health Organization; 1983:3–5. (PNSP 84-47).

16. United Nations. Data base on microcomputer diskettes (DISTAT). Version 1. New York: UN; 31 May 1988.

17. United Nations Secretariat, Department of International Economic and Social Affairs, Center for Social Development and Humanitarian Affairs and Statistical Office. Report of the expert group on development of statistics on disabled persons. New York: UN; June 1984. (ESA/STAT/AC.18/7).

18. United Nations Secretatiat, Department of International Economic and Social Affairs, Statistical Office and Center for Social Development and Humanitarian Affairs. Methods and objectives for development of data bases on disabled persons. New York: UN; Feb 1985. [Working paper].

19. Vega A. Rehabilitación: enfoque epidemiológico. 1990. [Unpublished document].

20. Vega A. Utilidad y aplicabilidad de la clasificación internacional de deficiencias, discapacidades y minusvalías (OMS). [Thesis for the degree of Specialist in Physical Medicine and Rehabilitation]. Caracas, Venezuela: MSAS-DSGDF.

21. Vicent-V P. Usos de la epidemiología en la vigilancia y control de las enfermedades en general. *Documentos del seminario sobre usos y perspectivas de la epidemiología*. Buenos Aires: PAHO; 1984:48–56. (PNSP 84-47).

22. White KL. La epidemiología contemporánea: perspectivas y usos. *Documentos del seminario sobre usos y perspectivas de la epidemiología*. Buenos Aires: Pan American Health Organization; 1983:211–217. (PNSP 84-47).

23. World Health Organization. Reports on specific technical matters: disability prevention and rehabilitation; Twenty-Ninth World Health Assembly. Geneva: WHO; 1976. (A29/INF.DOC/1).

24. World Health Organization. *International classification of impairments, disabilities and handicaps: a manual of classification relating to the consequences of disease*. Geneva: WHO; 1980. 205 pp.

25. World Health Organization. *Clasificación internacional de deficiencias, discapacidades y minusvalías: manual de clasificación de las consecuencias de la enfermedad*. Madrid: Instituto Nacional de Servicios Sociales; 1983.

26. World Health Organization. Meeting of principal investigators for testing the classification

of impairments, disabilities and handicaps. Voorburg, Netherlands: WHO; June 1985. (DES/ICIDH/85.23).

27. World Health Organization, Regional Office for Europe. Disability concepts: a position paper prepared in connection with the United Nations Decade of Disabled Persons. Second draft. Copenhagen: WHO; December 1986.

28. World Health Organization, Regional Office for Europe. Better opportunities for disabled people; report on Regional Office activities in disability prevention and rehabilitation, 1983–1988. Copenhagen: WHO; 1989. (EUR/ICP/RHB 016).

29. World Health Organization, Regional Office for Europe, and Government of the Netherlands. Standardization in measurement of impairment, disability and handicap as a consequence of disease: report of a working group, Voorburg, Netherlands, 1983. *Mon Bull Health Stat* [Netherlands Central Bureau of Statistics]. 1984;3(2).

Chapter 2

ADVANCES IN REHABILITATION OF PERSONS WITH SPINAL CORD INJURY

William H. Donovan

Spinal cord injury (SCI) affects approximately seven to ten thousand individuals per year in the United States, and its incidence is quoted as 20–40 per million population in many countries. It affects males four times more than females, and although it occurs in all age groups, the mean age is 29, the median age 25, and the mode age 19.[49]

Etiologies of this condition vary from nation to nation, but in developed countries the distribution is generally as follows: motor vehicle accidents, 48%; falls, 21%; sports, 14%; acts of violence, 15%; and other, 3%.[49]

The last two decades have witnessed many advances in the treatment of patients with spinal cord injury. This chapter will discuss some of these advances according to the time frames when the treatment is given and according to the system affected.

TREATING THE SPINAL CORD

Considerable attention has been given recently to reports that methyl prednisolone appears to reduce the effects of trauma to the spinal cord. Work recently announced and published reported that patients treated with methyl prednisolone within eight hours following spinal cord injury had fewer permanent impairments than did matched groups treated with a placebo or an opiate antagonist. Extremely large doses of methyl prednisolone were employed (i.e., 5.4 mg/kg for 23 hours, after a loading dose of 30 mg/kg). While the drug did not actually reverse the paralysis, the patients in the methyl prednisolone group showed more functional return than did the patients in the other two groups.[4]

Despite these encouraging results, caution must still be advised: some previous studies using methyl prednisolone showed no benefit, and other investigators reported increased complications in patients who received the larger of two dosage regimens.[5,11] Therefore, as this treatment becomes widely employed, it will be important to watch for complications such as gastrointestinal bleeding and infections.

Moreover, the necessary measures to prevent further damage to the spinal cord must not be forgotten, such as externally stabilizing the axial skeleton during rescue and retrieval and maintaining optimal function of the circulation and ventilation during acute care. It is quite apparent to those physicians practicing in this field, that improved rescue techniques, improved stabilization during transport, and improved circulatory and ventilatory support during transport and during acute treatment in the trauma centers have resulted in more patients with incomplete lesions than in the past. This, in turn, has led to improved functional expectations and accomplishments by these patients with incomplete lesions. These efforts must continue, even in the face of the reported improved results from the use of methyl prednisolone.

TREATING THE SPINE FRACTURE

Over the last two decades, significant developments have occurred that now offer better ways to maintain stability and proper alignment of the fractured vertebrae. These developments include externally applied orthoses and surgically applied metallic devices. Most injuries to the spine are initially unstable enough that the patient should not be allowed to sit during the acute period unless stabilization has been assured by internal or external means. Without such support the patient would be at risk for developing a permanently unstable spinal column, a nonunion, or a malunion at the fracture site and/or possibly further neurological damage. For many years, surgeons and spinal cord physicians have argued whether it is more important and necessary to provide internal or external support so that the patient can sit up earlier or to allow the fracture to heal spontaneously with the patient confined to bed.

It has been shown[10,12] that performing surgical stabilization so that the patient can get out of bed during the acute period reduces the overall hospital stay of paraplegic patients. And, generally speaking, the lower the level of injury along the spine, the more important it is to begin mobility training early. Patients with injury at lower levels of the spine, such as T12 thru L5, have greater normal use of their arms and better trunk balance than high level paraplegics or quadriplegic patients. Therefore, they have more mobility goals to accomplish, as well as the necessary motor control to begin working on these goals right from the start. They also have fewer pathophysiological changes such as orthostatic hypotension and respiratory compromise, and so can progress through an early mobilization program more quickly since they require less or no time to accommodate to such changes. Further, these patients with lower level injuries often will require internal stabilization before they can sit, given the greater body weight that is borne through the spine at these lower levels of the axial skeleton. This body weight and the muscles attached to that portion of the spine would create deforming forces if the patient were allowed to sit up before the internal fixation and subsequent healing provide stability.

In some instances adequate stabilization can be obtained just with external devices, such as a halo-vest or a SOMI brace for cervical injuries, or a thoracolumbar stabilization orthosis (TLSO) for thoracolumbar injuries. But in those instances in which the spinal fracture may be too unstable to maintain the proper alignment when any of these devices is used, internal stabilization is warranted. Such internal stabilization is usually provided in the form of wire fixation and fusion for the cervical spine and fixation with metal rods or plates with pedical screws and fusion for the thoracic and lumbar spine.

Ever since the Harrington rod was developed by Dr. Paul Harrington, investigators have sought to improve this instrument. While this rod is un-questionably satisfactory for stabilizing many spinal fractures, some surgeons have complained of loss of fixation or failure of the metal. Other rods such as the Luque rod and the Cottrell-Dubosset system,[27] also suffer from the disadvantage of the need to immobilize a long segment of the spine (usually at least five vertebrae), creating excessive forces at the segments immediately above and below the immobilized ones. Recently developed pedical screw devices[44] offer the advantage of providing solid fixation using fewer seg-ments, usually three vertebrae; they are particularly useful when only one vertebra or one motion segment is involved in the fracture.

While the use of internal stabilization devices to allow early mobilization is necessary for some paraplegics, this concept is also applicable to some quadriplegics, particularly those whose lesions are incomplete, i.e., Frankel C and D (Table 1). These individuals have preserved more neurological function and have fewer pathophysiological changes to which to accom-modate. Getting them out of bed sooner allows work on their rehabilitation goals to begin sooner and discharge to be accomplished earlier. However, when considering the patients with more complete injuries, such as those

---

Table 1. Frankel classification of degree of incompleteness.

A. *Complete*—all motor and sensory function is absent below the zone of partial pres-ervation.

B. *Incomplete, preserved sensation only*—preservation of any demonstrable, repro-ducible sensation, excluding phantom sensations. Voluntary motor functions are absent.

C. *Incomplete, preserved motor nonfunctional*—preservation of voluntary motor func-tion which is minimal and performs no useful purpose. Minimal is defined as pre-served voluntary motor ability below the level of injury where the majority of the key muscles test less than a grade of 3.

D. *Incomplete, preserved motor functional*—preservation of voluntary motor function which is useful functionally. This is defined as preserved voluntary motor ability below the level of injury, where the majority of the key muscles test at least a grade of 3.

E. *Complete return of all motor and sensory function*—may still have abnormal reflexes.

with Frankel A or B, the issue of early mobilization is not nearly so compelling, given that significant pathophysiological changes in these patients make the accomplishment of the necessary rehabilitation tasks more difficult. For example, a quadriplegic patient must accommodate to the difficulty of orthostatic hypotension caused by the blockade of sympathetic fibers and to the respiratory compromise caused by the total dependence upon the diaphragm for inspiration. Surgery with general anesthesia only adds another risk for respiratory compromise. It is recognized that conditions such as blood volume, oxygenation, nutritional status, and energy levels need to be adequate before intensive rehabilitation can begin. This takes time for all patients, but for quadriplegics it often will require more time.

Those complete patients who have not had surgery but who are mobilized early in a halo-vest device will be able to sit, but there is not much more that these patients can do in such a limiting orthosis. In contrast, for cervical injuries the period of immobilization (i.e., bed rest) required for conservative management in bed is usually only six weeks, followed by six weeks of sitting in an external support such as a SOMI brace, which is less confining than a halo-vest. During the initial six weeks in bed, one can work on achieving all the above-mentioned conditions that should be met before intensive rehabilitation can begin. This will make the mobilization process after six weeks go faster (Table 2). Not surprisingly, recent studies have

Table 2. Usual time required for sufficient natural healing to insure stability.

		Cervical	Thoracic	Dorsolumbar
		Anatomical region (site of lesion)		
1.	*Before sitting can begin*[a]			
	Duration postinjury of bedrest only	6 weeks	4 weeks	8–12 weeks
	External support needed in bed	Soft collar	Usually none	Possibly TLSO
2.	*Before unrestricted activity can begin*[b]			
	Duration postinjury of bedrest only + sitting[c]	12 weeks	6–12 weeks	12–24 weeks
	External support needed out of bed	Rigid collar/ brace	TLSO	TLSO

[a]During this time a patient who has not had an internal stabilization or is not wearing an external orthosis which can prevent abnormal movement should remain in bed for the duration indicated.
[b]After the duration shown in (a) has elapsed patients may be allowed out of bed but must wear the external orthoses indicated.
[c]Durations indicated include the time shown in (a).

reported that no difference was seen with regard to the total length of hospitalization (i.e., acute treatment plus rehabilitation) in quadriplegic patients who underwent surgical internal stabilization versus those who did not.[15,16,50]

ENHANCING MOBILITY

Over the last 10 years, we have seen the improvement of lightweight wheelchairs which are easier to propel, easier to lift, and easier to transport in and out of a vehicle by the patient or an attendant. Many models are currently on the market for use in everyday and sport activities.

In addition, improved control mechanisms for powered wheelchairs have been developed. Proportional control systems have made these wheelchairs safer and have eliminated the jerking of older systems using microswitches. Recently developed control systems also allow an individual to operate an environmental control system from the armrest of the wheelchair. For patients with higher lesions, sip and puff systems have been developed that not only allow for accurate maneuvering of the power chair but also allow one to interface with the environmental control system.

In the area of orthotic devices, polypropylene and other lightweight plastic materials have been available for some time, and, more recently, carbon fiber materials have come under active investigation. Engen and his colleagues reported the use of a carbon fiber modular bracing system which can easily be put together in a physical therapy training environment.[19,20] This system significantly reduced costs while simultaneously providing a stable and durable orthosis to individuals with SCI, particularly those who are not obese or those who weigh no more than 175–180 pounds.

Functional electrical stimulation (FES) has recently received considerable attention; it has found many clinical applications, and research on it is still being actively conducted.[9,13] Basically, under laboratory conditions, paraplegic patients have been able to walk using functional electrical stimulation devices consisting of surface electrodes placed over key muscles such as hip flexors, knee extensors, and dorsiflexors of the feet.[9] Balance, however, remains a significant problem for these patients and, more recently, hybrid systems have been developed where combinations of muscle stimulation and bracing have been employed.[18] Marsolais and colleagues,[36] are currently investigating the possibilities of implanted stimulators which are programmed telemetrically to activate and deactivate in a fashion that simulates a gait cycle. There is still much work to be done before a system will be available that will allow any kind of functional ambulation.

Currently, FES has been more widely applied for those patients who are incomplete and only require one or two muscles to be activated by the electric stimulation. At this time, it would appear that this limited stimulation (e.g., of the pretibial muscles on one side) has more application in these patients.[13]

Functional electrical stimulation has also been advocated for simply improving muscle bulk strength and endurance, bone deposition, and aerobic capacity.[42] However, in order for these changes to be retained, the treatment must be applied throughout the individual's lifetime; otherwise, atrophy of the musculature and demineralization of the bone will return.

TREATMENT AND PREVENTION OF COMPLICATIONS

Pressure Ulcers

Patients depend upon their wheelchairs for mobility; they also depend upon their wheelchair cushions. Because they have absent or diminished sensory awareness in their skin and/or they are unable to perform adequate pressure relief, they risk developing pressure necrosis over bony prominences such as the ischial tuberosities. In the last decade, better devices for measuring skin pressure, such the Texas Interface Pressure Evaluator (TIPE) by Krouskop and colleagues[31] and the Skin Pressure Evaluator by Reswick and Rogers,[43] have been developed. These devices represent a significant advance in the ability to lower the risk of pressure ulcers by measuring the amount of pressure over bony prominences. Since measurements often change depending upon the cushion material and the posture of the patient, these devices allow the best cushion to be selected for each patient. However, problems that affect the accuracy of measurements of pressures under a sitting surface by any device are still of some concern.[24] Unfortunately, there is no one cushion that is best for everybody, although three- to four-inch dual density foam is relatively inexpensive and suitable for many. For patients at greater than average risk, air-filled cushions and cushions with gel are often needed.

For those patients who have developed pressure necrosis, there now exist improved surgical methods using myocutaneous flaps that will cover the eroded and ulcerated areas. It is possible to transfer muscle and skin on an arterial pedicle and preserve the blood supply to the flap via the muscle's perforating arteries as well as the skin vessels. Although this has improved the success rate for the repair of ulcerated tissue, strict adherence to first surgical principles must be remembered at all times: the wound must initially be surgically debrided of all infected tissues; if osteomyelitis is present, it must be treated by surgical debridement and antibiotics must be administered for at least six weeks; and the wound must be clean in all respects before closure can be considered. In addition, the patient's nutrition must be optimized, and all factors that impair healing, such as anemia and hypoproteinemia, must be corrected.[17]

Spasticity

Improvements and advances also have occurred regarding the neurological complications that follow spinal cord injury—spasticity is one such complication. Over the last decade, we basically have had available three medications that can be taken orally: diazepam, baclofen, and dantrolene. Baclofen, the safest of the three, has a molecular configuration similar to gamma-aminobutyric acid (GABA).

More recently, clonidine has been described by Donovan and colleagues[14] and Nance and colleagues[38,39] as having a beneficial effect on spasticity. Dosages of 0.1 mg to 0.4 mg daily have been recommended. Hypotension and somnolence are uncommon side effects to be checked for when using clonidine in the SCI population.

In addition, the use of intrathecal baclofen, although still under investigation, promises to be a very desirable method of dealing with patients with intractable spasticity that does not respond to oral agents or other physical measures such as functional electrical stimulation, range of motion, proper positioning, and so on.

Morphine was first used intrathecally by Wang and colleagues in 1979.[52] Erickson and others later demonstrated its efficacy in the control of spasticity as well as pain.[21] Penn and Kroin then reported the beneficial effects of baclofen on spasticity when administered intrathecally.[41] Loubser and colleagues[34] have more recently confirmed the latter work, and have shown that the use of intrathecal baclofen for the treatment of severe spasticity secondary to spinal cord injury is effective and safe and appears to be free of complications and the phenomenon of tolerance. This modality for the treatment of spasticity, if it continues to prove successful, will be a considerable advance over other invasive methods, since it is reversible, nondestructive, and adjustable from hour to hour. It is ideal for incomplete patients, in whom any available motor or sensory function must be preserved, in addition to controlling the spasticity.

Pain

This is another significant problem that some patients with spinal injury experience. Pain of musculoskeletal origin is similar to that faced by the able-bodied population and may be treated similarly, that is, with physical modalities and nonsteroidal medications. However, the patient with spinal cord injury may also experience pain referred to as central deafferentation pain. This is often described as burning, stinging, or freezing in character and may be accompanied in incomplete patients by dysesthesias when the skin in the affected area is touched lightly. It is usually diffuse in its distribution, most often involving the feet, rectum, and genitalia. It can also be localized to just one or two dermatomal segments. While such pain is rather common, it will often respond to oral agents such as amitriptyline, valproic acid, carbamazepine, or phenytoin.[23,53] Occasionally, however, some patients will fail to respond to any of these oral agents. In some instances, myelography or magnetic resonance imaging (MRI) will disclose nerve roots entrapped in scar or glial tissue, particularly when the pain is dermatomal. Freeing up this tissue will sometimes improve the situation. However, when the pain generator lies within the spinal cord itself, as is more likely when the pain is diffuse, some patients have been helped by the use of a procedure called the dorsal root entry zone (DREZ) lesion.[40] Minute lesions are made by radio frequency or laser probe within the substantia gelatinosa in the dorsal horn of the spinal cord. Although this will usually result in a loss of sensation for one to two segments above the original level of injury, it has been found to be quite helpful in relieving the central pain of some patients, particularly the lower level paraplegic patients who can "adapt" to the loss of sensation in one or two dermatomes.

Genitourinary

The last decade or so has seen improvements in this area that have helped many spinal cord patients. The formation of stones in the kidney, ureter, and bladder is a relatively common problem, particularly in those patients who use indwelling catheters. In recent years, the development of lithotriptors has made stone removal much easier and safer, and in most cases has obviated the need for an open exploration of the bladder or renal pelvis. Depending on the location of the stone, lithotriptors may be introduced percutaneously into the renal pelvis or through the urethra into the bladder, and then can pulverize the stone by means of shock waves generated by an electric discharge in the irrigating solution (electrohydraulic lithotripsy) or by means of ultrasonic energy (ultrasonic lithotripsy).[6,8] The kidney stone is flushed out through a nephrostomy tube or is allowed to pass through the ureter, which is protected by a stent so that the ureter does not occlude. Stones may also be removed by using the extracorporeal shock wave lithotriptor (ESWL). When this treatment is carried out, the anesthetized patient is immersed in a water bath and hydraulic shock waves are generated by an electric discharge in the bottom of the tank. The shock waves are carefully focused on the stone by a hemiellipsoid reflector. The shock waves pulverize the stone and the pulverized material is allowed to pass through the ureter.[55] Again, sometimes a stent is employed to insure against obstruction.

Those patients who wish to empty their bladders by spontaneous voiding and avoid the use of an indwelling catheter, may be hindered by the presence of detrussor sphincter dyssynergia (DSD). This phenomenon (the simultaneous contraction of the detrussor and the external urethral sphincter) often is responsible for incomplete emptying of the bladder (thereby increasing the risk of recurrent urinary tract infection) and for the development of high voiding pressures (thereby increasing the risk for reflux of urine into the ureter, hydronephrosis, and deterioration of the bladder, manifested by trabeculations and diverticulae). DSD can sometimes be alleviated by sphincterotomy, particularly in those patients with high voiding pressures, since a good voiding pressure is needed to expel the urine even after the sphinc-terotomy is done.

Intermittent catheterization (IC)—i.e., catheterizing the bladder, emptying it, removing the catheter, and then repeating this procedure every four to six hours—has proven to be quite an improvement in the care of spinal cord injury patients, particularly during the early post-injury period when it is desirable to maintain sterile urine. By eliminating the need for an indwelling catheter (IDC), intermittent catheterization has increased the chances of keeping the urine sterile (IDCs, routinely used in years past, were always associated with chronic bacteriuria). However, long-term intermit-tent catheterization is not always practical for all patients, such as those who must rely on family members to catheterize them. IC creates an ad-ditional need, and this means the patient cannot be independent in this area, a situation that runs counter to the general philosophy of rehabilitation, poses additional care burdens on the family, and interferes with the patient's lifestyle. For these patients, an IDC may be chosen as a last resort, keeping in mind that a high urine output must be maintained in patients who resort to an IDC.

IC is also impractical for those patients who have severe bladder hyper-reflexia with a small bladder capacity. Even when such patients can cath-eterize themselves, they are unable to store the urine generated by the kidneys during a four-hour period and will leak urine between catheteriza-tions. In some instances, this hyperreflexia and small bladder capacity can be reversed with anticholinergic medication, but some patients do not tol-erate the side effects of these drugs (e.g., dry mouth, blurry vision, etc.). Although anticholinergics can decrease bladder contractility, currently there is no satisfactory way to improve bladder contractility for those patients with hyporeflexic bladders, nor is there a reliable way to decrease the tone of the external urethral sphincter. Laboratory work in animals has shown that baclofen does reduce the tone of this sphincter. However, it does not appear to decrease the tone sufficiently to eliminate the DSD nor to improve voiding dynamics, since baclofen also decreases detrusor contractility.[34]

The artificial urinary sphincter has been available for about 10 years and has helped some people; it is recommended primarily for patients with acontractile or hypocontractile bladders.[54] These devices have not been free of problems: they can become infected and may have to be removed, or they may fail to provide the individual with continence while the bladder is filling or ease of emptying the bladder when it is full. In some instances, patients cannot strain or crede effectively and are unable to push urine out, and therefore may need to use IC despite having the artificial sphincter. However, even in such instances, patients usually retain the advantage of remaining continent for the four-hour period between catheterizations.

Urodynamics, which consists of the simultaneous measurement of the bladder and the abdominal pressures, the electrical activity of the external urethral sphincter, and the urinary flow rate whenever the patient voids, also has been a significant advance that has occurred in the last decade.[46] This investigative tool has allowed the clinician to ascertain whether the patient is in danger of developing the complications relating to DSD, as mentioned above. Generally speaking, if on urodynamic testing it is found that the patient has voiding pressures greater than 80 cm of water or even voiding pressures greater than 40 cm of water that are sustained for a prolonged period of time (more than two minutes for several contractions), he is in danger of developing deterioration of the bladder. In such circumstances, the patient should not be simply allowed to void and wear an external collector. Such patients are better off remaining on anticholinergics and using intermittent catheterization if they can catheterize themselves, or undergoing a sphincterotomy to decrease the obstruction caused by the external sphincter. Urodynamics has removed some of the guess work, allowing clinicians to make better clinical judgments.

An effective external collecting device for females still needs to be developed. Although devices have appeared from time to time, none of these has met with a high degree of patient acceptance;[29] it is to be hoped that there will be more to report in this area five years from now.

Sexual function is also significantly affected by a spinal cord injury, regardless of the level of lesion. The manifestations of dysfunction, however, are different in patients with sacral reflexes (e.g., bulbocavernous) than they are in those without them.

The technique of electroejaculation, using a probe inserted into the rectum which stimulates the release of sperm from the seminal vesicles, has been improved in recent years. This technique has been available to veterinarians for at least a half century, but it has only recently found application in patients with spinal cord injury.[2] It has recently been demonstrated that the sperm reduction and loss of motility that are usually found in spinal cord injury patients, particularly in those with complete lesions, can be improved in some cases through repeated ejaculations by the rectal probe electrode ejaculation method, which increases the number and motility of sperm.[28] Cases of satisfactory impregnation by artificial insemination using the spinal cord injury patient's own sperm, have been reported. Success, although still low, is improving.[45]

Because many men with spinal cord injury have difficulty attaining and maintaining erections, interest has focused on ways to retain an erection that will prove satisfactory for intercourse. One method that has had some success involves the use of an externally applied device that creates a vacuum around the penis.[37] Another method consists of surgically placing an implant, such as a semirigid silicone device or an inflatable device, within the corpora cavernosa. Complications, consisting mainly of erosions, have been high (25% according to some reports), particularly with the semirigid device.[51] The inflatable device works with a pump that can be placed in the scrotum or at the end of the device just under the glans.[26] While inflatable devices have had some problems, particularly erosion or migration, many patients have used them successfully. A third way to achieve erections consists of the injection of medication into the corpora cavernosa, i.e., directly through the skin into one corpus. Initially, papaverine and/or phentolamine were used,[25] and these drugs can produce an erection that can be maintained for approximately two hours. When the dosage is excessive, however, priapism can occur, and this has necessitated the evacuation of clots from the corpora to resolve the priapism.[35] More recently, prostaglandin E-1 has been reported to produce erections that last a similar amount of time but do not result in priapism and are less dangerous.[32]

Bowel

Incontinence of bowel also has been a difficult problem to solve for many spinal cord patients. Recently, incontinence bags that are suitable for bed-bound patients and are applied around the anus have been used (Drainable Fecal Incontinence Collector; Hollister, Libertyville, Illinois); the adhesive material is well tolerated. While methods currently employed that rely upon timed evacuation using suppositories, digital stimulation, and/or laxatives are effective for many people, for some these procedures are not consistently satisfactory and fecal incontinence does occasionally occur. Better devices and methods to control fecal incontinence in patients with spinal cord injury are needed.

Cardiovascular

One of the potentially serious cardiovascular complications for patients with lesions above T6 is autonomic dysreflexia (AD). AD is a mass reflex consisting of a noxious afferent input and sympathetic efferent output from the cord. It is usually associated with visceral dyssynergia, such as between the bladder and the urethral sphincter or between the evacuating colon/rectum and the anal sphincter.[22] Other viscera that can cause AD include the uterus, especially during the second stage of labor; the stomach, accompanied by pylorospasm; and the gall bladder and the ureter, e.g., when passing a stone. Common methods utilized to avoid autonomic dysreflexia of bowel and bladder origin include the use of topical anesthetics to decrease the noxious afferent input and the use of agents such as alpha receptor blockers (e.g., phenoxybenzamine), agents that work directly on the smooth muscle of the vasculature (e.g., hydralazine), or ganglion blockers (e.g., mecamylamine). More recently, a calcium channel blocker, nifedipine, has been found to be extremely effective for both the prevention and treatment of AD.[33] Nifedipine 10 mg may be taken orally for preventive purposes or may be taken sublingually for rapid onset. When used sublingually, the capsule must be punctured and the liquid or powder dissolved under the tongue. Action occurs within 5 to 10 minutes and lasts long enough for a rapid investigation as to the cause of the dysreflexia (e.g., plugged catheter, a full recto-sigmoid, etc.). Other rapid-onset, short-acting agents that have been used for some time include amyl nitrate (inhaled) and nitroglycerine (sublingual). Other effective agents include clonidine (oral or transdermal) for prophylaxis and diazoxide (I.V.) for emergencies.

Respiratory

Improvement in the respiratory area primarily has been in the recognition of a) fatigue as a cause of respiratory failure among quadriplegics and high paraplegics, b) the importance of preventive measures such as flu vaccines for these patients, and c) the value of early respiratory therapy for the acute spinal cord injured patient, including intermittent positive pressure breathing (IPPB), chest physiotherapy, and assisted cough. The need for assisted ventilation should be recognized early, before hypoxia becomes severe or chronic. Weaning from assisted ventilation is not indicated and should not be done until the strength of the patient's diaphragm has returned to an extent that ensures ventilation without fatigue. This generally means that the vital capacity must be 1.5 liters or greater, and the lungs must be clear and able to oxygenate the patient to at least a pO_2 of 80 on room air. In addition, the patient should be weaned by gradually increasing the time off the ventilator rather than by progressive reduction of the rate of intermittent mandatory ventilation (IMV). This latter method is commonly employed appropriately for neurologically intact patients who develop respiratory failure due to intrinsic lung disease. But it must be remembered that the cause of respiratory failure in most patients with spinal cord injury, if it occurs, is muscle paralysis and not lung disease. Therefore, weaning must be accomplished in a fashion similar to muscle training, where the muscle gradually increases in strength through paced exercise and is not allowed to fatigue. This is accomplished best by gradually increasing the time off the ventilator when the above conditions have been met.

For those patients who remain ventilator dependent, portable ventilators also have been improved. Newer ventilators are quieter and more portable, fit underneath a wheelchair, and allow the individual to leave his room and participate more actively in rehabilitation. This has been a significant help to high quadriplegics by allowing them access to the community. Electrophrenic respiration (EPR) continues to be a valuable asset to those who are candidates for it and who can afford it. Both phrenic nerves of the apneic patient must respond to the electric stimulus. It is wise to wait at least 6 to 12 months before implanting the units to be sure there is no potential for spontaneous recovery.[7]

Bone

Heterotopic ossification (HO) remains a problem for a few patients with SCI (about 6%).[48] Most patients who develop this complication can avoid joint ankylosis, even when the heterotopic bone is present in large amounts, as long as gentle range of motion (ROM) is continued from the outset on a regular basis. If the affected joints (usually the hips and knees) are immobilized and range of motion is not performed, severe disability will arise from the ankyloses, interfering with positioning in bed or the wheelchair. Any patient with HO severe enough to impede ROM should be treated with etidronate disodium (EHDP). On doses of 20 mg/kg/day for two weeks, then 10 mg/kg/day for one year, many patients will show some amelioration of the HO.[48] Additional measures have recently been advocated as a result of success seen after orthopedic procedures such as total hip arthroplasty. These measures include the use of nonsteroidal anti-inflammatory drugs[47] and radiation therapy.[1] Further controlled studies using these regimens on patients with SCI are needed, but they hold promise for reducing morbidity.

ASSESSMENT

Methods of scoring performance and measuring outcome have been available for some time for SCI patients. More recently, the functional independence measure (FIM) has been introduced and has been found easier to employ and less cumbersome than prior measures.[30] It lacks sensitivity for measuring improvement among high-level injuries, but is valid for use by paraplegics.

PREVENTION

Finally, no discussion of the advances in rehabilitation would be complete without mentioning improvements in prevention. The goals for all of us must surely be to help reduce the incidence of spinal cord injury by supporting those measures designed to accomplish this. It is gratifying to see that awareness programs which alert the public to the dangers of using drugs and alcohol, particularly while driving, have had some impact. The lowering of the speed limits, the wearing of lap and shoulder belts, the use of reliable infant seats, the installation of air bags, and the lobbying by relatives whose loved ones have been the victims of trauma to the spinal cord have all helped prevent or lessen this serious catastrophic disability. It is important, of course, that laws that are passed be enforced, particularly those regulating speed limits, those concerned with driving while intoxicated, and those requiring the wearing of seat belts. In addition, further efforts must be made to educate people to avoid diving into shallow water. Other preventive steps that should be encouraged in the future include structuring the environment to help prevent falls by the elderly and gun control or at least gun regulation, since gunshot wounds account for 15% of all spinal cord injuries.[56]

REFERENCES

1. Ayers DC, Evarts CM, Parkinson JR. The prevention of heterotopic ossification in high-risk patients by low-dose radiation therapy after total hip arthroplasty. *J Bone Joint Surg* [Am]. 1986;69A:1423–1430.
2. Bennett CJ, Seager SW, Vasher EA, McGuire EJ. Sexual dysfunction and electroejaculation in men with spinal cord injury: review. *J Urol.* 1988;139:453–457.
3. Bracken MB, Collins WF, Freeman DF, et al. Efficacy of methylprednisolone in acute spinal cord injury. *JAMA.* 1984;251:45–52.
4. Bracken MB, Shepard MJ, Collins WF, et al. A randomized, controlled trial of methylprednisolone or nalaxone in the treatment of acute spinal cord injury. *N Engl J Med.* 1990;322:1405–1411.
5. Bracken MB, Shepard MJ, Hellenbrand KG, et al. Methylprednisolone and neurologic function one year after spinal cord injury. *J Neurosurg.* 1985;63:704–713.
6. Branne GE, Bush WH. Ultrasonic destruction of kidney stones. *West J Med.* 1984;140:227–232.
7. Carter RE, Donovan WH. Reflections of impact of electrophenic respiration in the management of high quadriplegics. *SCI Digest.* 1981;3(3):37–43.
8. Clayman RV, Surya V, Miller RP, et al. Percutaneous nephrolithotomy: extraction of renal and ureteral calculi from 100 patients. *J Urol.* 1984;131:868–871.
9. Cybulski GR, Penn RD, Jaeger RJ. Lower extremity functional neuromuscular stimulation in case of spinal cord injury. *Neurosurgery.* 1984;15:132–146.
10. Davies WE, Morris JH, Hill V. An analysis of conservative (non-surgical) management of thoracolumbar fractures and fracture-dislocations with neural damage. *J Bone Joint Surg* [Am]. 1980;62A:1324–1328.
11. DeMaria EJ, Reichman W, Kenny PR, et al. Septic complications of corticosteroid administration after central nervous system trauma. *Am Surg.* 1985;202:248–252.
12. Dickson JH, Harrington PR, Erwin WD. Results of reduction and stabilization of the severely fractured thoracic and lumbar spine. *J Bone Joint Surg* [Am]. 1978;60A:799–805.
13. Dimitrijevic MD, Malazic M, Erdman M. Modification of gait in ambulatory spinal cord injury patients. Paper presented at the 9th Annual Scientific Meeting of the American Spinal Injury Association. Houston, Texas; 1983.
14. Donovan WH, Carter RE, Rossi D, Wilkerson MA. Clonidine effect on spasticity: a clinical trial. *Arch Phys Med Rehabil.* 1988;69:193–194.
15. Donovan WH, Cifu DX, Sandin KL, Kopaniky DR. Neurologic and skeletal outcomes following closed cervical spinal cord injury. Paper presented at the 29th Annual Scientific Meeting of the International Medical Society of Paraplegia. Ramat Gan, Israel; 1990.
16. Donovan WH, Cifu DX, Schotte DE. Neurologic and skeletal outcomes in 113 patients with closed injuries to the cervical spinal cord. *Spine.* [In press].
17. Donovan WH, Garber SL, Hamilton SM, Krouskop TA, Rodriguez GP, Stal S. Pressure ulcers. In: DeLisa JA, ed. *Rehabilitation medicine—principles and practice.* Philadelphia: JB Lippincott; 1988:476–491.
18. Douglas R, Berno P, Isakov E. Ambulation using the reciprocation gait orthosis and functional electrical stimulation. Paper presented at the 29th Annual Scientific Meeting of the International Medical Society of Paraplegia. Ramat Gan, Israel; 1990.
19. Engen T. Lightweight modular orthosis. *Prosthet Orthot Int.* 1989;13:125–129.
20. Engen T, Lemkuhl D, Smith M. Inexpensive, lightweight, custom-fitted KAFO's for persons with paraplegia. Paper presented at the 15th Annual Scientific Meeting of the American Spinal Injury Association. Las Vegas, Nevada; 1989.
21. Erickson DL, Lo J, Michaelson M. Control of intractable spasticity with intrathecal morphine sulfate. *Neurosurgery.* 1989;24:236–238.
22. Erickson RP. Autonomic hyperreflexia: pathophysiology and medical management. *Arch Phys Med Rehabil.* 1980;61:431–439.

23. Farkash AE, Portenoy RK. The pharmacological management of chronic pain in the paraplegic patient. *J Am Paraplegia Soc.* 1986;9:41–50.
24. Ferguson-Pell MW. Seat cushion selection. *J Rehabil Res Dev.* 1990;27(2):49–73.
25. Gasser TC, Roach RM, Larsen EH, et al. Intracavernous self-injection with phentolamine and papaverine for the treatment of impotence. *J Urol.* 1987;137:678–680.
26. Gregory JG, Purcell MH. Penile prostheses: review of current models, mechanical reliability, and product cost. *Urology.* 1987;29:150–152.
27. Gurr KR, McAfee PC. Cottrel-Dubousset instrumentation in adults: a preliminary report. *Spine.* 1988;13:510–520.
28. Halstead LS, VerVoort S, Seager SW. Rectal probe electrostimulation in the treatment of anejaculatory spinal cord injured men. *Paraplegia.* 1987;25:120–129.
29. Johnson DE, O'Reilly JL, Warren JW. Clinical evaluation of an external urine collection device for nonambulatory incontinent women. *J Urol.* 1989;141:535–537.
30. Keith RA, Granger CV, Hamilton BB, Sherwin FS. The functional independence measure: a new tool for rehabilitation. *Adv Clin Rehabil.* 1987;1:6–18.
31. Krouskop TA, Noble PC, Garber SL, Spencer WA. The effectiveness of preventive management in reducing the occurrence of pressure sores. *J Rehabil Res Dev.* 1983;20(1):74–83.
32. Lee LM, Stevenson RWD, Szasz G. Prostaglandin E1 versus phentolamine/papaverine for the treatment of erectile impotence: a double blind comparison. *J Urol.* 1989;141:549–550.
33. Lindean R, Leffler EJ, Kedia KR. A comparison of the efficacy of an alpha-1 adrenergic blocker in the slow calcium channel blocker in the control of autonomic dysreflexia. *Paraplegia.* 1985;23:34–38.
34. Loubser PG, Narayan RK, Sandin KJ, Donovan WH, Russell KD. Continuous infusion of intrathecal baclofen: long term effects on spasticity in spinal cord injury. *Paraplegia.* [In press].
35. Lue TF, Hellstrom WJG, McAninich TW, Tanagho EA. Priapism: a refined approach to diagnosis and treatment. *J Urol.* 1987;136:104–108.
36. Marsolais EB, Kobetic R. Implantation techniques and experience with percutaneous intramuscular electrodes in the lower extremities. *J Rehabil Res Dev.* 1986;23(3):1–8.
37. Nadig PW, Ware JC, Blumoff R. Noninvasive device to produce and maintain an erection-like state. *Urology.* 1986;27:126–131.
38. Nance PW, Shears AH, Nance DM. Clonidine in spinal cord injury. *Can Med Assoc J.* 1985;133:41–42.
39. Nance PW, Shears AH, Nance DM. Reflex changes induced by clonidine in spinal cord injury patients. *Paraplegia.* 1989;27:296–301.
40. Nashold BS. Current status of the DREZ operation. *Neurosurgery.* 1984;15:942–944.
41. Penn RD, Kroin JS. Long-term intrathecal baclofen infusion for treatment of spasticity. *J Neurosurg.* 1987;66:181–185.
42. Ragnarrson KT, Pollack S, O'Daniel W, Edgar R, Petrofsky J, Nash MS. Clinical evaluation of computerized functional electrical stimulation after spinal cord injury: a multicenter pilot study. *Arch Phys Med Rehabil.* 1988;69:672–677.
43. Reswick JB, Rogers JE. Experience at Rancho Los Amigos Hospital with devices and techniques to prevent pressure sores. In: Kenedi RM, Cowden JM, Scales JT, eds. *Bedsore biomechanics.* Baltimore: University Park Press; 1976:301–310.
44. Roy-Camille R, Saillant G, Mazel C. Internal fixation of the lumbar spine with pedicle screw plating. *Clin Orthop.* 1986;203:7–17.
45. Seager SW, Halstead LS, Ohl DA, et al. Electroejaculation and its utilization for fertility evaluation in 266 spinal cord injured men. Paper presented at the 29th Annual Scientific Meeting of the International Medical Society of Paraplegia. Ramat Gan, Israel; 1990.
46. Shah PJR. The assessment of patients with a view to urodynamics. In: Mundy AR, Stephenson TP, Wein AJ, eds. *Urodynamics.* Edinburgh: Churchill Livingstone; 1984:53–61.
47. Sodemann B, Persson PE, Nilsson OS. Prevention of heterotopic ossification by nonsteroid anti-inflammatory drugs after total hip arthroplasty. *Clin Orthop.* 1988;237:158–163.
48. Stover SL. Heterotopic ossification after spinal cord injury. In: Block RF, Basbaum M, eds. *Management of spinal cord injuries.* Baltimore: Williams & Wilkins; 1986:284–301.

49. Stover SL, Fine PR, eds. *Spinal cord injury—the facts and figures*. Birmingham, Alabama: University of Alabama Press; 1986:13–15.
50. Tator CH, Duncan EG, Edmonds VE, Lapczak LI, Andrews DF. Comparison of surgical and conservative management in 208 patients with acute spinal cord injury. *Can J Neurol Sci*. 1987;14:60–69.
51. Van Arsdalen KN, Klein FA, Hackler RH, Brady SM. Penile implants in spinal cord injury patients for maintaining external appliances. *J Urol*. 1984;131:59–62.
52. Wang JK, Nauss LA, Thomas JE. Pain relief by intrathecally applied morphine in man. *Anesthesiology*. 1979;50:149–151.
53. Watson CP, Evans RJ, Reed K, et al. Amitriptyline versus placebo in postherpetic neuralgia. *Neurology*. 1982;32:671–673.
54. Webster G, Stephenson TP. Artificial urinary sphincters. In: Mundy AR, Stephenson TP, Wein AJ, eds. *Urodynamics*. Edinburgh: Churchill Livingstone; 1984:373–380.
55. Wickham JEA, Webb DR, Payne SR, et al. Extracorporeal shock wave lithotripsy: the first 50 patients treated in Great Britain. *Br Med J*. 1985;290:1188–1189.
56. Young JS, Burns PE, Bowen AM, McCutchen R. *Spinal cord injury statistics: experience of the regional spinal cord injury systems*. Phoenix, Arizona: Good Samaritan Medical Center; 1982.

Chapter 3

REHABILITATION OF CHILDREN WITH BRAIN INJURY

Daniel Halpern

The customary management of children with brain dysfunction has focused on the peripheral results of the dysfunction, since these were the clinical manifestations with which the physician and other professionals treating the case were presented. As interest and attention have progressed, approaches have evolved in an increasingly "central" direction. The earliest approaches emphasized bony and soft tissue surgery and orthotic devices; these approaches are still widely used and, within well-defined limits, are generally helpful. Later, authors focused on sensory stimulation of the skin, muscle, tendons, and bony structures, with the intention of influencing spinal cord, midbrain, or labyrinthine reflexes. However, the relevance of these approaches to the rehabilitative process is questionable, partly because they have all failed to consider the primary role of the brain itself in any behavioral process and partly because no experimental evidence has been able to demonstrate clearly that the varying elements of existing knowledge incorporated into these therapeutic approaches make them effective in altering the capabilities of the individual.

In the past two decades, much information and understanding has been amassed concerning the manner in which the brain organizes behavioral responses to internal and external stimuli. The model has been developed of discretely organized systems that integrate and modulate stimuli and responses in specific behavioral and cognitive areas of human function.[66] These systems are generally anatomically dispersed and interact with one another in a characteristic manner. Alterations in the function of one system may influence that of any of the other systems. The systems that are significant in rehabilitation practice are motor control; mastication and deglutition; emotional and affective behavior; attentiveness, memory, and learning; sensation and perception; speech and communication; and cognition and abstract thinking.

In the child with a brain function disorder, major disparities may be present in the capability of one or more systems to carry out their usual functions. Therefore, the rehabilitation program must be guided by the qualitative and quantitative status of each of these functional systems, rather than an arbitrary developmental sequence derived from normal developmental schedules.

THE ROLE OF DEVELOPMENT

The process of growth and differentiation proceeds along certain well-defined paths, allowing the acquisition of new levels of function.[25,41] This process has its own biological determinants, but it is also influenced by experience. Normal growth and development depend upon this interaction between the biological structure and the experience associated with the individual's interaction with the environment. Thus, development is basically a learning process superimposed upon a substrate of inherent reactive or behavioral patterns that, biologically considered, in normal individuals may be phylogenetically derived.

In children with cerebral palsy or other childhood brain injury, the biological aspects have been altered from the norm by anatomical and neurophysiological changes wrought by the noxious event. Although the consequences of these changes can be modified to some extent by medical or surgical intervention, for the most part they are predetermined by the nature, location, and extent of the alteration and its effect on the operation of the systems involved. The symptomatic abnormalities that follow these changes are determined by the residual structure, the biologically predetermined functions allocated to that structure, and any prior learned activities based within those structures. Functional capacity is determined by the capability of the remaining central nervous system to learn, based on the residual systems governing (1) the learning process in general, (2) the remaining structure that supports the specific activity being considered, and (3) the experience to which the individual is exposed. The ultimate functional capacity, or developmental potential, of children with cerebral palsy or other brain dysfunctions depends upon the functional integrity of each of the neural systems, together with their interconnecting pathways, and the quantity and quality of the individual's exposure to the learning experience. Development in the brain-injured individual does not necessarily follow the same precise sequence as in the normal individual. In children who have suffered brain dysfunction, the fact that the process may be slower than normal is less important than the fact that it is qualitatively different.

REQUIREMENTS FOR OPTIMUM LEARNING

The extent to which learning is possible determines the progress that can be accomplished by a therapeutic program. We are often most concerned with motor behavior specifically, but social behavior, emotional responses, attentiveness, insight, attitudes, problem solving, and communicative behavior are all subject to the same principles and their evaluation is of equal importance. Their adaptation to the individual's requirements and abilities must be included in the habilitation/rehabilitation program. In instances where brain injury has occurred, the potential for change depends upon the ability of the residual, *relevant* brain structure to carry out the necessary organization of the desired function. In short, evaluation of the potential for rehabilitation, or habilitation, of children with brain dysfunction implies addressing these questions: First, to what extent are the neural systems required for the function intact? Secondly, to what extent are the neural systems required for general learning intact? Thirdly, what are the functional characteristics of the residual central nervous system and how do they affect symptomatology and functional capability? Both manifested deficiency of function and abnormal activity (negative as well as positive symptoms) must be addressed at the same time. To evaluate the degree of disability, and to plan an appropriate therapeutic program, therefore requires an understanding of the manner in which the central nervous system organizes the relevant neurophysiological functions and, in particular, the characteristics of the learning mechanisms. With this understanding as a basis, the clinical and functional evaluation will provide a picture of capabilities and deficiencies, as well as any idiosyncratic qualities of the residual central nervous system. A therapeutic program may then be designed that takes advantage of the capabilities that remain in the functional and learning areas, attempts to maximize areas of function that may be weakened, and either bypasses or uses a substitute for those functional or learning activities that are permanently limited or irretrievably destroyed. Equally important, the evaluation process allows the limits of functional ability to be established, marking the boundaries within which goals may be set. While deficiencies in our knowledge exist, enough has been achieved in recent years to provide a sound scientific basis for therapeutic and rehabilitative programs.

INTERVENTIONS

Where evaluation indicates that motor capabilities will not be alterable by a learning process, surgical interventions and prosthetic/orthotic assistance have been commonly used. There is ample evidence that they can minimize or modify the symptomatic sequelae of the neural deficiency. This is accomplished almost entirely by the selective ablation or interruption of structures or processes participating in the undesired symptomatology. Orthopedic procedures for the treatment of spasticity have become standardized,[64] and the usefulness of surgery to release or strengthen a muscle or tendon is well documented. Attempts to substitute the action of a spastic muscle for a flaccid one have been made, but have proved of limited value. Sharrard described transfer of the iliopsoas through a window in the ilium to supplement the gluteus medius.[64] Unfortunately, the transferred muscle loses much of its strength because of denervation, and the procedure has fallen into disfavor. A similar problem was found to follow the slide-release operation to the wrist and finger flexors of the forearm.

More recently, excision of lengths of bone has been advocated to diminish spasticity of the related muscles. The most commonly used procedures are excision of one row of the carpal bones for wrist flexor spasticity and femoral shortening for spasticity of the hamstrings or adductors of the hip. While both procedures are effective in reducing the spasticity of the targeted muscles, it should be noted that the antagonist muscles, which are often hypotonic to begin with, are further weakened by the diminution of effectiveness resulting from the altered length-strength relationships. In the case of femoral shortening, the secondary weakening of the quadriceps may have serious effects on the ability to ambulate. Several months of intensive therapy may be required to maximize knee extension or even to improve it to an adequate level.

In the presence of asymmetric spasticity of the spinal musculature, spinal fusion using Luque or Dwyer instrumentation has been extremely useful in correcting or preventing scoliosis.[7,50] However, if too great a proportion of spinal length is immobilized, and there is limitation in manual dexterity or range of motion of the major joints of the upper extremities, there is a possibility of loss of important self-care functions, such as dressing or toileting. In this situation, the Luque and Dwyer instrumentation allows the surgeon greater freedom of choice than the older Harrington procedures, which require longer segments to be immobilized. Prior to surgery, a period of training using a thoracolumbar-sacral orthosis for external immobilization may be helpful in avoiding such disastrous consequences. Either a technique for accomplishing these important activities may be learned before the permanent procedure is attempted, or the fusion-fixation procedure may be modified or deferred. In the worst case, the loss of function will not come as a surprise when it is irremediable.

Neurosurgeons have revived a modified version of Forster's[23] original posterior rhizotomy operation using modern electrodiagnostic techniques to selectively ablate afferent fibers contributing to the clinically observed pattern of spasticity.[12] While favorable results in reducing spasticity have been reported, it is still undetermined whether the improvement in function achieved is superior to that obtained by the older orthopedic soft tissue releases or by lengthenings. If the results are shown to be better, another question is whether the relative risk of the multiple laminectomies required is warranted when compared with that of the orthopedic procedures. In almost all the reports the procedure was used to treat lower extremity problems that have been addressed reasonably satisfactorily by the orthopedic procedures. Greater attention to upper extremity function is needed; while the orthopedic approaches[26] are known to be modestly useful, posterior rhizotomy to the segments of the cervical cord still must be validated.

An indication of the benefits to upper extremity function that may be obtained by interruption of proprioceptive afferents can be inferred from the usefulness of intramuscular neurolysis[15] in upper extremity spasticity. In this procedure, intramuscular phenol instillation is administered in a manner calculated to interrupt afferent elements of the nerve, together with some of the motor innervation.[33] The advantage of intramuscular neurolysis is that each muscle can be approached individually and the dose titrated to the needs of the individual. The procedure itself is minimally traumatic, and the anesthesia required is extremely light. The relaxation persists for an average of nine months.[34] An adequate therapeutic trial that includes specific training in utilization of the involved musculature can demonstrate whether there is enough motor control and capacity for learning manual skills to warrant a permanent procedure. The neurolysis may be repeated at nine-month or yearly intervals to prolong the learning experience. The disadvantages are that the procedure is temporary and that proper technique requires one to two hours for each muscular group.

As an adjunct to surgical procedures, orthoses have been useful. The most frequently used is a short leg-brace to control equinus. Recently, the all plastic ankle-foot orthosis (AFO), usually made of heat-molded polypropylene, has been in vogue. This orthosis does not have an ankle joint. While some have claimed its inherent elasticity is adequate, for individuals who are otherwise competent walkers the rigidity of the ankle inhibits a longer, more efficient, and more cosmetic stride because of the instability of the foot at heel-strike. Inserting a soft sponge rubber heel in the shoe can sometimes compensate for the whiplike motion in a manner similar to the action of a single-axis cushioned heel (SACH) in prosthetics. Inserting an ankle joint between the foot and leg sections is a better, but more expensive, solution. The older double upright bar with ankle joints provides better function for these individuals and as a rule is less expensive, but it is less desirable cosmetically.

Another problem with polypropylene ankle or foot orthoses is that an accurate fit to the medio-lateral aspects of the patient's heel is rarely achieved. Control of the rear of the foot is inadequate, stability during ambulation is compromised, and pes planus or varus is permitted to develop. The orthotist must compensate for this poor fit by cementing properly carved pelite or plastizote inserts on the medial or lateral contours of the orthosis where it contacts the calcaneus. Glass reinforced polyester material can provide a better fit, but the frequency of sensitivity of the patient to the resins or toxicity to personnel during the fabrication process has limited its acceptance by orthotists. A more suitable material and technology for this purpose is necessary. Nonetheless, the polyester can be handled relatively safely by using the same vacuum form molding as is used with the polypropylene, which minimizes exposure. A polyvinyl resin also has shown a lower incidence of toxicity.

Long leg-braces, or knee-ankle-foot orthoses (KAFOs), are useful in assisting knee extension while walking in individuals with a crouching posture during stance or ambulation. They are not preferred as a permanent solution because of their weight and inherent awkwardness, in addition to the difficulty they cause in independent dressing. However, they can be an extremely important aide during training for erect stance and ambulation. At first, with assistance in balance, stance may be practiced. Then, with the braces still locked, training may focus on learning proper weight shift, balance, and reciprocation, gradually introducing the dynamic sequence of knee flexion and extension during stepping to develop an efficient, low energy gait. Progression to ambulation training may be started when balance and weight shift are adequate. Later in training, the patient walks for increasingly prolonged periods with the joint unlocked. It is important during this type of training to be sure that both hips and ankles have a complete range of motion, and measures must be taken to minimize hypertonia of the hamstrings, and, less frequently, of the quadriceps.

Spinal braces are used as a teaching aid during the training process or to provide assistance in sitting erect in a wheelchair. For the young child with severe spinal hypotonia, a Hoke-type corset with a supportive metal H-bar in the back is extremely helpful. It should be shaped to provide an appropriate contour for the thoracic and lumbosacral torso with adequate lumbar lordosis, thus permitting a cosmetically appropriate erect sitting posture. The corrected posture is important so that the child becomes accustomed to the desired proprioception. This sense of correct posture is crucial for future training. All too often, if a floppy posture prevails in the early years, the child develops no perception of correct posture. Subsequent efforts to alter the poor posture are rejected, even if greater motor capabilities are achieved.

In older, more severely affected individuals, a polypropylene thoraco-lumbar-sacral orthosis (TLSO) of the bivalved type may be used to improve posture in the wheelchair. This method provides better control of posture than does the use of multiple straps or lateral supports attached to the wheelchair. It also affords a stable foundation for training of upper extremity function. Such an orthosis cannot be used to restrain severe dystonic posturing, which may be elicited either by intention to move or by a multiplicity of uninhibited reflexes. However, there is a place for such a restraint when it is used in conjunction with a careful, consistent inhibition training program. The patient's tolerance for equipment and procedures must not be exceeded, since antipathy to the device may break down compliance with the program. A distinction must be made between obligatory dystonia and that related to excitation in response to the novelty of the program or the devices used. Appropriate medications may be of help in these situations of excessive responsiveness.

Similar considerations apply to the acquisition of adequate head control. A hinged head halter,[35] has been described by the University of Minnesota group and has been extremely useful for either head or spinal postural control when used in accordance with appropriate behavioral training principles. For more severely affected individuals, it may be alternated with a device that supports the head for longer periods of time. A modified well-fitted Philadelphia collar may be used for positive head support, together with a TLSO, if needed, for spinal support. The collar can be removed separately during training sessions and the head halter substituted. Manual assistance may be provided by the therapist if erect posture can only be maintained successfully for moments. The head halter provides tactile sensory cues to elicit erect head or spinal posture for brief periods of time, and its use can be increased as ability improves. Bizzi and his colleagues have carried out a number of interesting studies on the mechanisms involved in achieving head posture.[5]

Wheelchair positioning for severely affected individuals has been emphasized periodically. Multiple straps attached to side and back supports immobilize the patient in the most cosmetic position. The discomfort of this immobilization, plus the unrelieved pressure of sitting, has stimulated attempts to develop a form-fitting seat to distribute the pressure better. However, except in the smallest individuals, the superincumbent weight distributed evenly over the maximum sitting area still exceeds tolerated capillary-venous pressure. Solutions based upon mechanically operated alternating pressure devices have been described[48] but are not commercially available. The alternative to immobilization is a compromise that allows some movement, but at the expense of poorer posture. A satisfactory and less difficult solution for most individuals is to tilt the back and seat of the chair backward 15–30°, effectively increasing the area over which pressure is distributed and at the same time decreasing pressure on the seat. Concern has been expressed that vestibular extensor reflexes might be increased, but this has not been observed in instances when the above principle was used. The tilted-backward position is also useful for individuals with hypotonia of the spinal musculature for the same reason, namely, that it decreases the deforming force of gravity. The head halter may be attached to the wheelchair to assist and promote active erect sitting posture.

Children with severe impairment of communication have been helped by visual or manual communication boards. The child selects subject matter by pointing, by eye movement, or by operating a trigger switch attached to a scanning device. The display can be in the form of words, phrases, letters for spelling, symbolic images (as in the Bliss system), or pictures (as in the Rebus system), depending upon the abilities of the child. With the advent of sophisticated computer technology, children with communication defects and severe motor impairment have been able to achieve considerable functional improvement.[40,68]

PHARMACOLOGIC CONSIDERATIONS

Recently, advances in the understanding of neurotransmitter activity have opened new possibilities of pharmacologic approaches to the rehabilitative process. These advances have improved our understanding of the neural processes involved in the employment of alternative pathways to effect an activity.[9] The most significant fact revealed in all the related literature is that while neurotransmitter manipulation may modify responsiveness to stimuli, either favorably or unfavorably, specific experience, optimally provided, is always a basic requirement for accomplishing the appropriate learning. An interesting observation in this work is that norepinephrine appears to play a role in the interaction between the cerebellum and cerebral cortex. Its administration after lesions to the cerebral cortex caused by surgery in animals or stroke in humans assists in the reappearance of functional motor activity. Dextroamphetamine has been used for the enhancement of norepinephrine effects in much of this work, although dopamine effects are significantly increased as well by this medication. The effects of dextroamphetamine[55,57] and related medications on attentiveness and improvement of defects that inhibit learning behavior—distractibility, perseveration, stimulus-bound responsiveness, and hyperactivity—are particularly dependent upon dopaminergic activity.[43,44]

Norepinephrine has been shown to have an important role in some aspects of processes involved in learning and problem solving.[56,57] Other important pharmaceutical applications are reported by Miczek,[55] who has shown that anticholinergic medications have a suppressive effect on learning based on aversive or avoidance response. Similarly, Vanderwolf[67] has demonstrated severe impairment of learning and memory following cholinergic and serotonergic blockade. While other areas of the brain participate in learning, and avoidance learning in particular, Blozovski[6] has shown that the limbic system plays a role in the mediation of this cholinergic-dependent avoidance learning. Medications like the phenothiazines, butyrophenones, and tricyclics affect noradrenergic, cholinergic, and serotonergic synaptic activity to varying degrees. Their utilization for behavioral management or for facilitated learning requires an understanding of the relative actions of the neurotransmitter, together with appropriate modification of teaching techniques. Since the anticholinergic effects act primarily on aversive learning, teaching techniques should emphasize positive reinforcement primarily and should not generate negative consequences to responses when these medications cannot be avoided. Careful training techniques must be accompanied by close observation of the responses and attitudes of the individual patient. A common teaching technique involves prompt feedback, or knowledge of results as a guide to improvement of the skill and as a motivating device. However, if the feedback is administered in such a manner that it may be construed by the patient as punitive, or negatively characterized, learning may be impaired. On the other hand, positive reinforcement may still be effective, provided these medications do not produce generalized sedation. The effects of the norepinephrine system on positive reinforcement may even be enhanced by the tricyclics. Those with low anticholinergic activity are to be preferred for situations in which attentive or inhibitory functions are deficient and other medications like the amphetamine group are not effective, or have temporarily lost their effectiveness. This information should not be construed to mean that feedback, or negative reinforcement, should always be avoided. If the cholinergic systems are intact, then feedback, even if negatively construed, may be a very helpful learning mechanism, as long as goals are realistic and motivation is maintained. This method provides a basis for learning skills by gradual or stepwise approximation.

The benzodiazepines appear to interfere with learning in a general way by virtue of their overall sedative effect or production of a state of diminished responsiveness. Therefore, when attempting to correct maladaptive or incorrect motor patterns, where negative reinforcement by feedback or negative instruction may be required, anticholinergics and benzodiazepine may be contraindicated. While the phenothiazines and butyrophenones have major effects on synaptic cholinergic levels, the butyrophenones block dopamine receptors and the tricyclic medications also have significant effects on norepinephrine, dopamine, and, in some cases, serotonin levels. The usefulness of the tricyclics in ameliorating aspects of hyperactivity or impulsivity may outweigh their anticholinergic properties. It is often possible to use one of the newer products in this family that have minimal undesired effects.

A broader understanding of the complex actions of these medications permits their more discriminating utilization. Functional improvement through training may be enhanced by avoidance of medications that would tend to interfere pharmacologically with the learning process and administration of those that might help it, when indicated. For example, hyperactivity that is part of the attention deficit syndrome and hyperactivity deriving from generalized irritability of the uninhibited midbrain reticular-activating system must be distinguished. In the attention-deficit disorder, responses are characteristically to stimuli that are irrelevant to the context or meaning of the situation—that is, to such elements as size, sequence, proximity, brightness, or motion rather than significance. Amphetamines, tricyclics, or methylphenidate may be useful in these individuals. On the other hand, those with diffuse excitability, restlessness, or irritability to nonspecific stimuli may do better with more general tranquilizers of the benzodiazepine or phenothiazine group, preferably one that has minimal anticholinergic activity.

THERAPEUTIC TECHNIQUES OR APPROACHES

Various methods and techniques have been described that purport to introduce stimuli to influence the nervous system at different sensory-motor levels.[3,8,61] Few experimental investigations have actually been carried out, and none have convincingly shown significant functional effects that stem from their stimulation characteristics.[58,63,71] Where positive results have been found, they can usually be ascribed to learning that occurred during the controlled (or sometimes serendipitous) experiential exposure that is a usual component of these procedures. This exposure is often introduced by the therapist as play, which is well recognized as favoring learning. However, what is learned may not always be what is intended, if basic principles of learning are not carefully followed.

Much consideration has been given to "developmental sequences." However, while these sequences are well established in normal individuals,[25,41] it must be recognized, as noted above, that the development of individuals with brain dysfunction follows a characteristically unique path. It is not simply slower than normal; therefore, it must be clinically evaluated for each patient. Each of the relevant functional systems of the central nervous system referred to above must be individually considered, as must the effects of their interactions on performance and learning in the system being observed, together with the effects on general ability to learn and to solve individual problems. The "normal" sequence is a general guide only. Where patients show a nascent ability to accomplish a useful motion or behavior, the fact that it may be out of the normal sequence or involve an "undesired reflex" should not prevent its being used and further developed through training to functional skill level. To the extent that an undesired reflex interferes with function, measures should be taken to diminish its impact. These measures may be inhibitory training, orthopedic or neurologic surgery, or peripheral or intramuscular neurolysis.

The notion of brain plasticity has also been proposed[4] as a unifying concept for rehabilitation. This topic subsumes such disparate processes as the training of vision in amblyopic animals, environmental enrichment, neural sprouting, catecholamine in animals after cortical lesions and in humans after strokes, training of facial movements in individuals after hypoglossal-facial anastamosis, sensory substitution, and the training of such unusual motor phenomena as voluntary ocular torsion of extreme degree. Yu has shown that another manner in which function may be recovered after a lesion is through disclosure of a preexisting alternative pathway, which may be accomplished by means of an appropriate teaching procedure.[72,73] All of these processes are dependent upon more or less carefully applied experiential exposure or behavioral training that results in effective learning.

The conclusion must follow that the most important means of altering the repertory of response of the central nervous system is the same for both the abnormal and the normal one, namely, through the learning process. The idea of plasticity, while valid as a truism, is of importance mainly as a philosophical or attitudinal approach in rehabilitation rather than a unifying theory of neurophysiology. The concept of plasticity does imply that a thorough understanding of basic neurophysiological mechanisms *at all levels* is important in directing the learning process for greatest efficiency by selecting the most effective training objectives and techniques on the basis of both general basic principles and specific individual neurophysiological and biochemical characteristics.

THE LEARNING PROCESS

Recent investigation into the psychological foundations of the learning process,[42,62] as well as experience in the training of high-level motor skills in the performing arts and athletics, emphasizes the importance of a number of cognitive activities in motor learning.[38] These studies indicate that a rehabilitation training program must include the following elements:

- attention focus and maintenance;[46,47,65]
- active repetition;[49,69]
- knowledge of results;[47,p.151]
- feedback;[59]
- memory.[65,66]

Reinforcement should be given, contingent upon the performance of the targeted activity, which may be a motor activity of the desired speed, strength, distance, or duration or a behavioral or cognitive activity. Reinforcement is defined operationally as a contingency to an action that increases the probability of repetition of that action on exposure to the same set of stimuli. The role of reinforcement, or reward as used in operant responses, or conditioning of behavior, is to confer significance on the response to which it is associated. As a result, attention is gained and directed, and motivation is increased. When skillfully used, these cognitive activities, which are essential for optimum learning, are enhanced. During the training process attention and feedback information may be focused on each of the subordinate or component elements of the motoric, behavioral, or attitudinal material to be learned[31,32] in order to build up a more complex motor pattern or skill.

OVERVIEW OF MOTOR ORGANIZATION

Because rehabilitation, or, in the case of young children, habilitation, focuses on motor function as a major aspect of the program, a brief overview of modern basic concepts of motor organization will be presented. The reader should be aware that a careful review of the basic neurophysiological literature concerning brain function will provide a greater depth of understanding, as well as improved ability to apply this information to the clinical situation in a constructive and imaginative manner.

The Role of the Cerebral Cortex

The motor cortex[19,20,21] either receives programming input directly or receives it indirectly from the premotor and frontal cortex,[70] frontal and prefrontal cortex,[24] limbic system,[1] and sensory and occipital cortex. Brooks[11] has emphasized that volitional motor programs are well-learned motions that can be performed without the need for sensory feedback after being learned, and that different types of movements can be chosen to meet varying circumstances, either in different situations or in the presence of dysfunction. The concepts discussed in these reviews and those to be mentioned later in connection with basal ganglia and cerebellar function reflect present-day knowledge of the organization of human motor activity and are basic to the rehabilitation of individuals with brain injury. Upper extremity movements and skills are reviewed by Humphrey.[40] Space does not permit even an abbreviated presentation of the fundamental concepts. Most studies support the idea that, in humans at least, the learning of skilled movements has at best only a tangential relationship to lower-level reflex activity. Grillner[27] has identified a mid-brain center integrating the reciprocation of quadruped walking, which needs to be triggered by cortical mechanisms. The balance and adaptation to inertia and irregularities of terrain that are required for independent walking are not included in this mechanism. The relationship of brain organization to spinal cord reflex activity is discussed by Evarts and Granit in some detail.[22] A distinction must be drawn between the learning of a movement and its performance. While subcortical structures have shown some capacity for altering performance in response to changes in stimuli, this has not been proven to be significant in humans if cortical participation is excluded by the lesion. On the other hand, a learned motor activity may include many elements in the neural hierarchy.

Spasticity, Dyspraxia, Stereotypy

The work outlined in the reviews cited above confirms and explains the clinical descriptions of deficiencies in motor function in terms of dyspraxias at different levels of motor organization. For the purpose of applying a specific training program to individuals with brain injury, it is useful to focus on the deficiencies in motor organization presented as dyspraxias at different symbolic levels. These are the following:

- complete apraxia or inability to carry out purposeful movement in the absence of paralysis;
- motor dyspraxia with stereotypy—associated irrelevant movements, or uninhibited reflex motions;
- motor dyspraxia—deficient motor sequences or synergies;
- ideomotor dyspraxia—functional purpose dyspraxia;
- constructional dyspraxia—visual spatial-perceptual-motor dyspraxia;
- ideational dyspraxia—symbolic purpose dyspraxia.

While spasticity represents a positive symptom of the defect in motor control, dyspraxia represents a negative component of the symptom complex. In this context, stereotypy may also be regarded as a positive symptom, since it is composed of muscle activity that would not normally occur.

Therapeutic management should be suited to each of these characteristic deficits. A motion is easier to learn if it is simplified and broken down into subordinate units. As the units are learned, they may be resynthesized during practice therapy sessions into a more complex whole. The translatory components may be trained by repetitions. Postural components will require training that emphasizes increasing duration of the contraction to meet the need of the movement pattern.

Flaccidity, associated with spasticity in the antagonistic muscles, may be considered an apraxia. Stimulatory or facilitatory stimuli may elicit a reflex contraction, which can be used as a basis for learning to achieve a voluntary contraction. The patient is instructed to attempt a volitional contraction simultaneously with the reflex. Initiation of reflex contractions resulting in stereotypic movements (by tapping or applying a rapid stretch to the muscle or tendon, or through vibratory stimuli[17,28] or functional electrical stimulation together with the command to activate the muscle) may succeed in eliciting enough response to permit a training program to be started.

The Role of the Basal Ganglia

The basal ganglia participate in the maintenance of postures that support active ongoing movements and take part in the coordination of automatic acts such as walking, climbing, and jumping.[13] Impairment of basal ganglia function gives rise to disturbances of posture, frequently with a predominance of flexion exaggeration, a plastic type of skeletal muscle rigidity, interference with initiation of movement, adventitious movements and postures, and slowness or loss of spontaneous reactive movements. DeLong and Georgeopoulos[14] have demonstrated that neurons in the basal ganglia participate in visually guided, slow "ramp" movements requiring accuracy, but are less active during ballistic or continuous motion. Nevertheless, the basal ganglia do appear to participate in rapid preprogrammed movements as well as slow ones.[13,p.1051]

Movement disorders associated with dopamine depletion include akinesia, or bradykinesia, adipsia, and aphagia—problems in which movement is diminished. Clearly, different systems act on the same structures. It has been suggested,[13,pp.1038,1041] for instance, that input from the nucleus accumbens may be responsible for control of these components, since lesions to this structure give rise to similar symptoms. Hagan and colleagues demonstrated that spatial learning deteriorates after catecholamine depletion in the rat brain.[29] Where these dopamine-dependent systems can be identified, the usefulness of appropriate medication should be explored.

The nucleus basalis of Meynert has been shown to provide a widely distributed acetylcholine contribution over large areas of the cerebral cortex.[18,60] A lesion to the nucleus basalis is followed by impairment of learning. More recently, a major direct gamma-aminobutyric acid projection pathway from the zona incerta of the thalamus to the cerebral cortex has been demonstrated. Lin et al.[51] described these pathways, which appear to be similar in their broad distribution to those of dopamine and norepinephrine, suggesting that they function largely in a state-regulating role rather than in the transmission of specific stimuli. Since this mode of action suggests a close relationship to cortical development and neural plasticity, future work in this area may have significance in the rehabilitation of children with brain damage.

While patients with spasticity may show problems in attentiveness, various attention deficit difficulties are common among patients with athetoid or dystonic cerebral palsy. Impulsive, stimulus-bound behavior and distractibility are quite common as a result of a lack of inhibition of responsiveness, similar to that seen in the motor sytem. Medications may be helpful.

While the dyspraxias may require facilitatory treatment and active motion training, the stereotypic motions and the dyskinetic and dystonic motor deficiencies require intensive inhibitory training. These procedures are discussed in some detail by Halpern.[31,32]

The cerebellum functions to regulate the accuracy and force of voluntary automatic and postural motor activity;[10,16,53] cerebellar contributions are noted during the preprogrammed phase of the movement, but not during the reflex phase. This means that some individuals may be able to learn a sequence of movements but not be able to carry them out in a functional setting if, for instance, postural or equilibratory activities are also required and prior training in integrating these two phases of motor activity has not been introduced. Such may be the case in certain patients with motor dyspraxia in whom interference with processing of postural information or control is present. This problem is frequent in individuals with athetosis, in whom automatic postural control in support of either an ongoing or an intended motion is characteristically deficient. Special attention must be paid to the postural requirements of both the axial and limb motor activities during the training program, and as these foundational activities are learned, they may be integrated into the functional activity. As mentioned above, in the case of individuals with ataxia, two alternative training modes may be offered. The first consists of breaking each motor act into simplified units and working on slow, careful motions while emphasizing close attention and accuracy. Maximum physical support should be provided to avoid the need for automatic postural activity while learning translatory control. The purpose is to make as much of the motion as possible take place under cerebral and basal ganglia control. On the other hand, since the cerebellum does not participate during intracortical reflex activity,[21] training the child to carry out certain motions by ballistic movements may enable him to bypass the problem. In the author's experience, both methods are helpful in selected situations. Deficiency in equilibrium responses is recognized as a specific syndrome in patients with cerebral palsy,[30] but may be amenable to special balance training.

Oral Motor Problems

In patients with brainstem lesions, difficulties in mastication,[54] swallowing, and related functions may present a serious problem.[52] Cinefluorographic study[45] can often clarify the nature of the deficient mechanism by demonstrating slowness of bolus transport, inadequate velar closure, vallecular or pyriform trapping, or silent tracheal aspiration. Some caution is needed in this type of study, since aspiration of large amounts of the barium sulfate mixture is undesirable. It is helpful prognostically to take an x-ray of the chest a day or two later if aspiration of the barium mixture during cinefluorography was detected. Clearing of the radiopaque material may signify that the aspiration was relatively minor and that an advance in the feeding program is relatively safe. Few studies have examined this issue, and further observation is needed. Positioning during swallowing is often important; Avart and Minassian have described seating arrangements to improve stability.

Speech pathologists have paid special attention to oral function, and these professionals coordinate a therapeutic feeding program together with the occupational therapist and rehabilitation nurse.[37] During cinefluorographic examination they can provide a comforting security to the child in the darkened radiological laboratory, and afterward their professional expertise is helpful in developing a therapeutic feeding program based on the findings.

THE PROGRAM

Beyond the relief of spasticity and the management of anatomic deformity, any changes in function will depend upon the learning capabilities of the residual brain tissue. In order to define learning ability and style, the clinical psychologist and neuropsychologist need to characterize the child's memory, attentive abilities, attitudes, motivation, and emotional state, all of which will influence behavioral responsiveness. The therapeutic program, its techniques, and its long-term and short-term objectives will be determined when this information is integrated with evaluation of the sensory, perceptual, motor, and communicative systems. It is in this role that the rehabilitation nurse and the physical, occupational, and speech therapist, as well as the parent and school teacher, have the responsibility to provide the experience appropriate to the learning ability and style of the brain-injured child and to the specific characteristics of the neural organization of the function being addressed.

The basic approach to the therapeutic management of individuals with excessive movement or tone applies to all patients with impairment of inhibitory ability, whether the motor patterns are spastic, athetoid, dyspraxic, or ataxic. The therapy program strongly emphasizes volitional inhibition of the aberrant motor activity, beginning almost always with the therapist providing assistance in the inhibition of the undesired components of the motion. Manually applied passive restraint is the simplest form of this assistance. The therapist not only can prevent the undesired movement, but is also in a position to sense any reduction in involuntary tone and to reinforce or reward it immediately or in accordance with a predetermined protocol.

Behavioral management should include training in specific muscular relaxation, gradually expanding to generalized relaxation. The individual can then usually tolerate gradually increasing levels of stimulation, within limits. Since individuals differ in their capacities, and most will not be able to learn complete relaxation, it is important to define the limits of stimulus amplitude—for ambient sound levels, visual noise, movement levels, and social noise—that can be tolerated by the patient without deterioration of attentional and motor control. With these background sources of stimulation, the specifically targeted motor and behavioral activities are individually identified for each child. Again, communication must be made at a level that is suited to the development of the child's understanding and language capability and in the sensory modality that is most useful for the individual. It is important to avoid the arbitrary prejudices of teachers, physicians, or therapists regarding which sensory modality is "best" or favoring "multisensory" approaches. For individuals with difficulty in focusing attention, communication presented in multiple forms may simply amount to excess noise and be counterproductive. Careful clinical observation of responses to trials of different modalities and formats of presentation, together with thorough neuropsychological evaluation to probe sensory-receptive ability and processing, will be most productive and should guide the elaboration and administration of the physical, occupational, and speech and language therapy. The effectiveness of educational or school programs will be enhanced by the application of similar behavioral measures, if the neurophysiological state of the child is objectively recognized in the learning environment. More importantly, techniques to manage the important experiential exposures of the child must be consistent in all areas. A similar emphasis should be placed by each member of the therapeutic team on the focus and maintenance of attentiveness to the relevant subject, on communication at an appropriate level and in the most suitable modalities, and on structured reinforcement for appropriate responses. This consistency in approach not only contributes to learning the target material, whether motoric, behavioral, or verbal, but also enhances learning how to learn.

REFERENCES

1. Adamec RE, Stark-Adamec C. Lower threshold of limbic-hypothalamic arousal to unexpected environmental changes or novel events. In: Doane BK, Livingstone KE, eds. *The limbic system.* New York: Raven Press; 1986:129–145.
2. Avart HN, Minassian S. Videofluoroscopic swallowing study: adaptive seating solutions. *Arch Phys Med Rehabil.* 1984;65:666.
3. Ayres AJ. *Sensory integration and learning disorders.* Los Angeles: Western Psychological Services; 1978.
4. Bach-y-Rita P, Lazarus JC, Boyeson M, Balliet R, Myers T. Neural aspects of motor function as a basis of early and post-acute rehabilitation. In: Delisa J, Currie D, Gans B, Gatens P, Leonard JA, McPhee M, eds. *Rehabilitation medicine—principles and practice.* Philadelphia: JB Lippincott; 1988:chap 10.
5. Bizzi EA, Polit A, Morasso P. Mechanisms underlying achievement of final head position. *J Neurophysiol.* 1976;39:435–444.
6. Blozovski D. Mediation of passive avoidance learning by nicotinic hippocampic-entorhinal components in young rats. *Dev Psychobiol.* 1985;18:355–366.
7. Boachie AO, Lonstein JE, Winter RB, Koop S, Vanden Brink K, Denis F. Management of neuromuscular spinal deformities with Luque segmental instrumentation. *J Bone Joint Surg [Am].* 1989;71:548–562.
8. Bobath K, Bobath B. The neurodevelopmental treatment. In: Scrutton D, ed. *Management of children with cerebral palsy.* London: Spastics International Medical Publications; 1984:6–18.
9. Boyeson MG, Feeney DM. The role of norepinephrine in recovery from brain injury. *Neurosci Abstr.* 1984;10:68.
10. Brooks VB, Thach WT. Cerebellar control of posture and movement. In: Brooks VB, ed. *Motor control.* Bethesda, Maryland: American Physiological Society; 1981:877–946. (Brookhart JM, Mountcastle VB, eds. *Handbook of physiology; section I, the nervous system:* vol 2).
11. Brooks VB. Motor programs revisited. In: Talbott RE, Humphrey DR, eds. *Posture and movement.* New York: Raven Press; 1977:13–49.
12. Cahan LD, Kundi MS, McPherson D, Starr A, Peacock W. Electrophysiologic studies in selective dorsal rhizotomy for spasticity in children with cerebral palsy. *Appl Neurophysiol.* 1987;50:459–462.
13. DeLong MR, Georgeopoulos AP. Motor functions of the basal ganglia. In: Brooks VB, ed. *Motor control.* Bethesda, Maryland: American Physiological Society; 1981:1017–1061. (Brookhart JM, Mountcastle VB, eds. *Handbook of physiology; section I, the nervous system:* vol 2).
14. DeLong MR, Georgeopoulos AP. Motor function of the basal ganglia as revealed by studies of single cell activity in the behaving primate. *Adv Neurol.* 1979;24:131–140.
15. Easton JKM, Ozel T, Halpern D. Intramuscular neurolysis for spasticity in children. *Arch Phys Med Rehabil.* 1979;60:155–158.
16. Eccles JC, Ito M, Szentogathai J. *The cerebellum as a neuronal machine.* New York: Springer-Verlag; 1967.
17. Eklund G, Steen M. Muscle vibration therapy in children with cerebral palsy. *Scand J Rehabil Med.* 1969;1:35–37.

18. Emson PC, Lindvall O. Distribution of putative neurotransmitters in the neocortex. *Neuroscience.* 1979;4:1–30.
19. Evarts EV. The motor cortex and voluntary movement. In: Brooks VB, ed. *Motor control.* Bethesda, Maryland: American Physiological Society; 1981:1104–1110. (Brookhart JM, Mountcastle VB, eds. *Handbook of physiology; section I, the nervous system*: vol 2).
20. Evarts EV, Fromm C. Transcortical reflexes and servo control of movements. *Can J Physiol Pharmacol.* 1981;59:757–775.
21. Evarts EV. Role of motor cortex in voluntary movements in primates. In: Brooks VB, ed. *Motor control.* Bethesda, Maryland: American Physiological Society; 1981:1083–1120. (Brookhart JM, Mountcastle VB, eds. *Handbook of physiology; section I, the nervous system*: vol 2).
22. Evarts EV, Granit R. Relations of reflexes and intended movements. *Prog Brain Res.* 1978;44:1–14.
23. Forster A. Resection of posterior nerve roots of the spinal cord. *Lancet.* 1911;2:76–79.
24. Fuster JM. Prefrontal cortex in motor control. In: Brooks VB, ed. *Motor control.* Bethesda, Maryland: American Physiological Society; 1981:1149–1178. (Brookhart JM, Mountcastle VB, eds. *Handbook of physiology; section I, the nervous system*: vol 2).
25. Gesell A, Amatruda CS, Knoblock H, Pasamanick B. *Developmental diagnosis.* 3rd ed. Hagerstown: Harper & Row; 1974.
26. Goldner JL. The upper extremity in cerebral palsy. In: Samilson RF, ed. *Orthopedic aspects of cerebral palsy.* London: Spastics International Medical Publications; 1975:221–257.
27. Grillner S. Locomotion in vertebrates: central mechanisms and reflex interaction. *Physiol Rev.* 1975;55:247–304.
28. Hagbarth KE, Ecklund G. The muscle vibrator—a useful tool in neurological therapeutic work. *Scand J Rehabil Med.* 1969;1:26–34.
29. Hagan JJ, Alpert JE, Morris RG. The effects of central catecholamine depletion on spatial learning in rats. *Behav Brain Res.* 1983;9:83–104.
30. Hagberg B, Sanner G, Steen M. The disequilibrium syndrome in cerebral palsy. *Acta Pediatr Scand.* 1972;226(Suppl):5–63.
31. Halpern D. Therapeutic exercise in cerebral palsy. In: Basmajian JV, ed. *Therapeutic exercise.* 4th ed. Baltimore: Williams and Wilkins; 1983.
32. Halpern D. Management of children with brain damage. In: Kottke FJ, Lehmann JF, eds. *Krusen's handbook of physical medicine and rehabilitation.* 4th ed. Philadelphia: WB Saunders; 1990.
33. Halpern D. Histologic studies in animals after intramuscular neurolysis with phenol. *Arch Phys Med Rehabil.* 1977;58:438–443.
34. Halpern D, Meelhuysen FE. Duration of relaxation after intramuscular neurolysis with phenol. *JAMA.* 1967;200:1152–1154.
35. Halpern D, Kotte FJ, Burrill C, Fiterman C, Popp J, Palmer S. Training of control of head posture in children with cerebral palsy. *Dev Med Child Neurol.* 1970;12:290–305.
36. Halpern D, Telegen A, Sineps D. Assessment and planning for children with speech problems. *Arch Phys Med Rehabil.* 1969;50:194–201.
37. Havlak D, Simonsen RJ, Goth K, Keyes A, Baber B, Dickenson P, Alexander K. Multi-disciplinary care of nutrition in the patient with head injury. *Arch Phys Med Rehabil.* 1982;63:520.
38. Hill LD. Contributions of behavior modification to cerebral palsy habilitation. *Phys Ther.* 1985;65:341–345.
39. Horsman L. Disabled individuals can talk to their computers. *Rehabil Lit.* 1983;44 (3–4):71–74.
40. Humphrey DR. On the cortical control of visually directed reaching: contributions by non-precentral motor areas. In: Talbott RE, Humphrey DR, eds. *Posture and movement.* New York: Raven Press; 1979:51–112.
41. Illingworth RS. *The normal child.* 9th ed. Edinburgh: E & S Livingstone; 1986.
42. Ince, LP. *Behavioral psychology in rehabilitation medicine: clinical applications.* Baltimore: Williams & Wilkins; 1980.
43. Iversen, SD. Brain dopamine and behavior. In: Iversen LL, Iversen SD, Snyder SH, eds. *Handbook of psychopharmacology; vol 8: drugs, neurotransmitters, and behavior.* New York: Plenum Press; 1977:333–384.

44. Iversen SD, Iversen LL. *Behavioral pharmacology.* 2nd ed. New York: Oxford University Press; 1981:151–165.
45. Jones RS, Kramer SS, Donner MV. Dynamic imaging of the pharynx. *Gastrointest Radiol.* 1985;10:213–224.
46. Keele SW. *Attention and human performance.* Pacific Palisades, California: Goodyear; 1973.
47. Klein RM. Attention and motor learning. In: Stelmach GE, ed. *Motor control: issues and trends.* New York: Academic Press; 1976:143–173.
48. Kosiak M. A mechanical resting surface: its effect on pressure distribution. *Arch Phys Med Rehabil.* 1976;57:481–484.
49. Kottke FJ, Halpern D, Easton JKM, Ozel AT, Burrill CA. The training of coordination. *Arch Phys Med Rehabil.* 1978;59:567–572.
50. Lascombes P, Fabre B, Fesler F, Schweitzer F, Previt J. Surgical treatment of spinal deformity due to cerebral disorders using Luque tube appliance. *Chir Pediatr.* 1989;30:271–276.
51. Lin CS, Nicolelis MAL, Schneider JS, Chapin JK. A major direct GABAergic pathway from zona incerta to neocortex. *Science.* 1990;248:1553.
52. Linden P, Mones R, Heroy J, Siebens AA. Dysphagia predicting aspiration. *Arch Phys Med Rehabil.* 1980;61:475–476.
53. Llinas RR. The cortex of the cerebellum. *Sci Am.* 1975;232:56–71.
54. Luschei EI, Goldberg LJ. Neural mechanisms of mandibular control: mastication and voluntary biting. In: Brooks VB, ed. *Motor control.* Bethesda, Maryland: American Physiological Society; 1981:1237–1274. (Brookhart JM, Mountcastle VB, eds. *Handbook of physiology; section I, the nervous system:* vol 2).
55. Miczek KA. Effects of scopolamine, amphetamine, and chlordiazepine on punishment. *Psychopharmacology (Berlin).* 1973;28:373–389.
56. Mohammed AK, Jonsson G, Archer T. Selective lesioning of forebrain noradrenaline neurons at birth abolishes the improved maze learning performance induced by rearing in complex environment. *Brain Res.* 1986;398:6–10.
57. Moore KE. Amphetamines: biochemical and behavioral actions in animals. In: Iversen LL, Iversen SD, Snyder SH, eds. *Handbook of psychopharmacology; vol 11: stimulants.* New York: Plenum Press; 1978.
58. Palmer F, Shapiro BK, Wachtel RC, Allen MC, Hiller JE, Harryman SE, Mosher BS, Meinert CL, Capute AJ. The effects of physical therapy on cerebral palsy. *N Eng J Med.* 1988;318:803–808.
59. Rack PM. Limitations on somatosensory feedback in control of posture and movement. In: Brooks VB, ed. *Motor control.* Bethesda, Maryland: American Physiological Society; 1981:252–253. (Brookhart JM, Mountcastle VB, eds. *Handbook of physiology; section I, the nervous system:* vol 2).
60. Ridley RM, Murray TK, Johnson JA, Baker HF. Learning impairment following lesion of the basal nucleus of Meynert in the marmoset: modification by cholinergic drugs. *Brain Res.* 1986;45:108–116.
61. Rood M. The use of sensory receptors to activate, facilitate, and inhibit motor response, automatic, and somatic in developmental sequence. In: Sately C, ed. *Approaches to treatment of patients with neuromuscular dysfunction.* Dubuque: William C. Brown; 1962.
62. Ross A. *Child behavior therapy.* New York: John Wiley; 1981:8–20, 90–104.
63. Scherzer AL, Mike V, Ilson J. Physical therapy as a determinant of change in the cerebral palsied infant. *Pediatrics.* 1976;58:47–52.
64. Samilson R, ed. *Orthopedic aspects of cerebral palsy.* Philadelphia: JB Lippincott; 1975. (Clinics in Developmental Medicine: nos 52/53).
65. Spitzer H, Desimone R, Moran J. Increased attention enhances both behavioral and neuronal performance. *Science.* 1988;240:338–340.
66. Thompson R, Crinella FM, Yu J. *Brain mechanisms in problem solving and intelligence: a lesion survey of the rat brain.* New York: Plenum Press; 1990.
67. Vanderwolf CH. Near-total loss of 'learning' and 'memory' as a result of combined cholinergic and serotonergic blockage in the rat. *Behav Brain Res.* 1987;23:43–57.
68. Vanderheiden G. Providing the child with a means to indicate. In: Vanderheiden GC, Grilley K, eds. *Non-vocal communication techniques and aids for the severely physically handicapped.* Baltimore: University Park Press; 1976.

69. White BL. Experience and the development of motor mechanisms. In: Connolly K, ed. *Mechanisms of motor skill development*. New York: Academic Press; 1970.

70. Wiesendanger M. Organization of secondary motor areas of the cerebral cortex. In: Brooks VB, ed. *Motor control*. Bethesda, Maryland: American Physiological Society; 1981:1121–1147. (Brookhart JM, Mountcastle VB, eds. *Handbook of physiology; section I, the nervous system*: vol 2).

71. Wright T, Nicholson J. Physiotherapy for the spastic child: an evaluation. *Dev Med Child Neurol*. 1973;15:146–163.

72. Yu J. Neuromuscular recovery with training after central nervous system lesions: experimental approach. In: Ince LP, ed. *Behavioral psychology in rehabilitation medicine: clinical applications*. Baltimore: Williams & Wilkins; 1980:402–419.

73. Yu J. Animal models of recovery with training after central nervous system lesions. *Int Rehabil Med*. 1982;4:190–194.

Chapter 4

PLASTICITY OF THE NERVOUS SYSTEM: IMPORTANCE IN MEDICAL REHABILITATION

Paul Bach-y-Rita

BACKGROUND

Neurorehabilitation has been a major part of the field of rehabilitation since 1890, when Frenkel described a detailed program that Licht[49] called ". . . the fundamental methodology of rehabilitation in chronic neurologic illness, namely daily exercises of active attempts by a patient to correct subnormal function by voluntary repetition." However, the scientific foundation for neurorehabilitation has never been sufficiently developed for a number of reasons, detailed elsewhere.[7] Thus, although the team approach to rehabilitation is now the most common approach to neurorehabilitation, it has not been adequately validated. I will discuss the concept of neurorehabilitation based on plasticity theory, as well as one such program, concentrating on late neurorehabilitation. This chapter is an expanded version of a handout prepared for a World Health Organization-sponsored lecture delivered in Beijing, China, in November 1988.

Spontaneous Recovery

Recovery from stroke and traumatic brain injury can be categorized as "spontaneous" recovery or recovery obtainable by interventions that influence neural mechanisms. The stages of recovery have been described by several authors, including Twitchell[72] and Brunnstrom,[26] and have been reviewed elsewhere.[9] In human studies, spontaneous recovery may be difficult to determine, since most patients receive assisted range of motion to the paralyzed extremities. Even in primate studies, Travis and Woolsey[70] demonstrated the importance of physical therapy to avoid contractures that would mask spontaneous recovery. When they provided passive limb, trunk, and neck movements 10–14 times per day in their brain-lesioned monkeys, they were able to demonstrate considerable return of function following extensive neocortical damage. As a result of this therapy, a totally decorticated monkey learned to right itself, get to its feet unaided, sit, stand, and walk alone. Results such as these had not been obtained in previous studies that had not included therapy.

FACTORS RELEVANT TO RECOVERY OBTAINABLE BY INTERVENTIONS

Neural Mechanisms

An analysis of the neural mechanisms involved in the damage and in the recovery process should lead to improved therapy methodologies. Three categories of considerations will be discussed here: neuroanatomical, neurophysiological, and neurotransmitter.

Neuroanatomical Considerations

Hierarchical organization of the brain. Phylogenetically and ontogenetically, the nervous system develops in a hierarchical sequence. Moore[55] noted that the entire central nervous system (CNS) can be divided into archi-, paleo-, and neomammalian parts. The archimammalian component is the central core and includes the autonomic and reticular systems of the neuraxis and the archicerebellovestibular system. The paleomammalian part includes the protopathic or protective systems, while the neomammalian portion represents the epicritic or exploratory component of the CNS. The majority of the neuronal processes projecting from the archi- systems do so bilaterally and are highly multisynaptic in character. The pathways of the paleo- system tend to cross (decussate) and exert their major influences contralaterally; they have fewer multisynaptic connections. The neocerebral systems appear to give humans laterality: they have the most numerous direct fiber connections between lower and higher centers and vice versa, and are the last to develop full functional capabilities, often years after birth. The neocortical structures that constitute 90% of the human brain mass are also the most subject to damage because of their exposed location and the fact that the blood vessels supplying these structures are principally terminal branches, thus allowing little opportunity for collateral circulation.[55]

The phylogenetically older levels of the CNS continually set and reset the background chemical environment, emotional status, and muscular tone, including balance and timing, that are necessary for normal stereofunctioning, for learning, and for manipulating the three-dimensional environment. The nuclear centers and fiber projections of all three systems (archi-, paleo-, and neo-) synapse with commissural interneurons so that the bilaterality of the brain is preserved, in spite of the evolutionary trend toward lateralization of function. Thus, even "hemiplegic" patients (with unilateral brain damage) reveal at least some bilateral dysfunction[55] (also see below).

Integrative structures.   Only a few reflexes in humans (e.g., myotatic, such as the patellar reflex) are simple two-neuron reflexes. The rest are more complex, including feedback circuits, ascending and descending collaterals, and commissural interneuronal connections. In most cases, thousands of neurons are involved in regulating the activity of a single cell. Almost all the ascending and descending fibers in the CNS white matter are long interneurons. Moore[55] considers that the majority of the pyramidal tract fibers are interneurons with integrative functions. Some synapse on other interneurons before synapsing on alpha and gamma motoneurons, while many are concerned with modifying incoming sensory information and/or relaying information to subcortical nuclear areas, including the cerebellum. Most pathways (the very recent ones less so) have numerous collaterals projecting to adjacent nuclear areas of the neuraxis, and the numbers of commissural neurons (which at all levels of the body transmit information from one side to the other) increase as the phylogenetic scale is ascended. These commissural interneurons play a role in bilateral coordination and are particularly important since most human activities (dressing, for example) are bilateral.[55]

Ipsilateral pathways.   Each half of the brain controls movement primarily on the opposite side of the body. However, in addition to contralateral control, the brain also demonstrates ipsilateral control (see below). Furthermore, increased ipsilateral control is developed following unilateral brain damage. Villablanca et al.[74] have shown this result in an adult cat model, and it is quite apparent in hemispherectomy cases. For example, Gardner[42] demonstrated that a considerable amount of motor control, including walking, returned in a patient following removal of a hemisphere (520 g of tissue!). Glees[43] reviewed animal and clinical hemispherectomy studies and pointed out that intellectual function and sensory and motor control for the whole body could be subserved by the remaining hemisphere. Although far from complete, the recovery was sufficient in some cases to allow bimanual function.

Brodal,[25] in an analysis of his recovery from a stroke, emphasized the ipsilateral defects that are not usually described in a clinical examination because they are not sought. The ipsilateral deficits have been documented by several research groups. Jebson et al.[46] noted that function of the "normal" hand revealed deficits in right and left hemiplegic patients, with the most significant effects being slowness in writing, eating, and emptying and filling cans. McClanahan and Vigano[50] studied an early (less than two months after injury) and late (more than one year) group of patients with right hemisphere lesions and demonstrated significant deficits in two gross motor tests requiring proximal limb speed and coordination (hand-arm tap and directed reaching), while fine motor tests showed few differences from controls. Most of the patients were unaware of the ipsilateral deficits. These researchers discussed their findings in terms of the anatomical data that revealed ipsilateral control of proximal limb muscles. Brinkman and Kuypers,[24] summarizing their work and the work of others, found that each half of the brain has full control over arm, hand, and finger movements contralaterally, but ipsilateral control mainly involves relatively proximal arm movements. While McClanahan and Vigano[50] did not find differences between patient groups and controls in two-point discrimination or sharp-dull sensory tests, they suggested that, since the gross motor tests have a component of directed reaching and perception of the relationship of body to objects, parietal cortex dysfunction could have contributed to the functional deficits. Similarly, Mountcastle et al.[57] have described parietal cortex cells that were active only during reaching within the immediate extrapersonal space, and have shown that some of them are related to ipsilateral arm movements.

Neurophysiological Considerations

Neurophysiological data related to recovery from stroke have been discussed extensively elsewhere.[5–11,17] A large part of this chapter is based on those publications.

Inhibitory mechanisms. The process of rehabilitation is closely related to selective function and to the precise coordinated movements that are disturbed by a brain lesion. For example, a child learning to write initially demonstrates electromyographic (EMG) activity in virtually all the muscles related to the hand. As ability increases, muscle activity decreases progressively until there is a minimum of activity, coordinated to produce just the motor control necessary for writing, which is relatively fatigue-free.[60] Similarly, reflexes that are normal shortly after birth (e.g., Babinski's) are inhibited and reappear only following brain damage.

Inhibition is much more important than is generally appreciated. Even the concept of "synaptic facilitation" has been seriously challenged by evidence that synaptic use may result in some cases in inhibition rather than facilitation. Bliss et al.,[21] based on conditioning experiments in isolated cortical slabs, concluded that the great majority of pathways examined must have contained synaptic functions that were less likely to transmit excitation the more often the pathway was used. Creutzfeldt[35] concluded that intracortical inhibition plays an essential, if not the exclusive, role in the elaboration of the peculiar response properties and "trigger features" of cortical neurons. His findings indicate that over a distance of 300–400 μm each cortical neuron is inhibited by its neighbors and that the individual cortical connections (he emphasizes the existence of a large number of intracortical fibers) are essentially and dominantly inhibitory. The cortical neurons are not isolated, but rather are included in a network of intracortical connections; the cortical inhibitory module is a cylinder of 500–1,000 μm diameter, and neurons in the center would be inhibited by other neurons in the cylinder. The cylinder is not a column; it is repeated continuously, with each neuron being at the center of such a cylinder. The organization is that of a network, rather than a mosaic.[35] Creutzfeldt notes that Phillips[62] has described a comparable network for the motor system. Throughout his analysis, Creutzfeldt[35] emphasized the parallel rather than the hierarchical processing of information.

Unmasking, which has been discussed in detail elsewhere,[6,7,41,75] may relate to the balance of excitation and inhibition and may involve increased receptor excitability at the synapses of surviving neural connections following the loss of some synapses due to brain damage.[12] Wall's[75] studies of sensory inputs to the spinal cord demonstrate how sensory loss can reveal neural connections that are heavily inhibited in the normal state. He suggests that this process may use diverse connections that had been laid down in the embryo but were inhibited during maturation. (Comparably, I have postulated that the take-over of muscle fibers when motor neuron loss occurs, such as in polio, may use vestigial pathways; in the embryonic stage muscle fibers are polyneuronally innervated, and although all connections except those from one motor neuron disappear shortly after birth,[15] vestigial remains of the polyneuronal pathways may serve as tracks for the growth of pathways from a surviving motoneuron to the muscle fibers denervated by motoneuron loss.)

Modification of reflexes. Until recently, reflexes, especially the primitive reflexes, were considered rather immutable. However, it is now known that even primitive reflexes such as the vestibular ocular response can be modified and even reversed with training.[51] Tendon transfer often relies upon this change. Weiss and Brown[81] first showed reflex modification to be possible with the transfer of the biceps femoris tendon to replace a paralyzed quadriceps in children with polio. Thus, the flexor muscle had to become incorporated into extensor patterns. While this was easily accomplished, a reversion to its flexor role could still occur, even a long time after surgery, if the patient was fatigued.

Modification of the reflexes is, of course, a natural phenomenon. The normal Babinski reflex of an infant becomes suppressed during development, but a brain lesion can unmask the suppressed reflex.

Neurotransmitters

One of the exciting new areas of stroke rehabilitation research is the role of specific neurotransmitters in functional recovery. These findings have emerged from the demonstration of the presence of large numbers of neuroactive substances, some of which are concentrated in specific parts of the brain. Much of the following is taken from a section prepared by P. Bach-y-Rita for the American Academy of Physical Medicine and Rehabilitation syllabus chapter entitled "Rehabilitation in Brain Disorders."[1]

In the past, the cellular organization of the brain was studied by classic histological and silver impregnation techniques. It is now possible to map chemically defined neuronal systems that do not necessarily correspond to those described by the morphological techniques. The chemical categorization, largely by classes of neurotransmitters, is leading to a greatly increased understanding of normal function, of the causes of some diseases, and of drug action mechanisms. In addition, some studies[17,65] are providing evidence on the effects of specific training on neurotransmitters, and thus on the relationship of neurotransmitters to brain plasticity. Several dozen currently known substances fulfill the criteria for neurotransmitters, and more are being discovered. In addition, there is strong evidence that a number of other naturally occurring substances, including the neuroactive peptides, amino acids, and cyclic nucleotides, also function as neurotransmitters or as modulators of neural function.

Certain substances have more or less invariable actions: gamma-aminobutyric acid and glycine inhibit, while glutamate and aspartate excite. For others, the effect depends upon the nature of the cell in which receptors are being tested. Thus, acetylcholine frequently excites but can also inhibit, whereas dopamine, norepinephrine, and serotonin almost always inhibit but have some excitatory actions. Most of the neuroactive substances are secreted at synapses; they are generally found in the highest concentrations in the presynaptic terminals, except for neurohormones and some neuromodulators. It is generally accepted (in spite of some contrary evidence) that transmitter molecules are stored within vesicles in the nerve terminal and that a calcium-dependent excitation-secretion coupling within the nerve terminal initiates the transient release of vesicular contents into the synaptic cleft. The receptors for all of the neurotransmitters studied to date are located on the surface of the cell. The only intracellular receptors are apparently those for steroid and thyroid hormones.[33]

Although synaptic transmission is the most accepted form of cell-to-cell communication in the brain, other means exist, such as hormonal and volume transmission.[13] Volume transmission, which has been postulated to be related to mass sustained function, both normal (e.g., sleep) and abnormal (e.g., epilepsy, cocaine addiction), has been discussed elsewhere.[12,17]

Among the most interesting neurotransmitters are the catecholamines, in particular dopamine and its metabolic products in the mammalian brain, norepinephrine and epinephrine. Dopamine, which comprises more than 50% of the CNS catecholamines, has a widely different distribution than epinephrine, and thus functions as more than a precursor. In parkinsonism, there are degenerative changes in the substantia nigra and partial destruction of dopamine neurons. Knowledge of the effects of disease processes on specific transmitter systems has led to effective use of L-dopa therapy for parkinsonism.

Another important catecholamine mechanism in the CNS is mediated by the locus ceruleus in the caudal pons. The fibers from this nucleus form five major noradrenergic tracks that virtually encompass the brain and cerebellum. A major effect of activating these pathways is the inhibition of spontaneous discharges, resulting in a slow type of synaptic transaction in which the hyperpolarizing response of the target cells is accompanied by increased membrane resistance.[33] Since the fibers from this small nucleus are so widespread (for example, from the locus ceruleus they sweep around the brain's frontal pole before coursing across the top of the brain), many injuries to the brain produce some destruction of locus ceruleus fibers. One consequence of damage to a terminal field projection site of the locus ceruleus is that a depression in locus ceruleus functioning occurs that affects areas remote from the primary injury site.[23] This phenomenon may be related to a shift from neurotransmitter production to protein synthesis in the locus ceruleus for repair purposes.[68] The depression in locus ceruleus functioning may be largely responsible for the transient behavioral dysfunctions observed after cortical injuries, since either amphetamine (but not apomorphine) or intraventricularly administered norepinephrine (but not dopamine) permanently accelerates recovery of function when a single dose is given shortly after injury.[23,39] Drugs that block norepinephrine activity also retard recovery of function.[23,29,40] It is particularly interesting to note that neither the retarded nor the accelerated recovery occurs in the absence of a concomitant rehabilitation program.[39]

Although the recovery of function after the transient symptoms is normally permanent, the brain is still in a vulnerable state. For example, unilateral sensorimotor deficits can be reestablished in recovered animals by administration of phenoxybenzamine (an alpha-adrenergic antagonist), but not by propranolol (a beta-adrenergic antagonist) or haloperidol.[23,40] These results indicate not only that norepinephrine is involved in maintaining the observed recovery but that certain drugs may be contraindicated following brain injuries.

Recent studies on catecholamines and other neuroactive substances suggest an exciting future for neuropharmacological therapies for stroke in combination with appropriate physical and other therapies. For example, Crisostomo et al.[36] have confirmed the Feeney et al.[39] findings in human stroke patients. Those who had active rehabilitation following a single small oral dose of amphetamine showed improvement in motor function.

The Role of Environment in Recovery of Function

Human and animal studies have revealed that the environment has an influence on recovery. For example, a large number of experiments that could be classed as rehabilitation studies have been undertaken with rats. The principal rehabilitation procedure has been manipulation of the environment.[77] These studies began with a pioneering experiment completed by Schwartz,[69] which demonstrated that allowing rats to experience an enriched environment for three months following occipital cortex lesions significantly improved their maze test scores. Rosenzweig and collaborators (summarized by Rosenzweig[65]) were able to induce significant changes in brain anatomy and chemistry in young and adult nonlesioned rats by giving them differential experience in one of three environments: standard colony cages (SC), a more enriched condition (EC) (which can be considered to be comparable to a rehabilitation program), or isolation in an impoverished environment (IC). The EC rats developed significantly greater cortical measures (tissue weight, total acetylcholinesterase activity, total cholinesterase, and cortical depth) than their restricted-environment litter mates. Most of these measures were significantly greater in the occipital region of the cortex than in other cortical areas. Furthermore, the EC effects on occipital cortical measures were also noted in rats blinded at birth.[66,67] The neuroanatomical effects of environmental complexity have been reviewed by Walsh.[76] Although in most experiments the EC was available 24 hours per day, a period of 2 hours per day was found to be as effective as 24 hours.[66]

The results with maze tests provide strong evidence that enriched experience promotes overall recovery of function. Good scores on the series of maze tests require a combination of sensorimotor capacities, motivation, learning, and memory. Unfortunately, a deficit in any one of these capacities results in inferior performance. Optimal recovery, at least for the rat, is not obtained simply by restoration of general health, and certainly not by protecting the individual from stimulation and opportunities for experience.[65]

Although stroke patients are not kept in environments comparable to the IC rats in these experiments, a patient receiving intravenous medication is kept relatively immobile to avoid displacing the needle and, in addition to this motor restriction, is in the sensory-deprived environment of a hospital room. Being placed in an intensive care unit compounds the environmental deficits: many, if not most, patients in intensive care units experience some periods of psychological disorientation.[59] Improving the environment in such units may reduce the incidence of psychiatric complications;[45] for example, over twice as many episodes of organic delirium were seen in an intensive care unit without windows as in a unit with windows.[82] The effects of these environmental factors on the mortality and morbidity of patients have yet to be determined.

In the postacute phase, patients kept in a rehabilitation ward are in unfamiliar, often hostile, environments, deprived of family and home. Rehabilitation facilities are often located in a basement or other harsh setting. These and other environmental factors may influence rehabilitation outcome. In fact, recent evidence has shown that the view through the window may influence recovery from surgery: Ulrich[73] found that surgical patients assigned to rooms with windows overlooking a natural scene had shorter postoperative hospital stays, received fewer negative evaluative comments in nurses' notes, and took fewer potent analgesics than matched patients in similar rooms with windows facing a brick building wall.

The appropriate environment for therapy is a subject of clinical importance. Whereas group activities and peer interactions may be appropriate for certain patients, other patients—and in particular certain therapeutic interventions—require a quiet environment and complete concentration. For example, electromyographic sensory feedback for developing neuromuscular control ideally requires quiet individual rooms owing to the high level of concentration necessary (see signal-to-noise ratio discussion below).

Psychosocial Factors

We have discussed the psychosocial aspects of recovery from brain damage elsewhere.[17] The following is extracted from that article.

Studies on how physically disabled persons perceive their disabilities[30,80] and how they assess the quality of their lives and the possibility of gaining abilities[79] revealed that stages of adjustment to disability, learned helplessness, and the perceived interference of disability with the attainment of goals may influence the perception as well as the desirability of partial or complete recovery of abilities. The family and the cultural milieu can also be considered key influences on the outcome of rehabilitation and/or on the desirability of recovery. Turner and Noh[71] reported that lack of social support is associated more strongly with depression than with other dimensions of psychological distress, and that the perception of support was more important for elderly persons' survival than the actual number of contacts or friends. Moos[56] has applied concepts of crisis theory to explain diverse responses of individuals to a health crisis. From this point of view, outcomes of a crisis will depend on how demographic/personal, illness-related, and physical and social environmental factors are integrated cognitively by individuals to produce a perception of the meaning of illness (cognitive appraisal), which consequently will trigger specific adaptive tasks and the development of coping skills.

Crisis theory[56] postulates that during times of disequilibrium individuals are very sensitive to outside influence; thus, actions and attitudes of health professionals and others who are significant in social contexts have a large impact on the rehabilitation process. Since staff attitudes may influence rehabilitation outcome, we consider that an understanding of the coping process and of the staff's role in it, as well as an element of optimism, can have a very positive effect.

The therapeutic environment also includes the home and social environments. This fact has been well recognized and has been incorporated into most long-term inpatient rehabilitation programs by means of the judicious use of home leave and weekend passes. In fact, a supportive family member may be able to undertake rehabilitation interventions that, although less technically developed than professional therapy, can achieve significant functional gains in the familiar and supportive environment of the home; in these surroundings, specific therapeutic activities may be more closely related to the patient's particular interests (see case discussed by Bach-y-Rita[5,pp.240–243]). Research into the effects of various therapy environments may lead to the most appropriate use of acute hospital bedside rehabilitation, rehabilitation units in acute hospitals, late (chronic) rehabilitation units, specific rehabilitation hospitals, community rehabilitation facilities, nursing homes, and home programs at different stages in the evolution of the stroke patient's recovery.

Time-Course of Recovery

The neurological and rehabilitation literature often states that virtually all the recovery from stroke that can be expected will take place during the first six months. Many laboratory and some clinical studies do not support this view, and the possibility exists that the cessation of recovery after six months results from a self-fulfilling prophecy; the clinician's attitude in this regard may influence the outcome (see "Mental Activity," below).

Laboratory studies have demonstrated that recovery of function continues to occur more than five years after a stationary lesion. For example, Harlow[44] found evidence of continuing recovery even in the sixth (last) year of his study of monkeys with brain injury. Blakemore and Falconer[20] noted a "remarkable" degree of late (after three to four years) recovery in their patients, and Levine,[48] in his study of war-injured soldiers, noted that "recovery from the effects of stationary lesions is continuous for a very long period of time and takes place for most and possibly all functions." In a more recent study, a patient with an extensive home rehabilitation program following a stroke at age 65 showed considerable recovery over a period of five years poststroke (see below).

Delay in initiating therapy after a stroke appears to reduce eventual functional recovery. For example, Black et al.,[19] in a study of recovery after cortical lesions in monkeys, found that monkeys in which therapy was delayed four months recovered 67% of preoperative function after six months of therapy, versus 82% recovery in the group in which therapy was initiated immediately. However, their study revealed other results that may also have clinical relevance, especially when the total amount of therapy that a patient can receive is severely limited by insurance coverage or for other economic reasons: When therapy was begun immediately after surgery, recovery of function after one week of therapy reached 9% of pre-operative function. When therapy was delayed four months, recovery after one week reached 50% of preoperative function.

In head injury patients, retrospectively matched for severity of the neurological damage, delay in initiating acute rehabilitation significantly increased (approximately doubled) the length and cost of rehabilitation, according to Cope and Hall.[34] The two groups consisted of those admitted before and after 35 days postinjury. The outcome at two years postinjury was comparable, although the trend suggested a better outcome in the early-admission group. A greater time difference in admission between the early and late groups might reveal differences in functional outcome.

In a study of the effect of rehabilitation on stroke outcome, Lehmann et al.[47] showed that significant functional gains obtained through rehabilitation were maintained at follow-up (an average of 28.7 months postdischarge). Furthermore, significant gains were possible among patients admitted six months and even a year after the onset of stroke. Thus, although prompt initiation of the rehabilitation program may be important, even a later program can produce significant functional gains.

Mental Activity

The human mind is capable of altering physiological functions. (No dualism is implied by this statement; the author considers mind to be a physiological function.) The broad area of behavioral medicine is based on this fact. But, in general, mind-body considerations are not sufficiently appreciated in designing treatment environments or the treatment itself. In medicine, this interaction is emphasized primarily in the study of placebos. For a new drug to be accepted, it must undergo rigorous testing, and the placebo effect must be subtracted from the "real" effect. But further consideration of the placebo effect highlights the enormous therapeutic power of the mind. Conversely, the physiologist Walter Cannon,[31] a pioneer in the field of homeostasis, was fascinated by voodoo death—the ultimate expression of the mind's ability to alter function. On the other hand, every clinician is aware of patients whose recovery seems inexplicable, but whose exceptional motivation and efforts (and often those of family members) are related to the positive outcome. This subject has been further discussed elsewhere.[5,17]

Plasticity in the Mature and Aged Brain

A large number of studies have revealed plasticity in the young brain. However, plasticity is a characteristic of normal brains of all ages. Recent studies suggest that dendritic trees of cortical neurons can grow extensively even in old age, and it would be expected that growth of synapses would accompany the expansion of the dendritic tree. In one of these studies, Buell and Coleman[28] showed that in layer-II pyramidal neurons in the human parahippocampal gyrus dendritic trees in nondemented aged persons (average age 79.6 years) were more extensive than in the brains of younger adults (average age 51.2 years). Most of the difference resulted from increases in the number and average length of terminal segments of the dendritic tree. Cells with shrunken dendritic trees were found in all brains, as reported by previous authors, but Buell and Coleman suggested that, in the nondemented aging brain, one population of neurons dies and regresses while another survives and grows. In another study, Carlen et al.[32] found that computed tomography scans revealed cerebral atrophy in the brains of eight chronic alcoholics; the four who then abstained and showed functional improvements also showed partial reversal of the atrophy. The investigators suggested that the partial recovery may have been due to regrowth of neuronal axons and dendrites that were damaged but not killed by ethanol use. These studies provide morphological evidence of plasticity in the mature and aged brain.

Learning Theory

At the end of the last century Bryan and Harter[27] analyzed the learning of telegraph operators (sending and receiving). The acquisition process for any primarily sensory skill, such as typing or telegraphic transmission, is remarkably similar. For each skill it is a slow process with several plateaus or periods of no learning. They considered that resumption of progress following a plateau was dependent on the organization of material into larger associated units, either perceptual or motor.

Miller[54] pointed out that only about six to eight elements can be held in the immediate memory at one time, and that it is immaterial whether the elements represent many or a few of the organism's receptors, or whether the units or "chunks" contain a few or many bits of information. Miller calculated the maximum capacity for transmission in several sensory systems and found that their various channel capacities were similar, with an average of 2.6 bits; that is, as the number of stimulus categories or the amount of stimulus uncertainty was increased, the amount of information transmitted reached this plateau. This corresponds to about six alternatives as a limiting number of values for the stimulus, beyond which the subject will be confused.

The rather rigid limits imposed by the inaccuracy of our absolute judgments of simple magnitudes can be expanded by the use of both simultaneous and successive discriminations. There are several ways by which the limits of the channel capacity for absolute judgments can be exceeded; for example, we can make relative rather than absolute judgments or we can arrange the task so as to permit a (temporal) sequence of absolute judgments, thereby involving memory.[54]

Absolute judgment and memory span are quite different kinds of limitations that are imposed on our ability to process information. Absolute judgment is limited by the amount of information (bits), whereas immediate memory is limited by the "items" or "chunks." The number of bits of information is constant for absolute judgments, and the number of chunks of information is constant for immediate memory.

In normal learning, more and more of the information extraction processes become automatic and unconscious, and the "chunking" process described by Miller[54] allows the number of bits per chunk to increase. For example, as a person learns to read, first individual letters are perceived, then words; as learning progresses, groups of words form a single "chunk." Does this process occur in the brain-injured patient relearning to function in his or her surroundings? Is the difficulty that a hemiplegic patient experiences in putting together the individual components of gait (which have been relearned in the rehabilitation program) into a smooth, coordinated movement related to deficits in "chunking?" Does the stroke patient learn by means of the alternating acquisition-consolidation phases (described since the last century), with each consolidation phase appearing as a plateau during which he/she is incapable of learning new material? If so, we will have to alter our concept of plateau. As used presently in the rehabilitation literature, it implies the end of learning, and upon reaching a plateau the patient is discharged. Further study of the learning process in a stroke patient may lead to therapeutic innovations such as the following: a) discharge to home or to a nursing home during consolidation (plateau) phases, with return to an active rehabilitation program when the patient enters an acquisition phase; b) more appropriate use of personnel, to avoid both staff and patient frustration; and c) inclusion of nursing homes in the therapeutic program, which may result in modifying their present (virtually exclusive) role as the final repository for therapeutic failures. Studies on the relevance of these and other learning theory concepts to stroke rehabilitation may offer considerable therapeutic benefits without requiring new theoretical breakthroughs.

BRAIN PLASTICITY AS A BASIS FOR RECOVERY FROM BRAIN DAMAGE

The neuroplasticity concepts discussed extensively in this chapter are important for an understanding of the potential for recovery following brain damage. A few additional comments will be added here before proceeding with a discussion of some developing programs of neurorehabilitation based on these concepts.

Polysensory Cells, "Multiplexing," and Neuronal Group Selection: Possible Mechanisms of Reorganization Following Brain Damage

Although brain regions and cells within individual brain regions are usually considered to carry out a particular function, there is a great deal of sharing of function and transference of functional representation of speech, motor control, and sensation. Papanicolaou et al.[61] have reviewed the data demonstrating hemispheric transfer and hemispheric sharing of the central representation of speech following damage to the left frontal cortex. Motor representation can vary from moment to moment at a particular cortical site, and function can be transferred from one hemisphere to another.[4,5] More than 80% of cells studied in the cat brain stem nucleus pontis oralis demonstrated sensory convergence.[2] I have considered the visual cortex to have multiple functions since our studies[58] showed that 47% of the cells that responded to light also responded to auditory and/or tactile (pinprick) stimuli. Wanet-Defalque et al.[78] note that metabolism is higher in the visual cortex of blind persons than in blindfolded sighted persons, whether at rest or doing an auditory or tactile task, and preliminary findings in young adults who experienced a brain injury several years earlier suggest higher metabolic activity in the visual cortex under all conditions.[22] Multiple functions of the visual cortex could include a sensory integration role; further, the same cells can participate in many functions. In 1967 I suggested that "subjective experiences may be products of a learning process in which afferent inputs from multiple sources are utilized."[3] The afferent information from a single receptor might take part in the production of several different sensations, and a single cortical cell may perform many functions.[4] Porter[64] has shown in monkeys that motoneurons innervating distally acting muscles are preferentially excited by convergent activity in corticomotoneuronal fibers; Phillips and Porter[63] had earlier found that the motor cortex projection area to a single motoneuron in the spinal cord could be up to 13 square millimeters, that areas were sometimes multiple, and that a colony for a given motoneuron commonly overlapped with colonies projecting to motoneurons of antagonistic as well as synergistic muscles.

Following a discussion of these findings, Evarts[38] postulated that recovery of function following damage to the focus for a particular movement may involve the establishment of new connections from cortical areas which in the intact animal are in the recruitment fringe (which may contain neurons that lie within the focus for a different movement). He noted that such fringe neurons have connections which allow them to assume control of new movements, given an adequate extension of their peripheral inputs and outputs within the spinal cord. Evarts considered that the motor reorganization that occurs following brain damage may involve the cerebellum, which may adaptively modify input-output relations and thereby compensate for changed information processing resulting from cerebral lesions. He suggested that recovery from restricted cortical lesions may involve a shift of control functions away from a damaged focus and into intact adjacent areas. Comparably, "multiplexing" and convergence are found in sensory systems[2] with widespread convergence on single brain stem cells; Murata et al.[58] demonstrated acoustic, pinprick, and visual convergence onto single visual cortical cells.

Sensory representation plasticity has been demonstrated by Wall in the spinal cord[75] and Merzenich in the somatosensory cortex.[52] Wall showed that afferents are present that provide a potential source of new input in the event of degeneration, and also noted a class of cells in the dorsal column nuclei that instantly switch their input upon the silencing of their normal input. With reversible cold block, the receptive fields immediately switched back and forth from one location to a widely separate location. Wall[75] considers that the brain-damaged patient learns to substitute alternative mechanisms for those he has lost. In his view nerve cells show a type of homeostasis so that, if they lose part of their input, they adjust their excitability to capture fully the excitatory effects of their remaining inputs. He suggests that the connections laid down in the embryo are more diffuse than those actually used in the adult brain and that, following brain lesion, suppressed connections may become de-suppressed; both sprouting and unmasking of ineffective connections offer the possibility of new connections after brain damage.[75] The recovery in an aged patient following extensive brain damage that included the destruction of about 97% of the pyramidal tract has been interpreted by Bach-y-Rita[5] as owing to the unmasking of connections to and from the remaining 3% of fibers.

Edelman's Theory of Neuronal Group Selection

Recently, Edelman[37] proposed a theory of neuronal group selection that can serve as a model for understanding mechanisms of recovery following brain damage. He introduces population thinking theory, which says the brain is dynamically organized into cellular populations containing individually variant networks, the structure and function of which are selected by various means during development and behavior. The units of selection are collections of hundreds of thousands of strongly interconnected neurons (neuronal groups), and they act as functional units. Several factors lead to the selection of combinations of neuronal groups. Those groups whose activities are correlated with signals arising from adaptive behavior are selected. During adult experiences, selection among populations of synapses becomes a key process. It is possible that new variations can occur within interacting neural networks and hierarchies of networks for the lifetime of the organization. Edelman's theories provide the basis for new thinking regarding brain plasticity and the mechanisms of recovery following brain damage.

A POSTACUTE NEUROREHABILITATION PROGRAM

We have developed a postacute neurorehabilitation program for the following reasons:

1. Concepts of neuroplasticity discussed in this paper and throughout the training program, as well as a review of some old clinical and experimental studies, suggested that the brain is sufficiently plastic to reorganize function even years after brain damage. A large number of persons with disabilities are potential candidates for late rehabilitation programs.

2. When a late neurorehabilitation program is initiated, after spontaneous recovery is no longer a factor, controlled studies of rehabilitation methodologies are more feasible. In fact, for the subjects in our research protocol, three semiannual baseline studies are performed and patients are not admitted unless they have shown no significant recovery over that time. Such controlled studies include objective measures such as brain images, positron emission tomography, magnetic resonance imaging, movement-related cortical potentials, and tests of motor function. Successful completion of these studies would lead to scientifically based, appropriately validated neurorehabilitation procedures.

Neuromuscular retraining methods (largely developed by Richard Balliet) emphasize external sensory feedback strategies to systemically increase patient proprioception, kinesthesia, and general awareness. Among the feedback modalities utilized are EMG feedback, functional electrical stimulation (FES), as well as various methods of therapeutic exercise (e.g., neurodevelopmental training, proprioceptive neuromuscular facilitation, Brunnstrom) and other behavioral techniques to retrain motor function. Common aspects of the neuromuscular retraining[14,18] include the following:

a. Active and passive normalization of muscle tone.
b. Establishment of improved laterality of identical muscles, including associated reaction.
c. Reduction of compensatory strategies, including undesired co-contraction of agonist/antagonist muscle groups.
d. Retraining of isolated movements or patterns in which each repetition is considered to be a discrete trial.
e. Establishment of reciprocal innervation.
f. Increase in the duration of active movement to sub-ballistic rates.
g. Application of slow, isolated motor control to functional task(s), emphasizing the concept of consistent correct behavior (ideally 75% correct response criteria) through increasingly complex tasks.

Other important components of the therapy program include the optimization of setting: one-on-one treatment, completely equipped individualized treatment rooms, and adequate treatment time (sessions of at least one hour). Emphasis is placed on training the patients to train themselves, with the help of significant others or friends. Active self-training methods that rely on simple but very specific therapeutic exercises are then applied in an extensive home program.

3. Cost-effective programs should take advantage of individual patient, family, and community resources to minimize the need for professional services. At present, approximately 95% of the therapy received by a typical patient is provided by the patient and/or a family member at no cost. Thus, appropriate neurorehabilitation may become accessible to a much larger percentage of the persons who could benefit from such services.

SENSORY SUBSTITUTION AS NEUROREHABILITATION

Adults who were born blind have used the remaining senses and brain mechanisms to develop motor, conceptual, and social behavior. However, the congenitally blind person has not had the experience of receiving and interpreting visual information and developing visual percepts. Such a person is an ideal model in which to study the development of visual spatial perception and behavior, especially since the experimenter can control all facets of the development, which can only occur with the use of the sensory substitution equipment. (In contrast, a hemiparetic patient can practice at home or in his hospital room following therapy sessions, and so there is less possibility to evaluate all of the factors that go into motor rehabilitation in these cases.)

Tactile vision substitution systems deliver visual information to the brain via the skin. The output of a small TV camera (controlled by the blind subject) is displayed on an area of skin, after transduction to a form of energy (delivered by vibrotactors or electrotactors) that can activate the skin sensory receptors. Blind persons not only develop the ability to perceive visual information, but use visual means of analysis (parallax, looming and zooming, monocular clues of depth and perspective, and subjective spatial localization). This model has served to provide a considerable amount of information on brain plasticity, perceptual mechanisms, and the coordination of sensory and motor factors in the development of a "perceptual organ," as well as other data.[4] It is also being used as a means to develop visual spatial concepts in congenitally blind children.[53] Tactile sensory substitution systems are under development for persons with other sensory losses (e.g., deafness, insensate feet and hands), as well as to permit sensory augmentation (e.g., in space suit gloves for extravehicular activities of astronauts).[16]

Although these studies have not yet led to practical instrumentation, successful development of such systems would enable neurorehabilitation for persons with sensory losses.

REFERENCES

1. American Academy of Physical Medicine and Rehabilitation. Syllabus chapter: rehabilitation in brain disorders. Chicago: AAPMR; 1985.
2. Bach-y-Rita P. Convergent and long latency unit responses in the reticular formation of the cat. *Exp Neurol.* 1964;9:327–344.
3. Bach-y-Rita P. Sensory plasticity: applications to a vision substitution system. *Acta Neurol Scand.* 1967;43:417–426.
4. Bach-y-Rita P. *Brain mechanisms in sensory substitution.* New York: Academic Press; 1972. 192 pp.
5. Bach-y-Rita P. Brain plasticity as a basis of therapeutic procedures. In: Bach-y-Rita P, ed. *Recovery of function: theoretical considerations for brain injury rehabilitation.* Bern, Switzerland: Hans Huber; 1980:225–263.
6. Bach-y-Rita P. Central nervous system lesions: sprouting and unmasking in rehabilitation. *Arch Phys Med Rehabil.* 1981;62:413–417.
7. Bach-y-Rita P. Brain plasticity as a basis for the development of rehabilitation procedures for hemiplegia. *Scand J Rehabil Med.* 1981;13:73–83.
8. Bach-y-Rita P, ed. Symposium on rehabilitation following brain damage: some neurophysiological mechanisms. *Int Rehabil Med.* 1982;4:165–199.
9. Bach-y-Rita P. The process of recovery from stroke. In: Brandstater ME, Basmajian JV, eds. *Stroke rehabilitation.* Baltimore: Williams & Wilkins; 1987:80–108.
10. Bach-y-Rita P. Brain plasticity. In: Goodgold J, ed. *Rehabilitation medicine.* St Louis: CV Mosby; 1988:113–118.
11. Bach-y-Rita P. Sensory substitution and recovery from "brain damage." In: Finger S, Levere TE, Almi CR, Stein DG, eds. *Brain injury and recovery: theoretical and controversial issues.* New York: Plenum Press; 1988:323–334.
12. Bach-y-Rita P. Thoughts on the role of volume transmission in normal and abnormal mass sustained functions. In: Fuxe K, Agnati LF, eds. *Volume transmission in the brain.* New York: Raven; 1991:489–496.
13. Bach-y-Rita P. Applications of principles of brain plasticity and training to restore function. In: Young RR, Delwaide PJ, eds. *Principles of restorative neurology.* London: Butterworths. [In press].
14. Bach-y-Rita P, Balliet RB. Recovery from stroke. In: Duncan PW, Badke MB, eds. *Motor deficits following stroke.* New York: Year Book Publishers; 1987:79–107.
15. Bach-y-Rita P, Lennerstrand G. Absence of polyneuronal innervation in cat extraocular muscles. *J Physiol.* 1975;244:613–624.
16. Bach-y-Rita P, Webster J, Tompkins W, Crabb T. Sensory substitution for space gloves and for space robots. In: Rodriguez G, ed. *Proceedings of the Workshop on Space Telerobotics.* Pasadena: Jet Propulsion Laboratories; 1987:51–57. (Publication 87-13, vol II).
17. Bach-y-Rita P, Wicab Bach-y-Rita E. Biological and psychosocial factors in recovery from brain damage in humans. *Can J Psychol.* 1990;44:148–165.
18. Balliet R. Neurorehabilitation of postacute brain injury: a key to optimizing functional motor recovery. In: Bach-y-Rita P, ed. *Traumatic brain injury.* New York: Demos; 1989:119–131.
19. Black P, Markowitz RS, Cianci SN. Recovery of motor function after lesions in motor cortex of monkey. In: CIBA Foundation, *Outcome of severe damage to the central nervous system.* Amsterdam: Elsevier; 1975:65–83.
20. Blakemore CB, Falconer MA. Long-term effects of anterior temporal lobectomy on certain cognitive functions. *J Neurol Neurosurg Psychiatry.* 1967;30:364–367.
21. Bliss TVP, Burns BD, Uttley AM. Factors affecting the conductivity of pathways in the cerebral cortex. *J Physiol.* 1968;195:339–367.
22. Blood K, Perlman S, Balliet R, Yuan J, Wilson M, Searles L, Sackett J, Lazarus J. Visual cortex hyperactivity during arm movements in brain injured individuals: evidence of compensatory shifts in functional neural systems. *J Neurol Rehabil.* [In press].
23. Boyeson MG, Feeney DM. The role of norepinephrine in recovery from brain injury. *Neurosci Abstr.* 1984;10:68.
24. Brinkman J, Kuypers HGJM. Cerebral control of contralateral and ipsilateral arm, hand and finger movements in the split-brain rhesus monkey. *Brain.* 1973;96:653–674.

25. Brodal A. Self-observations and neuroanatomical considerations after a stroke. *Brain.* 1973;96:675–694.
26. Brunnstrom S. *Movement therapy in hemiplegia.* New York: Harper & Row; 1970.
27. Bryan WL, Harter N. Studies in the telegraphic language: the acquisition of a hierarchy of habit. *Psychol Rev.* 1899;6:345–375.
28. Buell S, Coleman P. Dendritic growth in aged human brain and failure of growth in senile dementia. *Science.* 1979;206:854–856.
29. Burke RE. Group 1a synaptic input to fast and slow twitch motor units of cat tricep surae. *J Physiol.* 1968;196:605–630.
30. Campbell ME, Cull JG, Hardy RE. Disabled persons' attitude towards disability. *Psychology.* 1986;23:16–20.
31. Cannon W. Voodoo death. *Am Anthropol.* 1942;44:169–181.
32. Carlen SR et al. Reversible cerebral atrophy in recently abstinent chronic alcoholics measured by computed tomography scans. *Science.* 1978;200:1076–1078.
33. Cooper JR, Bloom FE, Roth RH. *The biochemical basis of neuropharmacology.* 4th ed. New York: Oxford University Press; 1982.
34. Cope DN, Hall K. Head injury rehabilitation: benefit of early intervention. *Arch Phys Med Rehabil.* 1982;63:433–437.
35. Creutzfeldt O. Some problems of cortical organization in the light of ideas of the classical "Hirnpathologie" and of modern neurophysiology. In: Zulch KJ, Creutzfeldt O, Galbraith GC, eds. *Cerebral localization.* Berlin: Springer; 1975:217–226.
36. Crisostomo EA, Duncan PW, Propst M, Dawson DV, Davis JN. Evidence that amphetamine with physical activity promotes recovery of motor function in stroke patients. *Ann Neurol.* 1988;23:94–97.
37. Edelman GM. *Neural darwinism.* New York: Basic Books; 1987. 371 pp.
38. Evarts E. Brain control of movement: possible mechanisms of function. In: Bach-y-Rita P, ed. *Recovery of function: theoretical considerations for brain injury rehabilitation.* Bern: Hans Huber; 1980:173–186.
39. Feeney DM, Gonzalez A, Law WA. Amphetamine, haloperidol and experience interact to affect rate of recovery after motor cortex lesion. *Science.* 1982;217:855–857.
40. Feeney D, Hovda DA, Salo A. Phenoxybenzamine reinstates all motor and sensory deficits in cats fully recovered from sensorimotor cortex ablations. *Fed Am Soc Exper Biol Abstr.* 1983;42:1157.
41. Finger S, Stein DG. *Brain damage and recovery.* New York: Academic Press; 1982.
42. Gardner WJ. Removal of the right cerebral hemisphere for infiltrating glioma. *JAMA.* 1933;101:823–826.
43. Glees P. Functional reorganization following hemispherectomy in man and after small experimental lesions in primates. In: Bach-y-Rita P, ed. *Recovery of function: theoretical considerations for brain injury rehabilitation.* Bern: Hans Huber; 1980:106–126.
44. Harlow HF. Higher functions of the nervous system. *Annu Rev Physiol.* 1953;15:493–514.
45. Heller SS, Franke KA, Malm JR, et al. Psychiatric complications of open heart surgery. *N Engl J Med.* 1970;283:1015–1019.
46. Jebson RH, Griffith ER, Long EW, et al. Function of "normal" hand in stroke patients. *Arch Phys Med Rehabil.* 1971;51:170–181.
47. Lehmann JF, Delatour BJ, Fowler RS, et al. Does rehabilitation affect outcome? *Arch Phys Med Rehabil.* 1975;56:375–382.
48. Levine J. Relative effects of occipital and peripheral blindness upon intellectual functions. *Arch Neurol Psychiatry.* 1952;67:310–314.
49. Licht S. Introduction. In: Licht S, ed. *Stroke and its rehabilitation.* Baltimore: Waverly Press; 1975.
50. McClanahan M, Vigano S. Evaluation of sensory motor function of the "uninvolved" upper extremity of patients with unilateral brain damage from stroke [Thesis]. Stanford, California: Division of Physical Therapy, Stanford University; 1978.
51. Melvill Jones G, Gonshor A. Goal-directed flexibility in the vestibulo-ocular reflex arc. In: Lennerstrand G, Bach-y-Rita P, eds. *Basic mechanisms of ocular motility and their clinical implications.* Oxford: Pergamon Press; 1975:227–245.
52. Merzenich M. Dynamics of neocortical processes and the origins of higher brain functions. In: Changeux JP, Kouislie M, eds. *The neural and molecular bases of learning.* J Wright and Sons; 1987:337–358.

53. Miletic G, Hughes B, Bach-y-Rita P. Vibrotactile stimulation: an educational program for spatial concept development. *J Visual Impair Blindness.* 1988;Nov:366–370.
54. Miller GA. The magical number seven, plus or minus two: some limits on our capacity for processing information. *Psychol Rev.* 1956;63:81–97.
55. Moore JC. Neuroanatomical considerations relating to recovery of function following brain lesions. In: Bach-y-Rita P, ed. *Recovery of function: theoretical considerations for brain injury rehabilitation.* Bern: Hans Huber; 1980:9–90.
56. Moos RH. Overview. In: Moos RH, ed. *Coping with physical illness.* New York: Plenum Medical; 1984:3–25.
57. Mountcastle VB, Lynch JC, Georgopoulos A, et al. Posterior parietal association cortex of monkey: command functions for operations within extrapersonal space. *J Neurophysiol.* 1975;38:871–908.
58. Murata K, Cramer H, Bach-y-Rita P. Neuronal convergence of noxious, acoustic and visual stimuli in the visual cortex of the cat. *J Neurophysiol.* 1965;28:1223–1239.
59. Nadelson T. Psychiatric aspects of the intensive care of critically ill patients. In: Skillman J, ed. *Intensive care.* Boston: Little, Brown; 1975:36–60.
60. Paillard J. The patterning of skilled movements. In: *Handbook of psychology,* vol 3. Baltimore: Williams & Wilkins; 1960:1679–1708.
61. Papanicolaou AC, Moore BD, Deutsch G. Reorganization of cerebral function following lesions in the left hemisphere. In: Bach-y-Rita P, ed. *Traumatic brain injury.* New York: Demos; 1989:105–118.
62. Phillips CG. Cortical localization and sensorimotor processes at the "middle level" of primates. *Proc R Soc Med.* 1973;66:987–1002.
63. Phillips CG, Porter R. *Corticospinal neurones: their role in movement.* London: Academic Press; 1977.
64. Porter R. Corticomotoneuronal projections: synaptic events related to skilled movements. *Proc R Soc London [Biol].* 1987;B231:147–168.
65. Rosenzweig M. Animal models for effects of brain lesions and for rehabilitation. In: Bach-y-Rita P, ed. *Recovery of function: theoretical considerations for brain injury rehabilitation.* Bern: Hans Huber; 1980:127–172.
66. Rosenzweig M, Bennett EL, Diamond MC, et al. Influences of environmental complexity and visual stimulation on development of occipital cortex in rats. *Brain Res.* 1969;14:427–445.
67. Rosenzweig M, Krech D, Bennett EL, et al. Effects of environmental complexity and training on brain chemistry and anatomy: a replication and extension. *J Comp Physiol Psychol.* 1962;55:429–437.
68. Ross RA, Jah PH, Reis DJ. Reversible changes in the accumulation and activities of pyrazine hydroxylase and dopamine beta hydroxylase in neurons of the locus ceruleus during the retrograde reaction period. *Brain Res.* 1975;92:57–72.
69. Schwartz S. Effect of neonatal cortical lesions and early environmental factors on adult rat behavior. *J Comp Physiol Psychol.* 1964;57:72–77.
70. Travis AM, Woolsey CN. Motor performance of monkeys after bilateral partial and total cerebral decortication. *Am J Phys Med.* 1956;35:273–310.
71. Turner RJ, Noh S. Physical disability and depression: a longitudinal analysis. *J Health Soc Behav.* 1988;29:23–27.
72. Twitchell TE. The restoration of motor function following hemiplegia in man. *Brain.* 1951;74:433–480.
73. Ulrich RS. View through the window may influence recovery from surgery. *Science.* 1984;224:420–421.
74. Villablanca JR, Gomez-Pinilla F, Sonnier BJ, Hovda D. Bilateral pericruciate cortical innervation of the red nucleus in cats with adult or neonatal cerebral hemispherectomy. *Brain Res.* 1988;453:17–31.
75. Wall PD. Mechanisms of plasticity of connection following damage in adult mammalian nervous systems. In: Bach-y-Rita P, ed. *Recovery of function: theoretical considerations for brain injury rehabilitation.* Bern: Hans Huber; 1980:91–105.
76. Walsh RN. Effects of environmental complexity and deprivation on brain anatomy and histology: a review. *Int J Neurosci.* 1981;12:33–51.
77. Walsh RN, Greenough WT, eds. *Environments as therapy for brain dysfunction.* New York: Plenum Press; 1976.
78. Wanet-Defalque MC, Veraart C, DeVolder A, Metz R, Michel C, Dooms G, Goffinet A.

High metabolic activity in the visual cortex of early blind human subjects. *Brain Res.* 1988;446:369–373.

79. Weinberg N. Physically disabled people assess the quality of their lives. *Rehabil Lit.* 1984;45:12–15.
80. Weinberg N, Williams J. How the physically disabled perceive their disabilities. *J Rehabil.* 1978;44:31–33.
81. Weiss PA, Brown P. Electromyographic studies on recoordination of leg movements in poliomyelitis patients with transposed tendons. *Proc Soc Exp Biol.* 1941;48:284–287.
82. Wilson LM. Intensive care delirium: the effect of outside deprivation in windowless units. *Arch Intern Med.* 1975;130:225–226.

Chapter 5

SEXUALITY ISSUES AND REHABILITATION STRATEGIES FOR PHYSICALLY DISABLED ADULTS AND CHILDREN

Theodore M. Cole and Sandra S. Cole

Sex! The word connotes pleasant thoughts such as love making, fun, and warmth. Disability! The word conveys the concepts of loneliness, ugliness, incapacity, and pain. Sex and disability! The emotional reaction to these two terms together might include such ideas as impossible, frustrated, withdrawn, vulnerable. The linking of these two words may require rehabilitation professionals to alter attitudes—both their own and those of others—in order to facilitate the healing process.

Physicians are trained to understand pathology and physiology, but not necessarily contemporary sexual attitudes and behaviors. Moreover, the sexual information they do possess may be the result of personal preferences and feelings as much as scientific knowledge. The net result is that physicians are sometimes poorly prepared to hear and treat sexuality complaints.

Patients and their families may contribute to this problem if they are unwilling to discuss the sensitive issue of sexuality within a health care setting. The presence of a physical disability may not be a strong enough reason to leave behind years of socialization that have taught them that they cannot talk about sex to the doctor. That same sentiment may be transmitted to the next generation, completing the cycle and contributing to a continuation of silence about sexuality and disability. The physician is in a unique position to facilitate productive discussion of this aspect of rehabilitation if sexuality is treated like any other important facet of living—an appropriate area of concern for physicians and patients alike.

DEFINITIONS

Sexuality

To the extent that sexuality is a genital function, some physical disabilities may affect sexual function. Most, such as blindness, deafness, or myocardial infarction, do not. Some may produce a degree of sexual dysfunction without affecting the genitals. An individual with a disfiguring burn may want to be accepted, but instead may withdraw and cover up. It is clear, therefore, that sexuality is both defined and expressed by how people deal with it. Sexuality influences and is influenced by physical disability. Cole and Glass define sexuality as an "avenue towards intimacy."[7] A life without intimacy may be painful to the person with the physical disability and may add to the problems presented to the clinician.

Sexual Health

If one understands the above concepts, one can appreciate the concerns a handicapped person may have about expressing sexuality—about his or her sexual health. The clinician must consider all of these concerns in order to intervene usefully on behalf of the patient. The clinician should understand how to initiate questions and interventions related to sexuality. The rehabilitationist is best advised to give consideration to his or her own sexuality in order to become more effective in dealing with the sexuality of other people. Unlike other scientific areas, one cannot effectively employ a body of knowledge about sexuality without understanding one's own sexuality. The rehabilitationist should avoid imposing a view of sexuality upon the patient which, although meaningful to the rehabilitationist, may be outside of the value system of the patient.

For the patient, sexuality is a health issue. It is part of the whole person and it is a natural function. As with physical disability, however, previous life experiences can interfere with natural functions. The medical model, which includes eliciting a thorough history and performing a complete physical examination, is a useful construct when dealing with the subject of sexuality.

What is considered sexual health for one person may not apply directly to another. Sexual health is individual. However, some common denominators—such as self-esteem, freedom from prohibitive attitudes and ignorance, and a willingness to risk intimacy with another person—do exist. Sexual health also involves a level of physical ability which, although personal and individual, is nonetheless essential. Unfortunately for disabled people, there is very little information available to help them achieve this physical or emotional competence or even to help them become educated in the matter. Consequently, many disabled people have incomplete or erroneous information about their physical abilities.

SEXUAL DYSFUNCTIONS

Sexual dysfunctions may be divided into two groups: primary and secondary.[11] Primary, or organic, dysfunctions are the direct result of bodily dysfunctions or pathology, such as endocrine disturbances, specific brain disorders, genetic disorders producing infertility, neurological diseases, and the like. Primary sexual dysfunctions can also be caused by external factors that alter bodily functions, such as medications (see Table 1). Thus, tranquilizers, antidepressants, antihypertensives, street drugs, and a host of other medications have the potential for creating primary sexual dysfunctions in men and women.

Secondary sexual dysfunctions may be caused by internal or external conditions that are a result of the disability. Included in this group are secondary dysfunctions such as cognitive loss caused by brain injury or psychiatric problems (such as in bipolar disorders) and sexual dysfunctions produced by simple mood disorders, such as might accompany depression, alcohol abuse, etc. In addition, secondary sexual dysfunctions linked to the patient's situation and medical problem may be produced in the partner of the patient, for example, a spouse who refuses sexual activity because of fear that it might stress the patient's heart and lead to a heart attack.

As Griffith et al. point out, a traumatic brain injury can affect all aspects of a partner's customary sexual function.[11] It imposes additional stress on intimacy, which may already be strained, constrained, embarrassing, dysfunctional, abusive, or mistrusting.

Lack of understanding can lead to dysfunctional relationships between the patient and important members of the family. Prior affectionate relationships may suffer and be replaced by avoidance or distaste. Unaccustomed sexual behavior from a known or long-term partner can be very dysfunctional. The interactions of sexual dysfunction in the family can even spread to include nonsexual relationships. Children may be caught up in a stressful family situation caused primarily by a sexual dysfunction related to an organic cause. Additional secondary sexual dysfunctions may result from cultural influences or religious beliefs that are confounded by the disability.

Health care professionals should avoid contributing to secondary sexual dysfunctions. Unknowingly, they may desexualize the disabled person by putting him or her into an uncomfortable and dependent situation. Significant dependency can lead to feelings of infantilism and can reduce the patient's self-esteem and weaken gender identity. It is well documented that health care environments frequently fail to recognize or make allowances for the intimacy needs of patients and their families. A need that is avoided may be perceived as a need that is lost. Not being viewed as a sexual person can convey the message that sexuality has been lost. When this perception is conveyed by the health care team, the patient and the family may receive a pervasive negative message. The problem can be further augmented by community attitudes, which may be unaccepting or unsympathetic towards the sexual correlates of disease or injury. The task of reentering the community of origin may be greater than the patient or family can manage. A caring community can unwittingly create a sense of pity that strikes down feelings of self-esteem and self-worth.

Common Female and Male Sexual Dysfunctions

The following is a brief discussion of sexual responses and dysfunctions to orient the reader to the normal physiologic responses that may show primary or secondary dysfunction in the presence of physical disability.[13,14,18]

Kolodny, Masters, and Johnson[14] describe four phases in the sexual cycle. For both sexes, an excitement phase is followed by the plateau, orgasmic, and resolution phases. The excitement phase is that time when the person becomes aware of being sexually stimulated. It results in cardiovascular and muscular responses. Penile erection occurs in the male and vaginal lubrication in the female. Continued stimulation leads to the second phase.

The plateau phase is the period between excitement and orgasm. It affects the cardiovascular system and leads to congestion of the external sexual organs.

Orgasm is the third phase and may occur if stimulation during the second phase is sufficient and the person is receptive. Men most frequently experience one orgasm, whereas women may experience multiple orgasms. Most commonly, the male ejaculates during orgasm and the woman experiences a sense of rhythmic contractions of the pelvic muscles. Immediately after orgasm a refractory period ensues. It may be brief or prolonged depending upon the individual and the level of the sexual stimulation that is experienced. Further sexual stimulation will not produce further sexual arousal during the refractory phase. Its duration is frequently shorter in younger than in older people.

Resolution is the fourth phase, during which time the body returns to its prearoused state.

In both men and women, sexual dysfunction is often equated with the inability to achieve orgasm. However, as can be seen from the description of the sexual cycle, there are many opportunities for the cycle to be interrupted, producing a temporary sexual dysfunction. Educating people about these events is a simple way of treating apparent sexual dysfunctions. Transfer of information can help what might otherwise be construed as a sexual dysfunction to be better understood as an interruption or distraction from the sequence of events that the person desires.

Cole and Cole[6] point out that sexuality, intimacy, and genital function can be separated, but they are usually interconnected. Defining common genital dysfunctions is helpful for understanding how they cause or are caused by personal or interpersonal problems. Genital aspects of sexual function can have an impact upon the entire personality, and changes in genital function will frequently affect the personality structure of the individual.

Male Sexual Dysfunctions

The more common male sexual dysfunctions are premature ejaculation, primary erectile dysfunction, secondary erectile dysfunction, and retarded ejaculation. Sexual dysfunctions that are more closely linked to the moment of orgasm are relatively easier to treat.

The term premature ejaculation describes the situation in which the man ejaculates before he wants to. The interval between the onset of stimulation and ejaculation varies widely, and an acceptable interval is unique to each individual and to the circumstances. However, it is agreed that ejaculation before vaginal penetration is a significant dysfunction.

Primary erectile dysfunction occurs when a man has never been able to have or maintain an erection for the purpose of sexual intercourse. He may have had erections during masturbation and may have noted erections upon awakening from sleep. This dysfunction can result from primary organic disease or secondary causes such as anxiety, sexual trauma in early life, sex role confusion, feelings of sexual inadequacy, or prohibitive religious or moral beliefs.

Secondary erectile dysfunction occurs in men who were previously able to have erections for sexual purposes but are now unable. Erection may occur during early sexual stimulation but disappear when penetration is attempted. Some men report erections occurring with one partner but not with another. Secondary erectile dysfunction can be caused by primary sexual dysfunctions, such as those brought on by medication, but more commonly results from personal stress or from interpersonal or relationship problems.

Retarded ejaculation occurs when a man's ejaculatory reflex is inhibited while erection is maintained. Some men report ability to ejaculate through manual stimulation, but are unable to ejaculate during penile-vaginal intercourse. This situation is usually evoked by individual or interpersonal problems.

Female Sexual Dysfunctions

Preorgasmia is a term describing a woman who has never experienced an orgasm by any means. Primary or organic causes can sometimes explain this problem, but the difficulty usually lies in problems related to the family environment, childhood sexual trauma, or religious upbringing.

Secondary nonorgasmia is often situational. A woman may experience orgasm with masturbation but not be able to achieve orgasm during sexual intercourse. Some women experience a physical orgasm but do not enjoy the psychological component. This term also describes women who have experienced orgasm in the past but are not currently able to experience it.

Dyspareunia is the term used to describe disabling vaginal or vulvar pain during intercourse. Medical conditions can produce this pain, as can secondary causes related to interpersonal struggles.

Vaginismus is an involuntary spasm of the muscles of the pelvic floor that surround the outer third of the vagina. It is often associated with sexual fears and anxieties about intercourse and its causes can be found in the woman's earlier psychosexual development or in her inability to form sexual relationships. Vaginismus prevents penetration of the vagina by the partner's erect penis.

THE SEXUAL HISTORY

Why should the patient's sexual disability be evaluated? Sexual health is a part of overall health. Asking appropriate questions can lead to a proper diagnosis, which is the basis of effective intervention. Specific diagnosis of sexual dysfunction is made in the same way as other medical diagnoses, that is, on the basis of a history and physical examination. Appropriate questions must be asked in a sensitive manner that facilitates accurate answers. According to Kolodny, Masters, and Johnson,[4] more than 50% of North American adults experience sexual dysfunction during their lives. The actual frequency may be far greater. Many of these sexual problems, primary as well as secondary, are real, problematic, and treatable. In many cases, brief therapy or simple sex education may be all that is needed. However, the rehabilitationist may need to be able to provide more extensive therapy for patients with severe physical disabilities.

How to Ask Questions about Sexual Function

The medical model is useful here. Asking questions about mobility, self-care, weakness, and sensory loss is a comfortable way to begin asking questions about sexuality. Through this approach issues of intimacy may be integrated with the medical history. We do not recommend segregating sexual questions from other medical questions, since separating them may convey the message that sex is not a health issue or that it is to be dealt with outside of the usual medical investigation.

Nonetheless, it is true that discussions of sexuality are emotionally laden and are best carried out in a confidential and discreet manner. Often, the clinician can gain permission to ask personal questions by asking directly for permission. When the patient understands that there is a relationship between the question and the disability under consideration, the answers generally flow freely and conversation is made easier.

Sometimes health professionals are reluctant to begin a discussion of sexuality for fear that they will be expected to provide answers to patients' questions or problems. It can be explained to the patient that during the taking of the medical history information is gathered in order to arrive at a correct diagnosis; appropriate therapy follows. It is best to conduct the interview privately with the patient.

Observation of patient reactions that seem to interfere with obtaining the sexual history can be helpful in making a diagnosis. Indifference expressed by the patient may be a clue to a significant problem that is being consciously or unconsciously concealed. Denial of sexual concern may be more an indication of a need to hide problems than a true expression of their absence. However, at no time should one pursue questioning over the objections of the patient. In such cases, further discussion can be reserved for another time that is more comfortable or acceptable. Similarly, the questions should not place patients in conflict with their religious or moral beliefs. Questions can be frankly and simply asked without conveying a sense of endorsement or encouragement for any particular sexual activity or belief. In some few cases, patients may react with frank hostility to questions about sexuality. In these circumstances, it is best to avoid becoming defensive or engaging in lengthy explanations of sexuality-related questions. Anger and hostility usually reflect serious underlying emotional problems that may need sophisticated counseling or therapy.

The language of sex may be a stumbling block. The use of strictly medical terms may be as inappropriate as use of only lay terms. The clinician may learn that the patient's sex-related words and language are different from his or her own. In this case, he or she should learn how to use language that is comfortable and communicates most effectively with the patient. Practice in this regard may help the clinician or rehabilitation professional to be more effective.

It is also useful to conduct a second interview with the patient's partner present. Comparing answers in the two situations may lead to insights about sexual problems or the manner in which the couple is accustomed to handling them.

Where to Begin?

There is no more understandable place to begin than with questions about genital function. When asking questions about the urinary tract or when talking about menstruation, it is a simple step to ask at the same time about sexual function. Even sensitive or specific questions about sexual activities can be easily approached in this context. It should be remembered that nocturnal erections in the male are evidence of an intact reflex pathway and help differentiate between functional or physiological problems when men do not have erections while awake or under erotic conditions. Other specific questions help to identify normalcy or abnormality of genitourinary function; for example, Does ejaculation occur with orgasm? Does orgasm occur with erection? Is ejaculation anterograde or retrograde? Is the semen volume unusual?

In the case of women, questions about vaginal intercourse, pain, and arousal are appropriate. With sexual arousal, vaginal lubrication in the female is the physiological counterpart of penile erection in the male. The woman may detect its presence by digital examination of the vagina or vulva. Questions about her orgasm may lead to insights about her sexual activity.

The orgasm is known by many names, and it is highly emphasized by many people. However, it is not of primary importance to everyone. Some may rate their own orgasms as relatively unimportant.

Similarly, information about masturbation is part of the complete history. Masturbation is an activity that, although commonplace to some, is personally or morally unacceptable to others. It is not wise for the clinician to interfere with these moral positions, but it is important to know about the attitudes and patterns of sexual expression of the patient. Answers to specific questions about these and other issues can guide the examiner to a better understanding of the degree of sexual expressiveness that the patient allows himself or herself, which plays an important role in determining the sexual options that are available and/or acceptable to an individual or couple.

Descriptions of attempts at sexual intercourse are important to obtain. By listening carefully to the descriptions, one may gain insights about the likelihood of success. It should not be surprising to hear people use the word intercourse to describe activities other than penile penetration of the vagina. Some people include manual or oral stimulation within their definition of intercourse, whereas to others, vaginal penetration is essential to the term intercourse. Questions of this type must be asked without judgment. To be judgmental is to limit the usefulness of the interaction between the clinician and the patient. For example, one may not assume that a widowed patient has no outlet for sexual intercourse. Nor may one assume that a married person is exclusively heterosexual.

A wide variety of important medical issues are associated with sexual activity. Their presence or fear about them may exert a powerful influence on the sexual interest, activity, and satisfaction of the patient or the patient's partner. In the last half of the twentieth century, sexually transmitted diseases have become a major concern and public health issue, AIDS being the most dramatic and fearsome of the group.

It is also important to ask about the use of medications. Table 1 lists some of the most common medications that are known to have the potential for affecting sexual responsiveness in both men and women. Alcohol is one of the most commonly used drugs that interferes with sexual responsiveness. When used in excess, it has a profound depressant effect upon libido and sexual performance.

The extent of the sexual concern of both members of the partnership must be determined. Sex may be an overriding concern to one, but a minimal concern to the other. This disagreement by itself may constitute a basis for

Table 1. Drug causes of organic impotence.

Major tranquilizers
  Phenothiazines
  Butyrophenones
  Thioxanthenes
Antidepressants
  Tricyclics
  MAO inhibitors
Minor tranquilizers
  Benzodiazepines
  Mephenesin-like drugs
Sedatives and hypnotics
Anticholinergic drugs
  Antispasmotics
  Antiparkinsonian drugs
  Antihistamines
  Muscle relaxants
  Antiarrhythmic (disopyramide)
Antihypertensives
  Diuretics
  Vasodilators (questionable)
  Central sympatholytics
  Neurotransmitter depleters
  Alpha- and beta-adrenergic blockers
Drugs with abuse potential
Miscellaneous
  Cimetidine
  Clofibrate
  Cyproterone
  Estrogens
  Progestins
  Digoxin
  Indomethacin
  Lithium
  Methylsergide
  Metoclopramide
  Metronidazole
  Phenytoin

Source: E.R. Griffith, S. Cole, and T.M. Cole, "Sexuality and sexual dysfunction," in M. Rosenthal et al., eds., *Rehabilitation of the Adult and Child with Traumatic Brain Injury*, 2nd ed. (Philadelphia: F.A. Davis Publishers, 1990), p. 208, Table 15–1. Reprinted with the permission of the publisher.

sexual problems or may magnify a sexual dysfunction. Information of this type is best obtained in a private interview with the patient and a second private interview with the partner.

Genitourinary function may not be the only source of problems. Associated injuries or diseases may also require investigation. For example, bone fractures, soft tissue injuries, pain syndromes, limitation of joint motion, or disfiguring injuries may lead to functional or cosmetic derangements that affect the patient's sense of self-worth and self-acceptance. An individual whose tracheotomy interferes with easy communication may regard speech problems as a major sexual handicap. Difficulty in controlling oral secretions in a public setting may be similarly regarded. It is apparent that these obvious and easily appreciated problems may decrease the individual's willingness to seek or accept sexual activity. The alteration of somatic sensation, such as may occur with central or peripheral neurological injury or disease, can alter erotic experiences and make skin painful to touch.

Today, sexual abuse is recognized to be a more common occurrence than was previously believed. A history of rape, incest, or physical abuse may not be easily elicited. Some people have buried the event in their subconscious mind because it was so traumatic and unacceptable. Yet these experiences, forgotten or remembered, can have a profound and lasting effect upon sexual health during adulthood. These issues are very difficult and deserve the attention of careful and experienced sexual therapists.

Living arrangements may have an important effect upon sexuality, especially when privacy and personal comfort are compromised. Similarly, independence and dependency, as well as role reversal and role acceptance, may have an importance that is not always immediately obvious. Some people have great difficulty in accepting a change from an independent to a dependent role.

Fear of pregnancy may also interfere with sexual activity or pleasure. Conversely, a desire to become pregnant may place overriding demands or expectations upon each sexual experience so as to make it unpleasant. Clearly, therefore, a very broad construct of sexuality in its many manifestations must be kept in mind as the clinician explores this most private, personal, and vulnerable area of human behavior.

PHYSICAL EXAMINATION

The physical examination necessarily includes examination of the genitals. However, not all alterations or dysfunctions of the genitals are accompanied by sexual dysfunctions. Since sexuality is not equated with genitality, it follows that abnormalities of the genitals are not always experienced as loss of sexual capability. The body is capable of being eroticized in many areas other than the genitals. Two important points to remember are that sexuality is a broader concept than genitality and that sexual expression encompasses more than sexual intercourse.

Five aspects of the physical examination deserve special attention:

Motor system.   Strength, range of motion, coordination, mobility, and muscle tone can all affect the body, thus influencing sexual activity. Capacities can be identified and impairments can often be treated. Motor losses do not necessarily preclude sexual expressiveness or receptivity.

Sensation.   Variations in normal sensation may be perceived as quite inhibiting to sexual satisfaction. Partial or complete loss of sensation or a change of sensation may be disabling. Therapeutic approaches—including desensitization techniques, adaptive methods, and education—can overcome many of these problems. It is often said that the skin is the largest sexual organ of the body. The disabled person, therefore, may still have a very large body area over which to receive sexual pleasure.

Treating pain that interferes with sexual function is no different than treating pain that interferes with any other important bodily function. Pain and pain behavior are important constructs to understand and are not necessarily identical (see chapter 19). Vision, hearing, smell, and taste all play roles in sexual awareness, arousal, activity, and satisfaction. However, if one modality is impaired, other sensations may be substituted; e.g., loss of touch sensation may be compensated for by use of vision.

Losses of body parts and disfigurements.   Limb amputations can interfere with sexual function in that they produce cosmetic or functional problems. The ability to caress will be altered if an individual has lost hand function. Ability to move in bed and to control balance may be affected as a result of a lower limb amputation. The traumatic loss of facial parts, such as may occur after a burn or a severe laceration, may produce cosmetic and functional impairments. Counseling may be helpful. Here, just as in the rehabilitation of other disabling conditions, one can employ compensatory strategies or remedial training. Creativity and openness can help to solve many sexual problems, especially if guided by a skilled and interested health professional.

Cognition and perception.   One has only to consider the pervasive effects of cognition and perception to understand how vital they are to sexual communication. Rehabilitation strategies used to remedy cognitive and perceptual losses can also be applied to the sexual dysfunctions they may produce. Executive functions such as judgment, control, concentration, appropriateness, memory, and focusing are all involved in remediation. The course of rehabilitation may have a salutary effect upon sexual function.

Behavior.   Lastly, an overall impression may be gained from the patient's behavior during the examination. The examiner may witness the patient using many functions—communicative, social, intellectual, emotional—by watching body language, observing hygiene, and sensing social decorum, pacing, and affect.

LABORATORY EXAMINATION

As in the evaluation of any other medical problem, the laboratory examination complements the medical history and physical examination. Endocrinological tests, neurophysiological studies, and vascular evaluations may all help the clinician to understand the patient's sexual capabilities better. Urological procedures may shed light on genitourinary function. Nocturnal penile tumescence monitoring is easily done using snap-gage technology in the privacy of the patient's own home and bed. Electrodiagnostic studies, including needle examination of anterior and posterior sacral segments and nerve conduction studies, may help to diagnose alterations in neurological function. Noninvasive studies of blood flow in the penis may also be helpful, as may angiography, Doppler stethoscopy, and penile-brachial pulse ratios.

It is important to point out that, as one proceeds with the evaluation, education of the patient is essential. Asking a question about a sexual function may raise anxieties that can be effectively dealt with by simultaneously providing education.

CLASSIFYING SEXUAL AND PHYSICAL DISABILITIES

Type A Disabilities

Type A disabilities are those that are stable or progressive and occur either at birth, during early childhood, or before adolescence. Examples include congenital brain injury, limb amputation or deformity in early life, congenital loss of functions of special sensation, arthritis, metabolic disorders, and muscular dystrophies, to name a few.

Disabilities that occur at birth or develop prior to adolescence have a profoundly different effect upon the individual than those that occur after sexual maturation. The learning acquired during childhood and adolescence is nowhere more powerful than in the area of human sexuality and interpersonal relationships. A child disabled from an early age will experience the world differently than the able-bodied child. Not only are life's experiences different, but the child is regarded and treated differently by family members, friends, relatives, school mates, and society in general. These different growth experiences will lead to a different view about sexuality, which will continue a life of experiences different from able-bodied children.

As Easton points out, continuing effort is needed to address sexual issues with such individuals.[8] Not only do they experience the self-consciousness of adolescence, but their disability may prevent customary or normal interactions with children. Thus, the child may redirect his or her energy into other areas, such as success at school, verbal skills, etc. The child may be delayed in reaching emotional independence, and gaps in the maturation of the personality may occur which affect subsequent life experiences. These many needs may combine to sap the energy of the child and to direct what remains toward the demands of the physical disability (e.g., independence and mobility), leaving the child with a secondary handicap: the inability to take care of social and sexual needs. Robinault states that the clinician can take the role of healer, educator, and counselor.[17] The role of healer is created by access to medical arts, the role of educator by the diversity in which the child lives, and the role of counselor by the many options for sexual education and expression that are available and practical in our society.

Helpful Tips for Management by the Clinician

1. The inclusion of sexuality in the assessment of the child generates an opportunity to gather additional information about the child in his or her environment—attitudes, behaviors, and experiences. It also provides an opportunity for the clinician to provide factual and healthy sexual education to the child and the parent. Obviously, the clinician should operate within cultural and familial beliefs and not place the child in conflict with his or her family.

2. Able-bodied adolescents have a superficial understanding of the world and of sexuality. Handicapped children may be even more limited. The clinician should understand that when a child presents himself or herself as knowledgeable about sexual matters, it should not be concluded that such knowledge has the same meaning as it would for an adult.

3. Aggression is a well-known phenomenon among children. It can express itself in sexual ways and should be understood to be fundamentally similar to adolescent nonsexual aggression.

4. A sexual history provides a unique opportunity to offer useful information on anatomy, physiology, and appropriate behavior in public and private. The child may need frank information on how to ward off unlawful advances, which occur more often to the disabled than the able-bodied child. The perceived vulnerability of disabled children is known to contribute to their sexual violation. The disabled child may not have many opportunities to interact with peers and thus may not learn language and life experiences through adolescent conversation. Other people will have to supply the missing information so that the child is not further handicapped by lack of vocabulary. Interest shown in sexuality also gives the clinician opportunity to interact with the child's family. Families often appreciate the assistance of the clinician, since they may not have the skills necessary to assist their children in this area.

5. The clinician is in an excellent position to estimate the need for counseling of the child's family. Sexual issues may place a great strain on parents and family members and cause emotional decompensation.

6. The clinician should encourage a positive and constructive attitude towards the child's sexuality. There is no more damaging an experience for a child than to be neutralized or desexualized by health care professionals. Avoidance of sexual issues gives the negative and subtle message that the

disabled child is not expected to grow into an adult in all ways. Thus, a continued infantilization of the child may be fostered if adultlike behaviors are not expected.

7. It is helpful for the clinician to project the message that sex and sexual feelings are normal and natural. Some disabled children redirect their normal sexual energy and become focused upon mobility skills or academic issues to the exclusion of developing a well-rounded and full personality. Interpersonal skills may be sacrificed, and the child may become everyone's "best friend" and avoid intimate personal relationships.

8. The information that the clinician offers may be designed as much to help the individual understand the world as it is to change or instigate sexual behavior. Information does not necessitate action, and sexual education does not require that the child become sexually active.

9. Peer counseling has been found to be particularly useful in personal areas such as sexuality. Some communities have developed groups of disabled people who serve as peer counselors for other children and their families.

Type B Disabilities

These are disabilities that occur after sexual maturation or during adulthood. The individual had the opportunity to learn psychosexual and interpersonal behaviors and skills through the developmental steps of childhood and adolescence. Then, suddenly or slowly, the person's sexual functions were affected. Adjustment is necessary, just as it is for any other essential life function. Disabilities of adults can be sudden or insidious in onset and can be progressive or stable over the long term. The key feature here, however, is age at onset of the disability. Sexuality issues that disabled adults must deal with may relate to specific sexual activities, including intercourse. For those who are not achieving a satisfactory orgasm, advice on how to achieve it may be greatly appreciated. Moreover, fertility must also be addressed, since it is well known that disabled adults are not only interested but able to perform sexually. Examples of adult-onset disabilities include spinal cord injury, traumatic brain injury, disfiguring burns, limb amputations, multiple sclerosis, diabetic neuropathy, heart disease, stroke, cancer, and end-stage renal disease.

Helpful Tips for Management by the Clinician

1. The clinician should start discussion of sexuality early in the disability. The rehabilitation team can be helpful, but team members must give consistent and nonconflicting advice. It is necessary that the issues be discussed among the team members, just as for any other important life activity.

2. Team members should remind each other that it is important to view

the disabled person as a sexual being and to show respect for and sensitivity to personal issues. They should reinforce gender identity and help overcome fear of sexual abandonment.

3. In view of current public health problems, it is wise to provide up-to-date and accurate information about safe sex and avoidance of sexually transmitted diseases and sexual violence. If resource materials are available, they should be offered to the patient and the sexual partner or spouse. If materials are not readily available, the rehabilitation team has the responsibility to provide accurate and supportive information. Specific information about fertility, birth control, pregnancy, delivery, and parenting is appropriate and important.

4. Peer counseling should be provided to individuals and family members. If it is not available, it may be developed in the community under the guidance of the rehabilitation team.

5. A positive attitude towards sexuality should be expressed by discussing the expectation that sexual interests and behaviors will resume when the individual is medically stable. Adaptations and education are important in sexual adjustment just as they are in adjustment to an impairment of mobility.

6. Couple counseling should be made available where appropriate. Information on sexuality can be extremely useful when provided supportively to both members of the partnership, and thus the partner or spouse should be included in discussions whenever possible and considered when planning case management.

7. The clinician can help people learn the difference between fact and myth regarding sexual expectations and performance. Many people focus exclusively on genital activity in order to express themselves sexually. If genital function has been altered, they may conclude that sexual activity is impossible. A broad understanding of sexuality that goes beyond genitality will enable the clinician to couch a discussion of sexuality in a facilitative manner. It may be helpful to expand a patient's concept of sexuality by specifically including discussion of nongenital activities.

General Advice to Rehabilitationists

1. Provide accurate and supportive information that endorses sexuality as important and minimizes fear and feelings of inadequacy.

2. Use creative problem-solving techniques, just as one would for other aspects of physical disability. Encourage exploration and experimentation within the value system of the patient and the partner.

3. Remember that people are resilient. The topic of sexuality may be difficult to bring up, but it is appreciated when it is discussed with respect and thoroughness. Do not omit the topic, since omission may reinforce the patient's belief that it is neither expected nor possible. Discussions of sexuality can reflect dignity when carried out with genuine concern and respect.

REHABILITATION OF SEXUAL PROBLEMS AFTER PHYSICAL DISABILITY

Therapy for sexual problems should begin in the earliest phase of rehabilitation, which is the time the patient, the spouse, and the family are able to begin using the information. Information given early sets expectations for an ongoing dialogue. The early stage of disability, when the patient or the family feels vulnerable, is the time to initiate effective discussions of sensitive matters. After a myocardial infarction, a stroke, or a traumatic injury, the reinitiation of touch, contact, and affection by a family member who is encouraged to do so can exert a healing influence. In some disabilities, such as burn injury, changes in personality often occur in the early stages of recovery, and it is helpful to discuss with the family issues of intimacy and behavior that may be difficult to understand. Discussion of unpredictable behavior and personality changes can be integrated into counseling about rehabilitation and can help the family prepare for the special needs that will have to be met during the process of recovery.

Ongoing Assistance

Counseling is the most important modality. The disability may produce a sexual role reversal, as when a previously enabled person now requires assistance from a partner. The role of caretaker and lover can become confused. Alternatively, the able-bodied partner may feel a desire to abandon the disabled person or may feel frustrated and angry. Frequently, cultural or religious beliefs can play a role—sometimes helpful and sometimes not. Such beliefs may limit the partner's ability to provide confident support. Explaining about the illness or the injury can go far toward relieving these problems. Sexual sentiments are often accompanied by intense feelings of secrecy, guilt, or shame, and these feelings can further complicate the recovery process.

Traditional Medical and Surgical Treatments

The wide range of physical dysfunctions that can occur as a result of illness or injury afford many opportunities for the use of traditional treatments. Some treatments can have an impact upon sexuality, for example, chronic use of steroids by a patient with arthritis. Hirsutism, obesity, and acne can all adversely affect sexuality. Body alterations resulting from an orthopedic injury or a malignancy can interfere with the use of the body for closeness and intimacy. Some patients have pre-existing medical problems, such as diabetes or chronic lung disease, that can be made worse by a new disability. Depression and anxiety in the patient and family members frequently accompany disabilities. Treatment of all these problems can favorably affect sexuality.

Treatments for medical problems can themselves have secondary sexual concomitants that are undesirable. The treatment of hypertension may lead to impotence. The treatment of seizures may lead to a loss of sexual interest.

Surgery may play an important role in improving sexual function. Orthopedic deformities that inhibit the use of the body for physical closeness can be corrected. Surgery may be an effective way of reducing breast hypertrophy, as in the case of myelodysplasia. Plastic surgery may reduce cosmetic deformities of the face, thus facilitating closeness and intimacy. Surgical implantation of devices to restore erectile function in the male may have a role in the treatment of physically disabled people.

Functional Restoration or Adaptation

Treatments that restore motor or sensory functions play an important role in assisting a patient with sexual problems arising from illness or disability. Mobility, hygiene, positioning, movement, comfort, pain relief, and endurance are all aspects of physical functioning that are customarily treated in rehabilitation, and these same therapies, using customary rehabilitation techniques, may yield benefits to sexuality. Self-care, with a goal of independence and freedom of expression, can ameliorate sexual dysfunctions resulting from disability. Bladder and bowel management, oral hygiene, and ability to arrange clothing all offer possible gains in the area of sexuality. The speech pathologist may treat the aphasia of stroke and in so doing play an important and helpful role in the restoration of communication, a feeling of self-esteem, and consequently sexual function.

Specific Therapies

Adaptive aids have been traditionally accepted in rehabilitation and they are also helpful in the area of sexuality. These may include adaptation of the environment (the bedroom) or adaptation of the body (using a vibrator to give sexual pleasure to the genitals).

External erectile devices are helpful. An example is "banding," or the temporary use of a tourniquet around the base of the penis to produce vascular engorgement and thus erection. Such a device is noninvasive and is a safe method of establishing erection to enhance vaginal intercourse and sexual satisfaction. Respondents who use it report increased satisfaction and improved sexual relations. Explanation, instruction, and counseling prior to use is strongly recommended. Either the patient or the partner must have upper extremity function in order to use this device. Application is usually limited to 30 minutes because the constrictive band placed around the base of the penile shaft can produce injury if it is too tight for too long a time.[22]

Several invasive options exist for management of erectile dysfunction, including penile prostheses and intracavernosal pharmacotherapy. All procedures have potential complications. Implantation of penile prostheses requires hospitalization and surgery. Complications can include erosion or infection. Expense is also a disadvantage. However, successful results are highly satisfactory to the recipient and partner. Comprehensive counseling is recommended.

Direct penile injection of papaverine can produce erections sufficient for vaginal penetration and has been reported as highly satisfactory by some patients. However, in spinal cord-injured men, prolonged erection can occur and result in priaprism and other complications.

Electroejaculation

Electrical probes placed in the rectum that deliver a small, regulated electrical current can stimulate ejaculation. This method has proven highly successful, particularly in spinal cord-injured men. (The same technique has been used in animal husbandry for artificial insemination programs for many years.) Several medical centers in North America do the procedure, which has led to a number of pregnancies and full-term, normal births since the 1980s.[2,12]

In a well-established protocol, patients selected for electroejaculation will be seen by urologists. Their partners will work with gynecologists to prepare for artificial insemination. About 50% of spinal cord-injured men can obtain ejaculation regardless of the type of spinal lesion. This method yields the greatest success with thoracic lesions and complete lesions.

Vibromassage

Vibromassage or stimulation of the penis of a spinal cord-injured male with an electric vibrator can produce ejaculation with less medical involvement and expense. However, contraindications include autonomic dysreflexia in the quadriplegic person, atrial fibrillation, and tissue breakdown from vibratory pressure applied to one spot for too long. Therefore, physician-supervised trials are recommended, followed by artificial insemination of the sperm if ejaculation is possible (usually around 40% of spinal cord-injured men are able to ejaculate by this method).[20,21]

Fertility

Avoiding pregnancy can be difficult for spinal cord-injured women because of contraindications for the use of intrauterine devices and diaphragms due to lack of sensation. Oral contraceptives are usually discouraged because of the risk that venous thrombosis may develop and the inability to recognize leg pain. However, some physicians do recommend the use of oral contraceptives because the newer pills contain lower dosage levels of hormones, reducing the incidence of thrombophlebitis.

Recent research on the menstrual cycles of spinal cord-injured women indicates that consistent ovulatory cycles occur following the return of menses after injury. Reproduction is not permanently impaired. Natural family planning methods (with the exception of the basal body temperature, which is unreliable after spinal cord injury) may offer a viable alternative to artificial contraception when cycle length and menstrual symptoms are regular.[16]

Special attention must be given to the fertility concerns of women with disabilities. They will need clear instruction and information to understand the physiological changes that might affect fertility and pregnancy. Limitations of mobility, neuromuscular changes, pain, and loss of sensation all have an impact on the possibility for pregnancy and birth. Methods of managing hygiene and bowel and bladder function, avoiding infection, maintaining good nutrition, and stabilizing blood pressure need to be taught to the patient.[5,19]

SEXUALITY ISSUES FOR CHILDREN

When a child experiences a disability, it is essential that parents provide the child with information that he or she might otherwise not receive because of social isolation resulting from the disability. Parents and other adults should discuss with the child implications of the disability. They should give the child adequate information about his or her body and its function and convey realistic expectations for the future. Many factors work together in the imprinting of sexual values upon a young person, including role models, spontaneous experiences, family roles and rules and their violation, basic sex education and information, the ability to have and maintain relationships, and the child's own experiences in the daily living environment.[10,15]

When a disability is present, the situation produces changes in natural sexual development. For example, in an effort to protect the disabled child, it is common for families to withhold information about sexuality altogether. The parents may not understand the critical importance of information itself and, with good intentions, may overprotect the child from information or experiences (or both).[9] The result can be isolation, and it becomes more difficult for the child to interact with peers, particularly around sexual issues. The child does not even acquire the "language of sex" in order to converse, flirt, tell stories, or "brag." He or she may then experience further isolation from peers.

A disabled young child often experiences excessive touching because of necessary health care tasks by family members, personal care attendants, and health care workers. Commonly, the child is handled so frequently that he or she may not acknowledge or operate with a sense of separateness and ownership of his or her own body. Medical professionals or other care givers often do not stop to identify or negotiate necessary touching of a disabled person. This can sometimes result in a further loss of autonomy.[4]

In the early stages of development, children will naturally explore through touch. At the same time, through curiosity and by asking questions, they are learning sex roles and exploring the boundaries of responsibility, which develops their sense of social value. Likewise, they are learning the difference between public and private behavior. Most children explore masturbation out of natural curiosity, even those who appear to be disinterested or disgusted about sex.

Puberty is a time of confusion, embarrassment, self-consciousness, and difficulty in asking for information. At this time children are very vulnerable. They need special attention to be sure that they are equipped with the necessary information to understand the body changes they are experiencing during their maturation, as well as the codes and roles set by society for them as emerging men and women.

Adolescence is a time when children experiment with one another and practice adult behavior. They turn their attention to grooming, fashion, and activities that will prepare them for adult life. They watch others or television in an effort to learn about sex and sexuality. Much of their knowledge is gained through sexual acting out, even though they lack specific or accurate information regarding birth control, pregnancy risks, morals, or values. Boys and girls will need assistance in early adolescence to understand about spontaneous ejaculation and menstrual hygiene and to learn about appropriate and inappropriate touch.

A helpful tip to parents is to allow their children to grow and mature naturally, not to infantilize them further by dressing them in clothes appropriate to a younger age. Families are often intensely concerned about the sexual and emotional vulnerability of the child and hope that "nothing bad" will happen to him or her. The result can be, of course, that the young person does not learn how to behave as an adult and becomes further infantilized by society.

Lack of privacy and limitations of mobility may decrease the opportunity for disabled young people to practice and understand their emerging sexuality. In addition, opportunities to socialize, interact, and establish relationships may be adversely influenced by the unavailability of transportation and, most particularly, the inaccessibility of buildings for people with braces, crutches, and wheelchairs.[3]

The siblings of the child with a disability need to have specific information about the disability itself and its implications for the family. Needless to say, siblings may be asked to assist the disabled child in activities of daily living, and if they do not have a basic understanding of the situation, they could easily become antagonistic or hostile. It is important for siblings to be told, and to believe, that they will have the opportunity to live their own lives and that their needs are not "second place" to those of the disabled child.

Particularly when the disabled child has some intellectual impairment, siblings will need to be taught how to interact, how to encourage, how to be consistent, and how to give feedback. Siblings are at risk of stigma and rejection by friends and playmates. Thus, the disability can affect the body image and self-esteem not only of the disabled individual but of siblings as well.

Consistent information and encouragement from peers and family can generate respect, foster concern, and encourage positive interaction without guilt or resentment.

STAFF TRAINING

The rehabilitation staff may not be prepared to deal with the topic of sexuality without further training and preparation. Trying to facilitate specific sexual discussions can lead to discomfort among staff that is quickly sensed by the patient and the family. Training can help the staff to develop their facility for discussions of sexual problems.

The useful model for helping staff work in this area has been described by Annon.[1] It specifies four levels of staff involvement in sexuality issues that together are known as the PLISSIT model. The first level is permission (P), in which the clinician gives a clear message to the patient or family that the discussion of sexual issues is okay. Limited information (LI) is a level at which staff provide basic information about anatomy, physiology, and therapy that has a direct bearing on sexual function. At the next level the staff provide specific suggestions (SS) for interventions targeted to sexual issues; skills in counseling, advocacy, and education are needed here. Intensive therapy (IT) requires a level of sophistication that may make it the reserve of specialists in psychology and counseling, since the therapist will need to have had advanced training and to be able to provide interventions for difficult situations. This schema helps the rehabilitationist understand the level at which he or she is functioning and provides a framework for considering the need for referral to more in-depth therapy.

The in-service model is a very effective way to teach sexual counseling and therapy. It is appealing to the rehabilitation staff because it utilizes teaching styles with which they are familiar. Cases are presented and the treatment team engages in problem solving by first defining problems and then developing alternative solutions. Teaching or training of the patient follows, and monitoring of outcome is the final step.

REFERENCES

1. Annon J. *The behavioral treatment of sexual problems: brief therapy.* New York: Harper & Row; 1976.
2. Bennett CJ, et al. Sexual dysfunction and electroejaculation in men with spinal cord injury: a review. *J Urol.* 1988;139:453–457.
3. Cole SS. Disability/ability: the importance of sexual health in adolescence; issues and concerns of the professional. *SIECUS Rep.* 1981;May–July:3–4.

4. Cole S. Facing the challenges of sexual abuse in persons with disabilities. *J Sex Disability.* 1987;7(3):71.
5. Cole S. Women, sexuality, and disabilities. *J Women Ther.* 1988;7(2&3):277–294.
6. Cole TM, Cole SS. Rehabilitation of problems of sexuality in physical disability. In: Kottke FJ, Lehmann JF, eds. *Krusen's handbook of physical medicine and rehabilitation.* 4th ed. Philadelphia: WB Saunders; 1990:988–1008.
7. Cole TM, Glass DD. Sexuality and physical disabilities. *Arch Phys Med Rehabil.* 1977;58:585–586.
8. Easton J. Children, parents, and schools. Paper presented at Seminar on Sexuality and Physical Disabilities: Medical Aspects of Clinical Care. Ann Arbor: University of Michigan Medical Center; November 1980.
9. Gordon S. *Living fully: a guide for young people with a handicap, their parents, their teachers, and professionals.* New York: John Day; 1975.
10. Gordon S, Gordon J. *Raising a child conservatively in a sexually permissive world.* New York: Simon and Schuster; 1983.
11. Griffith ER, Cole S, Cole TM. Sexuality and sexual dysfunction. In: Rosenthal M, et al, eds. *Rehabilitation of the adult and child with traumatic brain injury.* 2nd ed. Philadelphia: FA Davis; 1990:206–224.
12. Hirsch IH, et al. Electroejaculatory stimulation of a quadriplegic man resulting in pregnancy. *Arch Phys Med Rehabil.* 1990;71:54–57.
13. Kaplan HS. *The new sex therapy.* New York: Brunner-Mazel/Times Books; 1974.
14. Kolodny RC, Masters WH, Johnson VE. *Textbook of sexual medicine.* Boston: Little, Brown; 1979.
15. Leight L. *Raising sexually healthy children.* New York: Rawson Associates; 1988.
16. Reame N. The menstrual cycle in women with spinal cord injury. *Am J Rehabil Med.* [In press].
17. Robinault IP. *Sex, society, and the disabled: a developmental inquiry into roles, reactions, and responsibilities.* Hagerstown, MD: Harper & Row; 1978.
18. Schover LR, Jensen SB. *Sexuality and chronic illness: a comprehensive approach.* New York: The Guilford Press; 1988.
19. Shaul S, Dowling PJ, Laden BF. Like other women: perspectives of mothers with physical disabilities. In: Deegan MJ, Brooks NA, eds. *Women and disability: the double handicap.* New Brunswick, NJ: Transaction Books; 1985.
20. Smith J. Making babies: the boom in men's fertility. *Spinal Network.* 1989;Spring:38–41.
21. Szasz G, Carpenter C. Clinical observations in vibratory stimulation of the penis of men with spinal cord injury. *Arch Sex Behav.* 1989;18:461–474.
22. Zasler ND, Katz PG. Synergist erection system in the management of impotence secondary to spinal cord injury. *Arch Phys Med Rehabil.* 1970;70:712–715.

Chapter 6

ADVANCES IN ELECTRODIAGNOSIS

Ernest W. Johnson

Awareness of advances in the uses of electrodiagnosis with standard equipment is essential to keep up-to-date in this specialized field. With careful technique and meticulous planning, all of the following electrodiagnostic methods can be used with the older electromyographic instruments.

NEEDLE ELECTROMYOGRAPHY

The five steps of the needle examination are well known: I) examination of the muscle at rest, II) insertional activity, III) minimal muscle contraction, IV) maximal muscle contraction, and V) distribution of the EMG abnormalities.

Measurements of significance in step I include fasciculation potentials and fibrillation potentials, as well as an evaluation of tremor rate. Fasciculation potentials are identified by their very slow rate of firing and their irregular rhythm. They are classified by their shape as simple or complex. Complex fasciculations are further divided into the usual polyphasic potentials, frequently seen in neuropathic and myopathic diseases, and repetitive discharge or myokymic potentials, frequently seen in Guillain-Barré syndrome and radiation myelopathy as well as in certain other neuropathic diseases.

Fibrillation potentials are important as indications of abnormal muscle cell membrane irritability. They are seen in denervation as well as a number of other abnormal states, including inflammatory diseases of muscle, upper motor neuron diseases such as stroke and spinal cord injury, muscle diseases (e.g., Pompe's disease), muscle injury, and abnormal muscle concentrations of potassium, as would be seen with hyper- and hypokalemia. The amplitude of the fibrillation potential will be reduced in atrophied muscle fibers; thus, the size may be helpful in deciding whether the condition under investigation is of remote or recent origin.

Insertional activity is the burst of injury potentials occurring as the needle electrode is moved through viable muscle. This burst of activity confirms that the needle is indeed in muscle tissue. In certain diseases (for example, myotonia and acute polymyositis), movement of the electrode provokes a prolonged burst of injury potentials. This is properly called increased insertional activity. However, when abnormal muscle irritability is minimal, such as would occur in the early stages of denervation, the needle electrode provokes several positive waves following the cessation of its movement through the muscle. We know now that the most common abnormality in this step is the appearance of several positive waves following the burst of injury potentials. The positive sharp wave is simply an artifactual recording of a single muscle fiber discharge. Thus, a positive wave could represent a spontaneous fibrillation, a single muscle fiber discharge (myotonia), or an end plate spike. Each of these is a discharge of a single muscle fiber that can be recorded as a positive wave with the tip of the exploring electrode in contact with the depolarized zone. Positive waves from an end plate zone can be differentiated from spontaneous fibrillation potentials by the rate and rhythm of the train of positive waves.[2] If they are a consequence of the tip of the needle in the end plate zone, the rate will be faster and the rhythm will be irregular (Figure 1). If the positive wave is being recorded from a fibrillation potential, the rhythm is usually regular and the rate is 2–10 per second. The most commonly misinterpreted potential in the needle electromyographic examination is the positive wave recorded from the end plate zone.

Step III, or the minimal contraction, is performed by examining a single motor unit potential and describing its shape, amplitude, duration, and rate of firing.

Note that the tip of the needle electrode is recording only a portion of the motor unit; that is, those few muscle fibers actually being recorded by the needle electrode tip. Thus, when one refers to a motor unit potential in the needle electromyographic examination, the actual potential is the algebraic sum of the few muscle fibers within the recording area of the electrode tip.

The Early Polyphasic in Radiculopathy

Aminoff[1] found the needle EMG exam the most helpful in diagnosing radiculopathy. Polyphasic potentials have been described within the first two to three weeks of the onset of radiculopathy. This interesting potential has been known for many years, but its shape has not been explained. We know that a reinnervation potential can occur four to six weeks after an episode of denervation. However, the early polyphasic can occur within the first week after a radiculopathy.

The current hypothesis to explain this interesting potential is the activation of two or more axons at the inflamed root level, thus resulting in a synchronous, but not exactly simultaneous, activation of those motor units at the needle electrode tip. The conducting axon activates the neighboring few axons by ephapsis. The resulting activity will appear at the needle electrode in the muscle at slightly different times for the different axons, since each axon has a unique rate of conduction. This results in the characteristic early polyphasic motor unit potential, which would be highly polyphasic, of normal amplitude, and of increased duration (Figure 2). It looks exactly like what one would believe it represents—that is, several motor units firing at almost the same time.

Myokymic Discharges

Myokymic discharges now are recognized in a variety of peripheral neuropathies and myelopathies. They represent ephaptic activation at a given area in the injured or diseased nerve, resulting in grouped discharges. They can be seen in anterior horn cell diseases, Guillain-Barré syndrome, and Bell's palsy, but they are most characteristic of radiation myelopathy.

Variation in Motor Unit Potentials

During step III, one can also examine the motor unit potential (MUP) in some detail, including the rate of firing, amplitude, shape, and variations, if they occur, during the continuing activation. Alteration in stability of the motor unit would be manifested by a changing shape and amplitude of the motor unit potential. These changes result from failure of neuromuscular transmission during repeated firing. This instability is seen in states of reinnervation as well as conditions affecting the neuromuscular junction, i.e., myasthenia gravis and myasthenic syndrome.

While the newer instruments have a trigger and delay line to facilitate this observation, older instruments are perfectly capable of demonstrating variation through close observation of repeated firing of the motor unit.[15]

Recruitment Frequency (Recruitment Interval)

Recruitment frequency represents the rate of firing of the first motor unit at the moment the second one is recruited (Figure 3). This recruitment pattern can also be described by the recruitment interval; that is, the interval between succeeding activations of the first unit at the moment the second one is recruited. The recruitment interval is the reciprocal of the recruitment frequency.

If the number of motor units available for that minimal effort is reduced, the first unit would fire more rapidly at the moment the second one is recruited. Thus, the recruitment frequency in neuropathy, when there are fewer motor units available, is increased and the recruitment interval reduced. An example would occur in early anterior horn cell disease if the anterior tibial muscle fires at 16–20 Hz instead of the 8–10 Hz seen in a

Figure 1. Monopolar needle electrode in end plate area. Note the end plate spikes and positive waves. (Each square = 10 msec, 100 μV.)

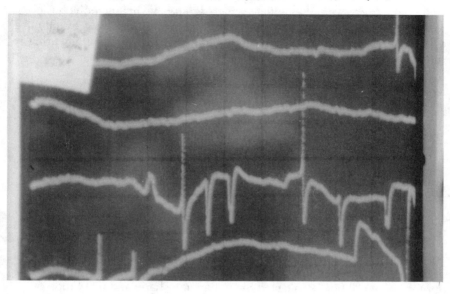

Figure 2. Early polyphasic motor unit potentials in extensor digitorum longus four days after onset of symptoms of paresis in an L5 radiculopathy. (Each slanted line = 10 msec; height = 200 μV.)

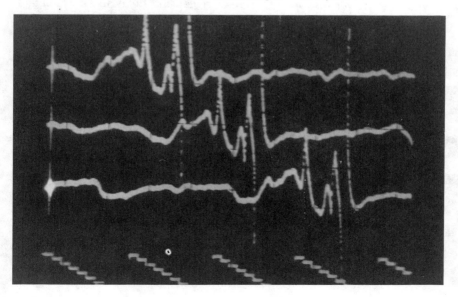

Figure 3. Recruitment frequency in extensor digitorum longus. Note that sweep goes left to right and bottom to top. Second MUP appears for the first time on right side of bottom trace. First motor unit is firing at 8 Hz at the moment of second motor unit recruitment.

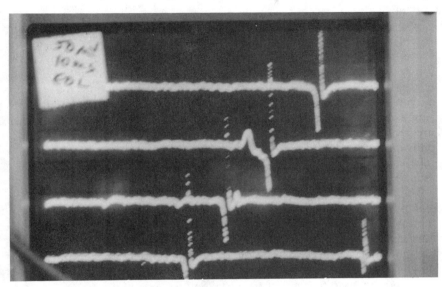

Figure 4. Decreased recruitment of motor units during maximal contraction of the flexor digitorum sublimus in a patient 42 years after acute anterior poliomyelitis. (Each square = 10 msec, 10 μV.)

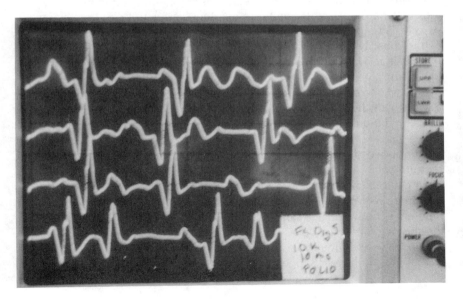

normal individual at the moment the second motor unit is recruited. This semiquantitative evaluation of early recruitment is fairly easily obtained in a cooperative patient and might be the earliest indication of weakness in radiculopathy or other neuropathic diseases when the manual muscle test is equivocal.

In myopathies, however, the reverse occurs; each motor unit is weaker, having lost muscle fibers. The first motor unit is firing more slowly for the same effort when the second motor unit is recruited. Thus, in myopathy the recruitment frequency is reduced and the recruitment interval is increased. This is further demonstrated by another important clue in early diagnosis of myopathic disease, namely, the difficulty in obtaining only a single motor unit on the screen for examination in step III. This electromyographic observation occurs when there is a need for two or three motor units to be recruited during the most minimal effort. Note that the earliest reliable electromyographic parameter in the diagnosis of myopathy is the reduced duration of the first recruited motor unit potentials.

The amplitude of the first recruited potentials is also an important parameter to evaluate in needle electromyography. If the low threshold and smaller motor units are reduced for some reason, the higher threshold units, which have a higher amplitude, would be the first recruited. Conversely, if the high threshold, high amplitude motor units are reduced, as in steroid myopathy or disuse atrophy, the recruitment pattern would be all small units first, and the condition could be mistaken for myopathy.

In step IV (maximal contraction), one attempts to evaluate the firing rate, amplitude, duration, and number of motor unit potentials occurring during a maximal effort (Figure 4). The recruitment pattern is difficult to evaluate, mostly because the motor units are overlapped in a full recruitment pattern. Also, it is helpful to use only a single joint muscle in step IV because it is extraordinarily difficult to contract maximally a two-joint muscle when the patient is reclining. Portions of an estimated 8–10 motor units will be in the vicinity of the tip of the needle, all firing at their maximal rate. This means the screen will be filled. Also, one should be aware that even if a quarter of the units are lost, a reduction in motor unit potentials would be very difficult to identify by the visualization on the screen or by the audio cue.

The above discussion suggests that the recruitment frequency in early recruitment is a better and more accurate measure of mild weakness than attempts to evaluate changes of pattern during a maximal contraction. For example, we know that in usual muscle grading (5, 4, 3, 2, 1, 0) the difference between a 5 and a 4 grade could be a loss of 40–50% of the motor units. Therefore, one could speculate that a muscle grade of 4 would be very difficult to evaluate, even though up to half the motor units in that muscle have disappeared.

STIMULATION STUDIES—LATE WAVES

F-Wave

A supramaximal stimulus with a cathode positioned proximally would result in a small late wave with a variable latency and shape (Figure 5). This is a motor response with the antidromic impulse traveling to the anterior horn cell and then the orthodromic impulse traveling back to the muscle. From 1% to 5% of the compound muscle action potential (CMAP) is an F-wave. This wave is a good indication of the state of the entire motor nerve,[5] which can be evaluated by:

- the shortest latency;
- the average latency;
- the difference between the minimal and the maximal latency;
- the number of responses per number of stimuli;
- the amplitude and the duration of the F-waves;
- the number of F-waves within one millisecond of the shortest latency;
- the number of F-waves with the same shape.

It is essential to evoke many F-waves. One is not enough. Some investigators use 8, while others recommend 16; Dr. Stalberg suggests 20 and another expert routinely evokes 32.[5,6,7]

A-Wave

This wave is usually intermediate between the CMAP and the F-wave. Supramaximal stimulation usually eliminates the A-wave. It is believed to derive from a reinnervating axon, resulting in a response which is slower than the M-wave but faster than the F-wave in most instances. However, some A-waves can have an even longer latency than the F-wave.

H-Wave

This is the electrical correlate of the muscle stretch reflex.[8] Tibial nerve stimulation in the popliteal space with a 1 msec duration and low voltage stimulus will evoke an H-wave in the soleus muscle. It represents the afferent and efferent arms of the stretch reflex with a single synapse. It is very reproducible, and a difference in latency from side to side of 1 msec or more suggests an S1 radiculopathy or a block somewhere along the pathway (Figure 6). The predicted mean latency can be derived from the formula:

.46 × the distance from the popliteal area to the median malleolus
plus 0.10 × the age in years
plus 9.14 (a constant).

Figure 5. F-waves showing each one is different shape and latency (anterior tibial nerve). (10 msec/200 µV per centimeter on photo.)

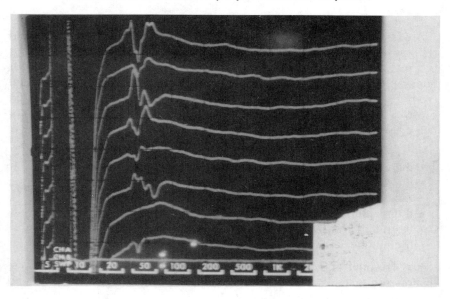

Figure 6. Superimposed H-waves showing delay in S1 radiculopathy.

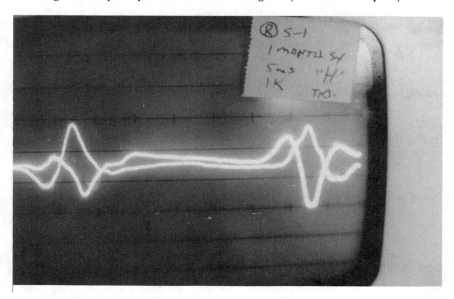

If the observed latency for both limbs is longer than the predicted mean, then the tibial nerve motor conduction or the sural nerve latency and amplitude should be measured, since an underlying peripheral neuropathy is likely.

More recently, the S1 spinal nerve has been stimulated and the efferent segment compared to the entire H-wave latency. In the normal individual it represents 47–48% of the pathway, while in S1 radiculopathy it is 45% or less. This result is observed because the S1 stimulation is beyond the point of compromise in an S1 radiculopathy.

One can also isolate the central loop of the H reflex by stimulating at the S1 spinal root with a long-duration, low-voltage stimulus. The S1 spinal nerve is stimulated 1 cm medial to the posterior superior iliac spine (Figure 7). The anode is placed on the anterior abdomen and the needle cathode is positioned deeply until its tip touches bone. The stimulus simultaneously activates both the efferent limb (orthodromic-motor) and the afferent limb (orthodromic-sensory) of the muscle stretch reflex. Resultant responses are two CMAPs, normally separated by 7–8 msec.

The soleus CMAP can be recorded from almost anywhere on the leg with a surface recording electrode, even over the anterior compartment (Figure 8). The amplitude of the H-wave is not a reliable diagnostic aid, since many influences can alter the amplitude and indeed obliterate the H reflex. The most common inhibiting influence is contraction of the foot dorsiflexors, the antagonist muscle group. The H reflex can also be recorded in the vastus medialis by stimulation of the femoral nerve.[8] Its detection could be of help in diagnosing an L4 radiculopathy. Also, the H reflex can be obtained in the flexor carpi radialis with stimulation of the median nerve.[14] A side-to-side difference of more than 0.8 msec is suggestive of a block in the pathway, for example, a C6 or C7 radiculopathy. In children two years or younger, the H-wave can usually be evoked in the muscle of all four limbs.

CARPAL TUNNEL SYNDROME

With conventional electromyographic equipment, one can stimulate on both sides of the carpal tunnel to determine the degree of blocking and slowing in the median nerve.[3,4] This should be done for both sensory and motor fibers.

Antidromic stimulation of the median nerve sensory fibers is done by stimulating at the wrist and recording with ring electrodes on digit 2 or 3. The stimulus is first applied at the wrist, 14 cm from the recording electrodes, and then repeated at mid-palm, 7 cm from the recording electrodes (Figure 9). The amplitude and duration of the sensory nerve action potential (SNAP), as well as the latency, are determined. In a normal individual the latency at mid-palm is about one-half that at the wrist and the amplitude is less than 30% larger than the sensory nerve action potential obtained by stimulation

Figure 7. A. Location of needle stimulation for S1 spinal nerve. **B.** Top trace: H-wave with stimulation of tibial nerve in popliteal space. Bottom trace: M-wave and H-wave with spinal nerve stimulation.

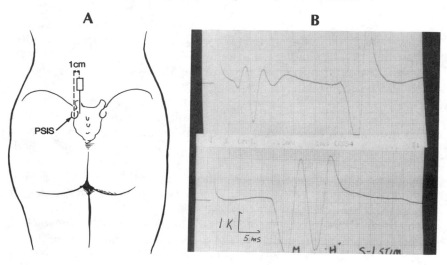

Figure 8. H-wave recorded from a surface electrode placed at various locations on the leg. Top trace: Surface recording over the extensor digitorum longus nerve. Middle trace: Surface recording over the anterior tibial nerve. Bottom trace: Surface recording over soleus nerve. Note that tibial nerve was stimulated in popliteal space for all recordings.

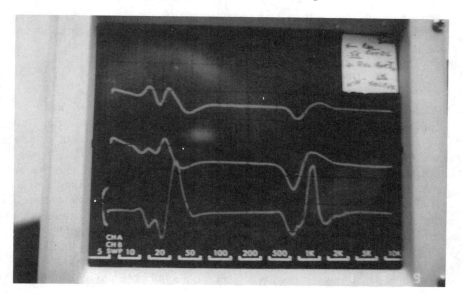

Figure 9. A. Electrode placement for antidromic sensory nerve action potential recorded from digit III. B. Normal values. C. Top trace: Mid-palmar stimulation (7 cm). Bottom trace: Wrist stimulation (14 cm). Note that there is substantial neurapraxia, a circumstance *not* apparent without mid-palm stimulation. (Horizontal marks = 1 msec; vertical marks = 20 μV.)

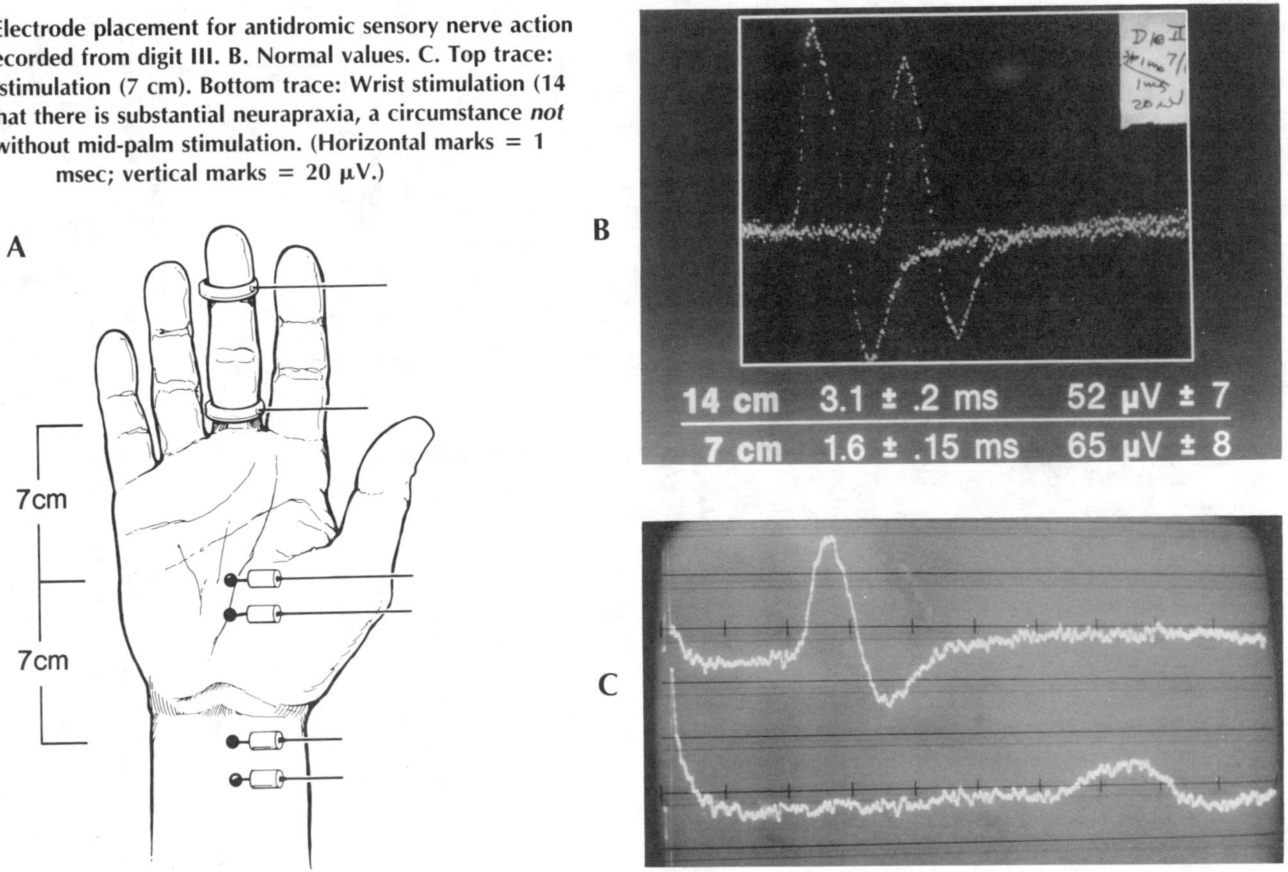

111

at the wrist. These results are the consequence of the stimulus and the recording electrodes being closer and minimizing temporal dispersion.

A phenomenon termed phase cancellation also influences the amplitude of SNAP when the stimulus is applied at some distance from the antidromic ring electrodes.[9] Theoretically, the recording ring electrodes should be 4 cm apart to minimize phase cancellation. This circumstance occurs when the negative phase of the SNAP partially cancels the positive phase of the SNAP when they overlap, causing an apparent reduction in the SNAP amplitude.

Wrist and mid-palmar stimulation of the median nerve motor fibers can also be done easily. The latency at mid-palm for the motor fibers is not helpful, but the amplitude of the CMAP will reflect the neurapraxic axons. In the normal individual the amplitude increase at mid-palm is usually less than 10% or under 0.5 millivolt.

Both motor and sensory studies on both sides of the carpal ligaments are necessary in order to establish the prognosis of carpal tunnel syndrome.[7,11]

Transcarpal Mixed Nerve Latency

With a surface recording electrode over the median nerve at the wrist, the stimulus is applied at mid-palm 8 cm distally. Latency in the normal individual is 1.8 msec, with a standard deviation of 0.2 msec (Figure 10). A similar latency is present when the ulnar nerve is stimulated and recorded in a like manner. A difference in latency between the ulnar and median nerve of greater than 0.2 msec is suggestive of carpal tunnel syndrome (CTS) if the measurements are done carefully.

As recorded with surface electrodes, the usual amplitude of the mixed nerve action potential is 100–150 μV for the median nerve and 40–60 μV for the ulnar nerve.[9] This difference in amplitude is a consequence of the location of the two nerves at the wrist—the median nerve is quite superficial, while the ulnar nerve is deep to the flexor carpi ulnaris tendon.

Bactrian Sign

With ring electrodes on the thumb, the median and radial nerves are stimulated simultaneously at the wrist, 10 cm from the recording electrodes. The antidromic latencies are usually 2.6 and 2.5 msec, respectively, and the amplitudes are 30 μV for the median and 12 μV for the radial.

In CTS the median sensory fibers are delayed in the carpal tunnel and the median SNAP will appear after the radial SNAP. Thus, a double or Bactrian hump will occur[7] (Figure 11).

If the latencies are normal but the amplitudes of both median and radial SNAPs are less than half of normal, a C6 radiculopathy is likely.

A more recent technique to study carpal tunnel syndrome is the deter-

Figure 10. Transcarpal mixed nerve action potentials (8 cm conduction). Top trace: Ulnar nerve. Bottom trace: Median nerve. Note that latency is increased for median nerve indicating mild carpal tunnel syndrome. (Each square = 20 μV; 1 msec.)

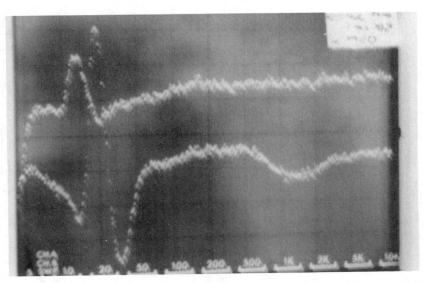

Figure 11. Top trace: Median and radial nerves stimulated simultaneously (Bactrian sign). Middle trace: Stimulated radial nerve (10 cm). Bottom trace: Stimulated median nerve (10 cm). (Each square is 1 msec; 20 μV. Antidromic sensory nerve action potential to digit 1.)

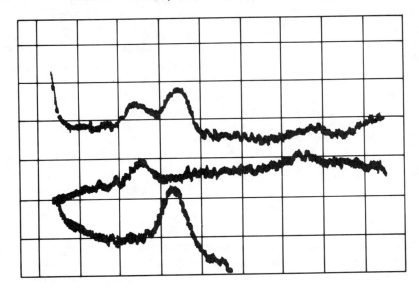

mination of the latency and amplitude of the first lumbrical muscle. In 3 out of 10 cases of CTS where the latency was normal to the abductor pollicis brevis, the motor fibers to the first lumbrical were blocked and slowed. The reverse has also been found.[3]

An interesting phenomenon is the relationship of the wrist shape to the likelihood of developing CTS. The side-to-side dimension at the distal wrist flexor crease is divided into the anterior to posterior measurement. A rectangular wrist is less likely to develop CTS and a squarer one is more likely.[6]

TARSAL TUNNEL SYNDROME

A less frequent clinical syndrome is tarsal tunnel syndrome. It is best diagnosed by the technique described by Saeed and Gatens.[13] The lateral plantar and medial plantar nerves are stimulated at the sole with surface recording over the tibial nerve (12 cm). The action potential of the mixed nerve is 12–15 μV. Slowing of conduction is easily demonstrated, as is a reduction in the amplitude of the mixed nerve action potentials.

PROGNOSIS IN RADICULOPATHY

After Wallerian degeneration has proceeded for four to five days, the distal (dying) axons are not excitable. This circumstance provides an excellent opportunity to determine the proportion of dead axons in radiculopathy.[1] Therefore, the prognosis of radiculopathy is established by stimulating the nerve to the muscle involved and comparing the CMAP with that of the contralateral normal limb. A reduction of 50% or more suggests a poor prognosis. If the axons are neurapraxic, the CMAP will be nearer in size to that of the contralateral[11,12] (Figure 12).

Lower limb muscles to be sampled to estimate prognosis for recovery from mononeuritic radiculopathy are:

- L4 vastus medialis
- L5 extensor digitorum longus
- S1 medial gastrocnemius

Upper limb muscles to be sampled are:

- C5 deltoid
- C6 infraspinatus
- C7 triceps
- C8 pronator quadratus[10]
- T1 abductor digiti minimi

In entrapment syndromes the same information can be obtained from the compound muscle action potential by stimulating proximally and distally to the entrapment. The intensity and distribution of the positive waves and

Figure 12. A. Electrode placement for surface recording from pronator quadratus. B. Top trace: Compound motor action potential 4 weeks after onset of paresis in C8 radiculopathy. (Vertical line = 2,000 μV; horizontal line = 4 msec.)

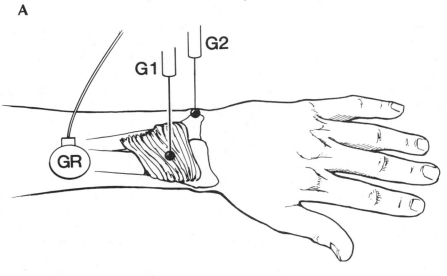

fibrillation potentials are less helpful in prognosis than the CMAP. Latencies do not help to determine the prognosis.

SPINAL NERVE STIMULATION

All spinal nerves can be stimulated distal to the confluence of the dorsal and anterior roots. This is done with a needle at the most proximal location at which a peripheral nerve can be directly stimulated. C8 stimulation is done with a needle 1 cm lateral and caudal to the C7 spinous process. The anode, a large flat electrode, is placed on the anterior shoulder directly opposite the needle cathode. Other spinal nerves can be stimulated cephalad and at the appropriate distance from the C7 spinous process.

REPETITIVE STIMULATION

Repetitive stimulation for a demonstration of neuromuscular transmission dysfunction is accomplished by 2/sec (2 Hz) stimulation in the following manner.

In myasthenia gravis a more proximal muscle should be stimulated, for example, the upper trapezius, the deltoid, or the nasalid on the nose. The disease is usually manifest with greater severity in the proximal muscles.

The neuromuscular transmission defect can be enhanced by heating the limb or by fatiguing the muscle with one minute of isometric exercise and repeating the 2/sec stimulation. Usually, the maximal decrement will occur by the fourth stimulation. This decrement will be most prominent from 45 seconds to 2 minutes after the fatiguing exercise.

In myasthenic syndrome (Lambert-Eaton syndrome) slow stimulations will give a varying result. However, high rates of stimulation will yield substantial facilitation, up to 1000%. A more comfortable way to demonstrate the facilitation is to apply a single shock supramaximally before and after 10 seconds of exercise. The CMAP will increase by tenfold or even greater.

In infantile botulism a similar presynaptic defect is present. Here, the application of high frequency stimuli (30–50 Hz) will show facilitation of 75–150%. The presynaptic defects are present in all the muscles so that one does not have to use a proximal muscle (as preferred in myasthenia gravis).

POSTPOLIO SYNDROME

The increasing weakness that some individuals experience 30–40 years after acute paralytic polio has been investigated electromyographically and most likely is the result of the failure of "hypermetabolic" motor units— enlarged motor units producing enlarged or giant potentials.[15] With the trigger and delay line on the electromyograph the firing motor unit will decrease in amplitude and vary in shape as the neuromuscular junction fatigues to failure (Figure 13). It is hypothesized that following acute polio these motor units sprouted axons which spread to and reinnervated neighboring denervated muscle fibers. The "hypermetabolic" motor units fatigue to failure sooner than do motor units of normal size. It is known now that these motor units apparently remodel throughout the person's life, so the presence of fibrillation potentials and positive waves does not really help in the establishment of coincident disease or progressive polio weakness.[15]

Figure 13. Postpolio syndrome in the biceps brachialis of a patient 37 years after acute poliomyelitis. There was reduction of amplitude and slowing of conduction in motor unit when it was stimulated repeatedly.

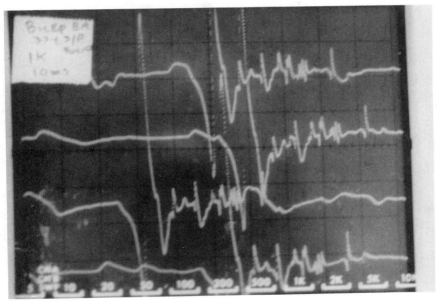

CONCLUSION

Meticulous application of electromyographic techniques will improve the data obtained from machines of any age.[2] The following procedures should be followed:

- Clean all electrodes and check the integrity of the leads.
- Place and secure the electrode carefully.
- Use the electrode paste sparingly but appropriately.
- Ensure that needle electrodes are sharpened and have appropriately exposed tips.
- Explain the test to the patient to get maximal cooperation.

- Plan the examination in a way to minimize discomfort.
- Unplug electrical appliances to avoid interference.
- Be deliberate in the orderly process of the electromyogram, making each step an intensive study.

If you are uncertain regarding the diagnosis, do not hesitate to repeat the examination after you have carefully reconsidered all of the possibilities.

REFERENCES

1. Aminoff M et al. Electrophysiologic evaluation of lumbosacral radiculopathies: electromyography, late responses and somatosensory evoked potentials. *Neurology.* 1985;35:1514.
2. Dumitru D, Walsh N. Practical instrumentation and common source of error. *Am J Phys Med Rehabil.* 1988;67:55.
3. Fitz W, Mysiw WJ, Johnson EW. Comparison of latency and amplitude of lumbrical I and abductor pollicis brevis in normal individual and carpal tunnel syndrome. *Am J Phys Med Rehabil.* 1990;69:198–201.
4. Gordon C, Johnson EW, Gatens PF, Ashton JJ. Wrist ratio correlation with carpal tunnel syndrome in industry. *Am J Phys Med Rehabil.* 1988;67:270–272.
5. Hong CZ, et al. Averaged F-wave conductive velocity of peroneal nerve. *Am J Phys Med Rehabil.* 1988;67:166.
6. Johnson EW, Gatens T, Poindexter D, Bowers D. Wrist dimensions: correlation with median sensory latencies. *Arch Phys Med Rehabil.* 1983;64:556–557.
7. Johnson EW, Sipski M, Lammertse TE. Median and radial sensory latencies to digit I: normal values and usefulness in carpal tunnel syndrome. *Am J Phys Med Rehabil.* 1987;68:140–141.
8. Kameyama O et al. Methodological considerations contributing to variability of the quadriceps H reflex. *Am J Phys Med Rehabil.* 1989;68:277.
9. Kimura J et al. Relationship between size of compound sensory or muscle action potentials and length of nerve segment. *Neurology.* 1986;36:6–7.
10. Mysiw WJ, Colachis SC. Electrophysiologic study of the anterior interosseus nerve. *Am J Phys Med Rehabil.* 1988;67:50.
11. Pease WS et al. Determining neurapraxia in carpal tunnel syndrome. *Am J Phys Med Rehabil.* 1988;67:117.
12. Pease WS, Cannell CD, Johnson EW. Median to radial latency difference test in mild carpal tunnel syndrome. *Muscle Nerve.* 1989;12:905–909.
13. Saeed M, Gatens P. Compound nerve action potentials of medial and lateral plantar nerves through the tarsal tunnel. *Arch Phys Med Rehabil.* 1982;63:304.
14. Schimsheimer R et al. The flexor carpi radialis H-reflex in lesions of the sixth and seventh cervical nerve roots. *J Neurol Neurosurg Psychiatry.* 1985;48:445.
15. Wiechers D. Acute and latent effects of poliomyelitis on the motor unit as revealed by electromyography. *Orthopedics.* 1985;8:870.

Chapter 7

THE LATE EFFECTS OF POLIOMYELITIS

Lauro S. Halstead

This chapter will explore some of the new health problems and challenges being faced by persons who had paralytic poliomyelitis or infantile paralysis years ago. It is based on studies and experience of persons in North America.

In 1987 there were more than 640,000 people in the United States who had experienced paralytic polio.[21] It is now believed that, 30 to 40 years after the acute episode, more than 50% of these people are having new health problems related to their polio,[32] including excessive fatigue, progressive weakness, pain, loss of function, and, less commonly, muscle atrophy. These problems escaped widespread attention until further regression from the plateau of neurological and functional recovery appeared at a much later age. The patients experiencing the problems are mostly middle-aged, but ranged from 24 years to 86 years in one survey.[16] Furthermore, the residual disabilities from polio may get worse as these persons age, compounded by common medical conditions that affect the elderly such as hypertension, heart disease, stroke, and arthritis.

POSSIBLE CAUSES OF POSTPOLIO COMPLICATIONS

Acute Polio and "Premature" or "Accelerated" Aging

Acute poliomyelitis, caused by one of three RNA viruses of the enterovirus group, invades the spinal cord of only 1% to 5% of the persons infected. Here, the virus's predilection for motor neurons in the lateral anterior horns produces a variable amount of paralysis. Regardless of the extent of paralysis, the virus typically infects over 95% of motor neurons, owing to its widespread dissemination throughout the central nervous system. After this invasion, cells either die or they shed the virus and regain a normal or near normal appearance. A possible explanation for motor neuron dysfunction recurring decades later is that these recovered motor neurons may remain more susceptible to insults later in life.

Once the virus has invaded the central nervous system, the extent of

119

neurological and functional recovery is determined by the number of motor neurons that (1) survive unimpaired, (2) recover and resume their normal function, and (3) develop terminal axon sprouts to reinnervate muscle fibers left orphaned by the death of their original motor neurons. This terminal axon sprouting enables either an uninvolved or a recovered motor neuron to adopt as many as 10 to 20 additional muscle fibers for every muscle cell innervated originally. Through this process, a single motor neuron that initially innervated 10 muscle fibers could conceivably innervate 100 to 200 fibers. As a result, the survivors of acute polio may be left with a few significantly enlarged motor units doing the work previously performed by many units. Because this mechanism of neurophysiological compensation is so effective, a muscle can retain normal strength even after 50% of the original motor neurons have been lost. However, the overworked anterior horn cells' control over a greater-than-normal percentage of muscle function may cause them to succumb "prematurely" to the aging process, resulting in pronounced weakness beginning as early as the fourth decade and steadily worsening with advancing age. Thirty to forty years after recovery, the giant motor units appear to lose their ability to sustain all of the terminal sprouts supplying so many muscle fibers. Consequently, the number of muscle fibers driven by each motor neuron declines, and the polio survivor experiences new weakness.

Residual Polio

Musculoskeletal disuse, musculoskeletal overuse, or motor unit dysfunction may act singly or together to produce progressive weakness, the cardinal symptom of postpolio complications. Their potential interactions and complications are illustrated in Figure 1. Musculoskeletal disuse leads to atrophy, weakness, contractures, and diminished endurance—complications thoroughly studied in other groups with sedentary lifestyles or neuromuscular lesions. Overuse, however, is less well understood, although studies suggest relationships between the number of motor units, muscle damage, and exercise intensity and duration.[19] But the extent to which a primary muscle defect is responsible for weakening some polio survivors remains unknown. Overuse has a cumulative effect over time; chronic mechanical strains on joints, ligaments, and soft tissues that have not been supported well for 30 or more years produce a self-perpetuating cycle of further complications. Recognizing overuse complications early and implementing effective interventions may avert severe postpolio disablement in middle or old age.

It is motor unit overwork, eventually causing neuronal dysfunction, that provides the most plausible theory for why new motor unit dysfunction can occur so many years after recovery from acute illness. The giant motor units characteristic of muscles reinnervated after acute polio increase the metabolic demand on the remaining motor neurons. According to this theory,

Figure 1. Schematic model showing three possible causes for the late neuromuscular and musculoskeletal complications of polio and their interactions.

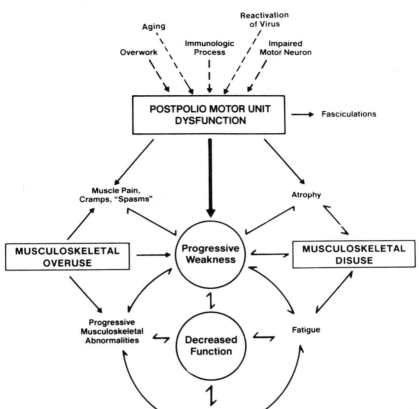

neurological dysfunction results from this increased metabolic load after a critical number of years. Several clinical studies and EMG data indirectly support the overuse theory.

Both Windebank and coworkers[32] at the Mayo Clinic and Maynard[20] found that in persons with similar neurological involvement, new weakness occurred more often in the weight-bearing muscles of the legs than in the nonweight-bearing muscles of the arms. And those limbs affected the most by the original disease were the most susceptible to new weakness. In subjects with about the same residual loss, Perry et al.[22] observed that, compared with asymptomatic polio survivors, symptomatic patients had a less efficient gait; both the intensity and duration of contraction of extensor muscles were increased. More recently, Agre and Rodriguez[1] found that symptomatic postpolio subjects had evidence of more severe original polio involvement by history, were weaker and able to perform less work than asymptomatic subjects, and recovered strength less readily than controls.

In electrophysiological studies, Wiechers and Hubbell[31] and Dalakas et al.[9] have found neuromuscular transmission abnormalities suggesting that the giant motor neurons may not be able to sustain indefinitely the metabolic demands of all their sprouts. As a result, individual terminals slowly deteriorate and reinnervated muscle fibers drop off. The more muscle fibers lost, the more apparent is the slowly progressive weakness.

Related to the overwork theory, the original viral attack of the anterior horn cells may have left some motor neurons functional but impaired, making them more vulnerable to dysfunction as time passes. Tomlinson and Irving[30] observed many smaller-than-normal neurons in the spinal cords of persons who survived long after the acute polio episode. Consistent with Bodian's findings,[5] their observation led them to conclude that the protein synthetic mechanisms of any cell invaded by polio are likely to be permanently damaged. Possibly, then, prolonged overwork with increased metabolic demand of the greatly enlarged motor units compounds injury to the motor unit sustained during acute infection.

Other Hypotheses

Although there is less evidence to support other hypotheses, they warrant mention as possible contributors to postpolio complications. Does premature aging of the polio survivor cause new neuromuscular changes? Normally, motor neurons do not die off in significant numbers until the seventh decade.[29] Polio survivors with fewer anterior horn cells to begin with, however, might suffer a disproportionate loss of clinical function if the relatively few giant motor units shrink or more anterior horn cells die. This hypothesis conceivably explains new weakness in some polio patients, but remains unsubstantiated by muscle biopsy changes such as group atrophy that would reflect the new loss of whole motor units. Furthermore, several studies have failed to show a positive relationship between the onset of new weakness and chronological age.[18,32] Instead, the determinant variable is the length of the interval between onset of polio and the appearance of new symptoms. If major motor neuron loss were occurring, new difficulties should steadily increase as the polio population ages.

Another hypothesis proposes immunologic involvement. Ginsberg et al.[14] recently described significant alternations in $CD4^+$ subsets in both symptomatic and asymptomatic postpolio subjects when compared with normal controls, supporting the possibility that immunologic factors may contribute to late disease progression. Dalakas et al.[8,10] have reported preliminary evidence of a lymphocytic response in muscle biopsies and IgG oligoclonal bands in the cerebrospinal fluid (CSF) of some symptomatic patients, whereas asymptomatic patients had no oligoclonal bands in their CSF. However, because these patients have not responded to immunosuppressant therapy, it remains uncertain whether such evidence of immunologic involvement can explain postpolio weakness.

Perhaps polio-related changes in the spinal cord are compromising motor neuron function. Pezeshkpour and Dalakas[23] observed active inflammatory gliosis, neuronal chromatolysis, and axonal spheroids in the spinal cords of polio patients who died of other causes many years after acute infection.

Finally, there is an intriguing suggestion by Rudman that "growth hormone (GH) menopause" may be a risk or precipitating factor in the development of postpolio syndrome (D. Rudman, personal communication). It has been shown that GH secretion drops off dramatically in approximately one-third of normal adults over the age of 40.[26] This results in a fall in somatomedin C (SmC), a substance which plays an important role in muscle cell protein synthesis, the proliferation of muscle satellite cells, and the regeneration of peripheral nerve sprouting. In a preliminary, unpublished survey, SmC was normal in a group of 12 asymptomatic older polio survivors and low in 9 of 10 symptomatic postpolio patients. A study is being planned to evaluate the effect of replacement GH on muscle size, strength, and endurance in symptomatic postpolio subjects (D. Rudman, personal communication).

PATIENT CHARACTERISTICS

Typical characteristics of postpolio patients with new health problems, originally identified in surveys,[13,16,18,32] have been confirmed by observation in the many postpolio clinics that have opened recently. The experience of one of these clinics, the Post-Polio Clinic at the Texas Institute for Rehabilitation and Research (TIRR) in Houston, is summarized in Tables 1 through 5. Most of the postpolio patients were women (66%), Caucasian (92%), married, well-educated, and employed outside the home. The majority of patients were middle-aged, the median age being 45 and the range between 24 and 86 years, and had contracted polio at a median age of seven years (range three months to 44 years). The median interval between onset of polio and onset of new health problems was 31 years. Although a similar interval has been found in other studies, it has ranged from two to eight decades.[9,18]

The factors most closely associated with risk for developing new problems are age and severity at onset of acute polio. The older the patient and the more severe the original symptoms, the greater the risk for developing new neurological problems 25 to 30 years later. Occasionally, however, a patient whose polio was apparently very mild initially and who had excellent clinical recovery still presents with typical postpolio symptoms.

Although postpolio symptoms usually begin insidiously, specific events that are more frequent among the elderly population often precipitate recognition of polio-related health problems. Such a precipitating event—a period of bed rest, weight gain, a fall, or a minor accident—would not cause as great a decline in health and function in persons who had never had polio. Another triggering mechanism is the development or exacerbation of unrelated medical problems, such as diabetes. The frequency of such problems increases with age.

What are the new, polio-related health and functional problems most often reported by polio survivors? Table 1 lists the most common new health and functional problems found in 132 consecutive patients seen over a one-year period at the TIRR Post-Polio Clinic. All patients were carefully evaluated to confirm the diagnosis of polio and rule out nonpolio causes for their new symptoms. Although specific complaints differ somewhat from one clinic to another, the Houston patients most often experienced a cluster of complaints: weakness, functional loss, pain, and fatigue. New atrophy, while relatively uncommon (28%), tended to occur only in conjunction with four or more other problems.

Weakness and Functional Loss

New weakness is usually prominent in muscles most severely involved in the original illness, but it may also occur in muscles believed to have been spared previously. Reduction in functional capacity tends to be directly proportional to muscle weakness. If functional reserve was already marginal, additional muscle weakness can result in marked functional incapacity. A patient's ability to compensate for random, scattered motor deficits by un-

Table 1. Most common new health and functional problems for 132 consecutive patients with confirmed polio.

Type of problem	Number	%
Health problems		
Fatigue	117	89
Muscle pain	93	71
Joint pain	93	71
Weakness:		
Previously affected muscles	91	69
Previously unaffected muscles	66	50
Cold intolerance	38	29
Atrophy	37	28
Cramps	24	18
Fasciculations	16	12
ADL problems[a]		
Walking	84	64
Climbing stairs	80	61
Dressing	23	17

[a]ADL = activities of daily living.
Source: Reprinted with permission from Halstead, L.S., "Late complications of poliomyelitis," in Goodgold, J. (ed.), *Rehabilitation Medicine.* St. Louis: CV Mosby, 1988, p. 322.

conventional muscle and joint movements may have adequately masked abnormal function until late-onset weakness of a critical muscle disrupted this delicate balance, resulting in a disproportionate amount of functional loss. Walking, standing, climbing stairs, and other activities requiring endurance may become more difficult if the legs are involved. Although polio survivors with presumably normal upper extremities may have been essentially "walking" with their arms for years, they may find ambulating, driving a car, transfers, or even dressing progressively more exhausting. Patients typically also find that recovering from strenuous activity takes longer than formerly. Exertion may also seriously compromise breathing, especially at night, in persons with initial pulmonary weakness.

Respiratory Impairment

In addition to weakness of respiratory muscles, impairment may be aggravated by decreased compliance of respiratory tissue, progressive scoliosis, recurrent pulmonary infection, and smoking. In the geriatric population, respiratory impairment from polio may be exacerbated by emphysema or chronic bronchitis resulting from a lifetime of smoking or exposure to occupational hazards. As in the acute phase of polio, respiratory failure is the most feared complication because it can ultimately lead to death.

At greatest risk for later serious pulmonary complications are those persons who had such severe respiratory involvement during the acute illness that they required ventilatory assistance. Also at high risk are those who developed deformities of the thoracic spine. Several preliminary studies suggest that as many as 18% to 38% of polio survivors who were successfully weaned off a respirator after the acute illness later required ventilatory assistance full or part time.[12] The long-term prognosis for those who were never weaned completely from a ventilator appears favorable.[3] More than half of patients interviewed 21 to 30 years after acute polio reported that the respiratory treatment they needed had not changed since one year after polio onset, 17% felt their impairment had improved, and 27% believed it had worsened. Only four persons needed more daily respiratory support than formerly.[3]

Fatigue

In addition to exhaustion related to physical exertion, postpolio patients also report generalized fatigue, described as a marked change in energy level, endurance, and sometimes mental alertness. Previously, everyday activities had been performed without any special effort. Postpolio fatigue usually occurs in the afternoon and early evening and often comes on so forcefully that patients talk about "hitting the wall." When this happens, they must stop what they are doing, rest, and take a short nap if possible.

Pain

When pain occurs, it is felt in the muscles or joints or both. Occasionally, pain takes the form of hypersensitivity and a sensation of crawling or cramping, especially at night. Otherwise, it is experienced as a deep, aching pain similar to the muscle pain experienced during acute polio. Physical activity and cold temperature tend to aggravate the pain. Although weight bearing often produces joint pain, it is rarely accompanied by swelling or inflammation.

The location of pain depends primarily on the patient's method of locomotion (Tables 2 and 3).[27,28] In many patients, muscle and joint pain appears to result directly from abnormal body mechanics that are compensating for muscle weakness and skeletal abnormalities. Consequently, the remaining innervated muscles carry increased work loads. Abnormal or excessive forces on unstable joints and supporting tissues increase the stress on them during daily activities. Strains accumulate silently over many years until they cross a critical threshold and produce painful muscles, joints, and ligaments.

DIAGNOSIS BY EXCLUSION

No serological, enzymatic, or electrodiagnostic test is able to distinguish symptomatic from asymptomatic postpolio patients. Despite the suggestion that the major pathologic process in postpolio syndrome is motor unit dys-

Table 2. Prevalence of chronic pain by method of locomotion in 114 postpolio patients.

Method of locomotion	Number	Number with pain	% with pain
Ambulatory, no brace (Independent)	67	56	(84)
Ambulatory with brace (Independent)	12	11	(92)
Ambulatory with crutches (Independent)	21	21	(100)
Wheelchair locomotion (Independent)	7	7	(100)
Wheelchair locomotion (Need personal assistance)	7	7	(100)
Total	114	102	(90)

Source: Reprinted with permission from Smith, L.K., and K. McDermott, "Addressing causes versus treating effects," in Halstead, L.S., and D.O. Wiechers (eds.), *Research and Clinical Aspects of the Late Effects of Poliomyelitis.* White Plains, NY: March of Dimes Birth Defects Foundation, 1987, p. 122.

Table 3. Location of chronic pain by method of locomotion in 114 postpolio patients.

Location of pain	Number	%
Independent ambulators with or without lower extremity orthoses	79	69
Back	37	(47)
Hip	19	(24)
Diffuse lower extremity	18	(22)
Other (neck, shoulder, knee, ankle)	31	(39)
Locomotion performance using crutches or wheelchairs	35	31
Neck and shoulders	18	(51)
Back	13	(37)
Gleno-humeral joint	11	(31)
Elbow	6	(17)
Wrist and hand	9	(26)
Other (lower extremity and head)	15	(43)

Source: Reprinted with permission from Smith, L.K., and K. McDermott, "Addressing causes versus treating effects," in Halstead, L.S., and D.O. Wiechers (eds.), *Research and Clinical Aspects of the Late Effects of Poliomyelitis.* White Plains, NY: March of Dimes Birth Defects Foundation, 1987, p. 122.

function, no existing objective method can predict whether progression will occur. Postpolio complications are thus diagnosed by exclusion of other medical, orthopedic, or neurological conditions that could be causing or aggravating the presenting symptoms. An interdisciplinary evaluation should be carried out by a team including a physician, physical therapist, and social worker, with referrals to other medical specialists as needed to rule out nonpolio-related causes. In addition to a careful history and physical examination, it is crucial to carry out appropriate laboratory studies, x-rays, electromyography and nerve conduction velocity (EMG/NCV) studies, psychosocial evaluation, and a functional assessment of gait, orthotic needs, and strength and endurance of key muscle groups. Standard screening tests such as an SMA 24 or thyroid panel have not proven to be helpful or cost-effective.

Patients who had respiratory impairment during acute polio or have a history of pulmonary disease should also undergo pulmonary function studies and measurement of arterial blood gases. Complaints suggesting respiratory impairment include shortness of breath, exertional dyspnea, daytime somnolence, early morning headache, sleep disturbance, and sleep apnea. Patients with nighttime sleep disturbances, especially dyspnea or apnea, and with elevated PCO_2 should undergo sleep studies, or at least evaluation of nighttime oxygen saturation, with ear oximetry.[12] Central and obstructive sleep apnea should also be differentiated by sleep studies.

The five criteria necessary for making a diagnosis of postpolio syndrome are listed in Table 4. The diagnosis of a prior episode of paralytic polio

Table 4. Criteria for the diagnosis of postpolio syndrome.

1. A prior episode of paralytic polio confirmed by history, physical exam, and EMG.
2. A period of neurologic recovery followed by an extended interval of functional stability preceding the onset of new problems. The interval of neurologic and functional stability usually lasts 20 or more years.
3. The gradual or abrupt onset of non-disuse weakness in previously affected and/or unaffected muscles. This may or may not be accompanied by other new health problems, such as excessive fatigue, muscle pain, joint pain, decreased endurance, decreased function, atrophy, and so forth.
4. Standard EMG evaluation demonstrates changes consistent with prior AHC disease; fibrillations, sharp waves, and increased percent of polyphasic potentials may or may not be present.
5. Exclusion of medical, orthopedic, and neurologic conditions that might cause the health problems listed above.

Source: Reprinted with permission from Halstead, L.S., "Post polio syndrome: definition of an elusive concept," in Munsat, T.L. (ed.), *Post Polio Syndrome.* Boston: Butterworth-Heinemann, 1990, pp. 23–38.

usually can be confirmed by examining the original medical records, eliciting a credible history of an acute febrile illness producing motor but no sensory loss, or noting whether other members of the patient's family or neighbors had a similar illness. One characteristic feature in the physical examination is the presence of focal, asymmetric weakness or atrophy. Electromyography should reveal changes consistent with chronic denervation and reinnervation characteristic of previous anterior horn cell disease. Other changes on routine EMG compatible with prior polio include increased amplitude and duration of motor unit action potentials; an increased percentage of polyphasic motor units, often of long duration; and a decrease in the number of motor units on maximum recruitment in weak muscles.

For establishing a diagnosis of postpolio syndrome, a specific pattern of recovery and neurological stability preceding the onset of new problems is so characteristic that its absence makes aging-related and other medical disorders much more likely explanations for the patient's symptoms. This pattern, depicted in Figure 2, includes a period of functional and neurological stability lasting at least 20 years.[17]

At least one of the new problems should be non-disuse weakness. One clue to non-disuse weakness is diminished function despite maintenance of the usual level and intensity of activity. Of the five criteria listed in Table 4, this one is often the most difficult to establish. A history of paralytic poliomyelitis does not exempt anyone from getting the chronic illnesses, diseases, or psychiatric disturbances that afflict the general population. Medical, orthopedic, or neurological conditions coexisting with postpolio problems may produce a similar set of overlapping signs and symptoms. Compression neuropathies, radiculopathies, degenerative arthritis, disc dis-

Figure 2. The natural history of polio based on data from patients evaluated in the Post-Polio Clinic, Houston, Texas.

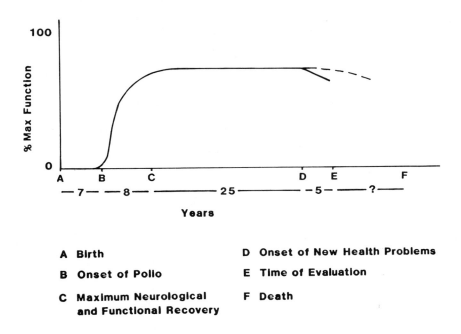

A **Birth**

B **Onset of Polio**

C **Maximum Neurological and Functional Recovery**

D **Onset of New Health Problems**

E **Time of Evaluation**

F **Death**

ease, obesity, anemia, diabetes, thyroid disease, and depression are some common examples. Furthermore, as shown in Figure 1, the original problem may be impossible to identify when, for example, weakness triggers a chain reaction of other complications, regardless of the underlying etiology. Nevertheless, because non-disuse weakness is such an important indicator of postpolio syndrome, and different etiologies dictate very different management strategies, a reasonable attempt should be made to differentiate postpolio weakness from other possible causes.

Amyotrophic lateral sclerosis (ALS) especially should be differentiated from postpolio syndrome because of the markedly different prognosis of the two. Despite some similarities between postpolio weakness and ALS, major differences found during clinical and laboratory evaluation (Tables 5 and 6) facilitate differential diagnosis.[7] Because some patients who had polio have been diagnosed as having ALS, certain clinicians have speculated that antecedent infection with polio might predispose one to developing ALS later in life.[24,25,33] It is now believed that ALS was misdiagnosed in some patients with a protracted course. Were these patients to be evaluated today, most would probably be diagnosed as having postpolio syndrome.[6]

Table 5. Comparison of clinical findings in patients with late polio and amyotrophic lateral sclerosis.

Patients	Weakness	Bulbar sxs	Fasciculations	Long tract signs	Sensory changes	Prognosis
ALS	often symmetrical, generalized	common	common	very common	absent	rapid, downhill course; death 3–5 years
Postpolio	asymmetrical focal	rare	occasional	very rare	absent	loss of strength at 1% per year

Source: Adapted from Dalakas, M.C., "Amyotrophic lateral sclerosis and post polio: differences and similarities," in Halstead, L.S., and D.O. Wiechers (eds.), *Research and Clinical Aspects of the Late Effects of Poliomyelitis*. White Plains, NY: March of Dimes Birth Defects Foundation, 1987, p. 74.

Table 6. Comparison of laboratory findings in patients with late polio and amyotrophic lateral sclerosis.

Patients	DNA repair	CPK	EMG	Muscle biopsy
ALS	abnormal	frequently elevated	fibs and PSW + + +, fasciculations + + +, MUP rarely > 10mV, fiber density ↑, jitter/ blocking ↑, neurogenic jitter often present[a]	group atrophy common; scattered angulated fibers; inflammation rare
Postpolio	normal	occasionally elevated	fibs and PSW +, fasciculations +, MUP often > 10mV, fiber density ↑ ↑ ↑, jitter/ blocking ↑, neurogenic jitter rare	group atrophy uncommon; inflammation in 40%

[a]PSW = positive sharp waves; MUP = motor unit potential.
Source: Adapted from Dalakas, M.C., "Amyotrophic lateral sclerosis and post polio: differences and similarities," in Halstead, L.S., and D.O. Wiechers (eds.), *Research and Clinical Aspects of the Late Effects of Poliomyelitis*. White Plains, NY: March of Dimes Birth Defects Foundation, 1987, p. 74.

TERMINOLOGY

Because diagnostic criteria remain nonspecific and pathognomonic tests are unavailable, a consistent diagnostic name has not yet been established for new health problems associated with prior polio. Indeed, several pathologic processes may interact at any given time to produce similar, overlapping symptoms (Figure 1). Use of a general rather than a precise diagnostic term takes into account the impossibility of determining a distinct origin for each new symptom. One heterogeneous term often used is postpolio syndrome, a diagnosis reserved for those patients whose symptomatology indicates motor unit dysfunction accompanied by variable musculoskeletal overuse. Not every polio survivor complaining of weakness, however, can be classified as having postpolio syndrome. This diagnosis should be made only after a trial of closely supervised exercise to rule out disuse weakness.

A more specific diagnostic term for postpolio complications is postpolio progressive muscular atrophy (PPMA). Only patients who show documented, objective evidence of neuromuscular deterioration and evidence on muscle biopsy of active denervation in the form of scattered angulated fibers qualify for this diagnostic category.[9] A less restrictive but similar term is postpolio motor neuron disease (PPMND).

MANAGEMENT

Health problems related to former polio must be managed to enable the person to continue functioning at home and work as independently as possible. The problems that warrant the earliest attention include muscle weakness, pain, respiratory failure, and psychological issues. In many cases, alleviating these problems will require changes in lifestyle that the physician must persuade the patient to accept.

Weakness

Depending on whether weakness is exacerbated by inactivity or overuse, a trial of progressive exercise or rest and support, respectively, should be instituted. Several studies[11,15] have shown improved strength in response to carefully supervised exercise programs for polio survivors with new weakness. However, since the effects of exercise on such muscles are unknown, long-term maintenance or strengthening exercises are recommended only for those muscles in which there is no clinical or EMG evidence of prior polio involvement. Exercising muscles initially damaged by polio may increase the risk of accelerating motor unit dysfunction and may produce overuse weakness.

For overuse complications the aim is to reduce mechanical stress, support weakened muscles, and stabilize abnormal joint movements. When patients have been pushing themselves and their muscles to maximum performance every day, a change in lifestyle that lessens stress and improves support of weakened muscles has often slowed the decrease in strength, prevented further deterioration, and, in some cases, actually reversed symptoms. However, even those patients who have overuse weakness can benefit from some kind of formal exercise program within the limits of comfort and safety. This program can range from gentle stretching and yoga to aerobic training. Alba and coworkers[2] found that 66% of 35 postpolio survivors were able to attain normal cardiopulmonary levels during exercise as measured on a Monarch arm ergometer, Quinton treadmill, or Collins chair ergometer. The remainder of the subjects were unable to obtain a normal range of work capacity due to focal or generalized fatigue in their extremities or improper biomechanical techniques during exercise. Therefore, when prescribing more vigorous exercise, any repetitious activity that appeals to the patient but does not cause undue pain or muscle fatigue may be selected. Weakness or discomfort that takes several hours to subside is a good indicator of excessive activity. Swimming is an ideal form of exercise for the postpolio patient; it not only avoids the stresses and microtrauma of other types of exercise but also readily accommodates concurrent musculoskeletal conditions such as the degenerative joint disease that become more prevalent with aging.

Pain

Pain management is designed to compensate for years of abnormal and excessive forces on unstable joints and supporting tissues. Conservative measures such as decreased activity, better support of unstable joints and weakened muscles, and improved biomechanics of the body during common daily activities, supplemented by low doses of anti-inflammatory medications, moist heat, and transcutaneous electrical nerve stimulation (TENS), usually help alleviate pain. Lifestyle modifications and improved biomechanics should be emphasized and the use of strong pain medications discouraged.

Cervical pillows, lumbar rolls, gluteal pads, dorsolumbar corsets, and heel lifts can help modify abnormal biomechanics. In addition, the musculoskeletal mechanics of sitting, standing, walking, sleeping, and other daily, repetitive activities at work must be corrected. The basic orthotic principles used in the management of other neuromuscular disorders also apply to relieving pain related to polio. Patients needing an orthosis that combines strength with lightness may benefit from the new plastics and lightweight metals if they can be convinced to trade in their old heavy braces. Frequently, patients prefer to repair and use these old braces than to start over again with new ones. Others may resist using any kind of brace support for cosmetic reasons.

Reductions in stress, activity, and weight are lifestyle changes that have the most impact on reducing pain. These strategies may be the most difficult to accomplish, however, because they often require developing behaviors that are very unlike the old, familiar ways of coping. It is essential to reduce the pace and intensity of discretionary activities.

Respiratory Impairment

Referral to a pulmonologist with experience in neuromuscular diseases is indicated for managing respiratory problems. Supplemental oxygen alone is sufficient to alleviate many patients' symptoms when nighttime desaturation has been documented. Others may experience marked improvement in both daytime and nighttime symptoms when given ventilatory assistance at night. The pneumo-wrap or raincoat and chest cuirass are the most practical means of providing nighttime ventilatory assistance. Alternatives that are not so readily available or practical include intermittent positive pressure with a Bennett mouth seal, nasal continuous positive airway pressure (C-PAP), and the iron lung. Few patients will benefit from a tracheostomy, which should be avoided if possible.[4] Every patient with impaired pulmonary function and a history of recurrent respiratory infections should receive flu vaccines yearly and pneumococcal vaccine (Pneumovax) at least once.

Psychological Issues

Emotional responses to experiencing new medical problems related to polio can be as traumatic and disabling as the physical problems. Although they may experience any combination of denial, anger, frustration, and hopelessness, postpolio patients generally fit into one of three distinct categories of psychological response: (1) those who do not regard themselves as handicapped, regardless of the extent of involvement and presence of obvious deformities; (2) those who feel disabled now, but who never did in the past, even during the acute illness; (3) those who feel that, because they are experiencing polio for the second time, they are "twice cursed."

Polio survivors may resist making lifestyle changes to accommodate weakness, fatigue, and other postpolio symptoms because they have worked so hard to overcome the initial paralysis and achieved a high level of functional performance and personal fulfillment. They no longer perceived themselves as handicapped and believed, even if some disability remained, that they had won; the long struggle with polio was over. When new limitations unexpectedly and abruptly develop 25 to 40 years later, these patients may still expect to regain lost function and feel better by persevering and working harder even though better advice may be to slow down.

To overcome the combination of denial, a personal history of successful coping, and reluctance to try something new, the physician can help the patient modify old coping mechanisms that are familiar. For example, the physician may suggest having an old brace repaired after the patient's first visit rather than prescribing a new one. Beginning with a minor, acceptable intervention may prepare the patient to make major changes later. A patient who has been ambulatory for 35 years may reject buying a wheelchair but agree to use a cane or take advantage of a wheelchair in an airport. The wheelchair may become more acceptable, however, as the patient learns that although the cane is helpful, it is insufficient to relieve symptoms. Polio survivors may also reject anything that publicly advertises handicapped status. Changes that enable them to retain some sense of control, such as displaying a handicap placard on the dashboard when desired instead of getting license plates for the handicapped, may enhance compliance.

PROGNOSIS

The pathological processes involved in postpolio syndrome are benign, unless there is severe pulmonary involvement or a swallowing disorder. Dalakas et al.[9] found an average loss of strength of 1% per year in 27 persons followed for a mean of 8.2 years. This represents the rate of natural regression, since no one in the group studied was being treated to combat or modify the weakness. If weakness is partially due to overwork of the motor unit, combined with musculoskeletal overuse, then interventions designed to reduce the metabolic demand on the overworked motor unit could conceivably alter this rate of decline. Many clinicians have reported that patients who conscientiously adjust their lifestyles do improve, often increasing strength and stabilizing function. Other patients experience profound weakness and diminished functional capacity, and, as a result, they are vulnerable to social isolation as well as a greater risk of developing osteoporosis, fractures, contractures, depression, and other disabling conditions.

REFERENCES

1. Agre JC, Rodriguez AA. Neuromuscular function: comparison of symptomatic and asymptomatic polio subjects to control subjects. *Arch Phys Med Rehabil.* 1990;71:545–551.
2. Alba A, Block E, Adler JC, et al. Exercise testing as a useful tool in the physiatric management of the post-polio survivor. In: Halstead LS, Wiechers DO, eds. *Research and clinical aspects of the late effects of poliomyelitis.* White Plains, NY: March of Dimes Birth Defects Foundation; 1987:301–314.
3. Alcock AJW, et al. Respiratory poliomyelitis: a follow-up study. *Can Med Assoc J.* 1984;130:1305–1310.
4. Bach JR, Alba AS, Bodofsky E, et al. Glossopharyngeal breathing and non-invasive aids in the management of post polio respiratory insufficiency. In: Halstead LS, Wiechers DO, eds. *Research and clinical aspects of the late effects of poliomyelitis.* White Plains, NY: March of Dimes Birth Defects Foundation; 1987:99–114.
5. Bodian D. Motoneuron disease and recovery in experimental poliomyelitis. In: Halstead LS, Wiechers DO, eds. *Late effects of poliomyelitis.* Miami: Symposia Foundation; 1985:45–56.
6. Brown S, Patten BM. Post-polio syndrome and amyotrophic lateral sclerosis: a relationship more apparent than real. In: Halstead LS, Wiechers DO, eds. *Research and clinical aspects*

of the late effects of poliomyelitis. White Plains, NY: March of Dimes Birth Defects Foundation; 1987:83–98.

7. Dalakas MC. Amyotrophic lateral sclerosis and post-polio: differences and similarities. In: Halstead LS, Wiechers DO, eds. *Research and clinical aspects of the late effects of poliomyelitis.* White Plains, NY: March of Dimes Birth Defects Foundation; 1987:63–80.

8. Dalakas M. Post polio syndrome: clues from muscle and spinal cord studies. In: Munsat TL, ed. *Post polio syndrome.* Boston: Butterworth-Heinemann; 1990:39–65.

9. Dalakas MC, Elder G, Hallett M, et al. A long-term follow-up study of patients with post-poliomyelitis neuromuscular symptoms. *N Engl J Med.* 1986;314:959–963.

10. Dalakas MC, Sever JL, Fletcher M, et al. Neuromuscular symptoms in patients with old poliomyelitis: clinical, virological and immunological studies. In: Halstead LS, Wiechers DO, eds. *Late effects of poliomyelitis.* Miami: Symposia Foundation; 1985:73–90.

11. Feldman RM. The use of strengthening exercises in post-polio syndrome: methods and results. *Orthopedics.* 1985;8:889–890.

12. Fischer DA. Poliomyelitis: late respiratory complications and management. *Orthopedics.* 1985;88:891–894.

13. Frick NM. Demographic and psychological characteristics of the post-polio community. Paper presented at the First Annual Conference on the Late Effects of Poliomyelitis. Lansing, Michigan; October 1985.

14. Ginsberg GH, Gale MJ, Rose LM, Clark EA. T-cell alterations in late postpoliomyelitis. *Arch Neurol.* 1989;46:487–501.

15. Grimby G, Einarsson G. Muscle morphology with special reference to muscle strength in post-polio subjects. In: Halstead LS, Wiechers DO, eds. *Research and clinical aspects of the late effects of poliomyelitis.* White Plains, NY: March of Dimes Birth Defects Foundation; 1987:265–274.

16. Halstead LS, Rossi CD. New problems in old polio patients: results of a survey of 539 polio survivors. *Orthopedics.* 1985;8:845–850.

17. Halstead LS, Rossi DC. Post polio syndrome: clinical experience with 132 consecutive outpatients. In: Halstead LS, Wiechers DO, eds. *Research and clinical aspects of the late effects of poliomyelitis.* White Plains, NY: March of Dimes Birth Defects Foundation; 1987:13–26.

18. Halstead LS, Wiechers DO, Rossi CD. Late effects of poliomyelitis: a national survey. In: Halstead LS, Wiechers DO, eds. *Late effects of poliomyelitis.* Miami: Symposia Foundation; 1985:11–32.

19. Herbison GJ, Jaweed MM, Ditunno JF. Exercise therapies in peripheral neuropathies. *Arch Phys Med Rehabil.* 1983;64:201–205.

20. Maynard FM. Differential diagnosis of pain and weakness in post-polio patients. In: Halstead LS, Wiechers DO, eds. *Late effects of poliomyelitis.* Miami: Symposia Foundation; 1985:33–44.

21. National Health Survey. *Prevalence of selected impairments (series 10).* Washington, DC: US Department of Health and Human Services. (In press).

22. Perry J, Barnes G, Granley JK. Post polio muscle function. In: Halstead LS, Wiechers DO, eds. *Research and clinical aspects of the late effects of poliomyelitis.* White Plains, NY: March of Dimes Birth Defects Foundation; 1987:315–328.

23. Pezeshkpour GH, Dalakas MC. Pathology of spinal cord in postpoliomyelitis muscular atrophy. In: Halstead LS, Wiechers DO, eds. *Research and clinical aspects of the late effects of poliomyelitis.* White Plains, NY: March of Dimes Birth Defects Foundation; 1987:229–236.

24. Pierce-Ruhland R, Patten BM. Repeat study of antecedent events in motor neuron disease. *Ann Clin Res.* 1981;13:102–107.

25. Poskanzer DC, Cantor HM, Kaplan GS. The frequency of preceding poliomyelitis in amyotrophic lateral sclerosis. In: Norris FH Jr, Kurland LT, eds. *Motor neuron diseases: research on amyotrophic lateral sclerosis and related disorders.* New York: Grune & Stratton; 1969:286–290.

26. Rudman D, Feher AG, Nagras HS, et al. Effects of human growth hormone in men over sixty years old. *N Engl J Med.* 1990;323:1–6.

27. Smith LK. Current issues in neurological rehabilitation. In: Umphred DA, ed. *Neurological rehabilitation.* 2nd ed. St. Louis: CV Mosby; 1990:509–528.

28. Smith LK, McDermott K. Addressing causes versus treating effects. In: Halstead LS, Wiechers DO, eds. *Research and clinical aspects of the late effects of poliomyelitis.* White Plains, NY: March of Dimes Birth Defects Foundation; 1987:121–134.
29. Tomlinson BE, Irving D. The numbers of limb motor neurons in the human lumbosacral cord throughout life. *J Neurol Sci.* 1977;34:213–219.
30. Tomlinson BE, Irving D. Changes in spinal cord motor neurons of possible relevance to the late effects of poliomyelitis. In: Halstead LS, Wiechers DO, eds. *Late effects of poliomyelitis.* Miami: Symposia Foundation; 1985:57–72.
31. Wiechers DO, Hubbell SL. Late changes in the motor unit after acute poliomyelitis. *Muscle Nerve.* 1981;4:524–528.
32. Windebank AJ, Daube JR, Litchy WJ, et al. Late sequelae of paralytic poliomyelitis in Olmsted County, Minnesota. In: Halstead LS, Wiechers DO, eds. *Research and clinical aspects of the late effects of poliomyelitis.* White Plains, NY: March of Dimes Birth Defects Foundation; 1987:27–37.
33. Zilkha KJ. [Untitled discussion]. *Proc R Soc Med.* 1962;55:1028–1029.

Chapter 8

POSTPOLIO SYNDROME: CONTRACTURES, DECONDITIONING, AND AGING

Richard R. Owen

INTRODUCTION AND HISTORY

Many people who had acute poliomyelitis begin experiencing new problems 10 to 30 years later. The complex of symptoms and signs has been called postpolio syndrome. Some investigators differentiate a more fulminant course of the condition as postpolio progressive muscular atrophy. The manifestations related to the signs and symptoms consist of: 1) progressive weakness and/or atrophy, 2) easy fatigability and poor endurance, 3) severe pain, 4) reduced flexibility and mobility often associated with pain, 5) additional musculoskeletal disability, 6) breathing difficulty, 7) sleep disorders, and 8) new neurological disorder. I believe that the syndrome and its effects vary depending on the location of the anterior horn cell involvement, the initial extent of paralysis, and the margin of function and flexibility related to mobility and daily activities. Acute, sustained overuse can result in a sudden diminution of strength that may seriously disable an individual. A change in lifestyle and activities may result in loss of a skill from underuse or underchallenge.

Our studies in Minnesota found that 41% of people who had acute poliomyelitis in the major epidemic year from July 1952 through June 1953 were now having additional problems that would fit the diagnosis of postpolio syndrome.[13] In a self-reported condition such as this, statistics may be difficult to assess because of the gradual onset of symptoms and signs and the varying expectations of individuals. The age at onset and the degree of initial involvement add to the reporting problems.

A conference was held in Chicago in 1981 to define the nature, origins, and incidence of postpolio syndrome. Publicity from this and later conferences made some people aware of the possibility of and an explanation for new, and often disturbing, symptoms. Unfortunately, an insufficient amount of information has been made available to primary care physicians, neurologists, and orthopedists, leading to disappointment and confusion for many people with postpolio syndrome who seek medical advice. Numerous regional, national, and international conferences on this condition have been held, and research is being conducted at many centers. In addition, major course presentations on postpolio syndrome have been made at the American Congress of Rehabilitation Medicine meetings.

A variety of surveys and studies since the 1981 conference have indicated a prevalence of 25% to 80% in people with polio residuals. Several health care centers have established specialized clinics for research on the condition and management of the disabling factors, where possible.

A number of theories have been proposed to explain the origins of the postpolio syndrome. The origins are probably multiple and interacting. Among the proposed theories are the following: 1) premature aging of diseased nerve cells, 2) latent or lurking poliovirus that is reactivated in certain individuals, 3) failure of the compensatory nerve structure that had previously aided in recovery, 4) the loss of marginal muscle function by underuse or undertraining, 5) the overuse of weakened musculature owing to impaired monitoring of fatigue in polio-involved musculature, 6) inadequate oxygenation from ventilatory muscle weakness, 7) inadequate oxygenation from heart and lung deconditioning, 8) sleep disturbance (apnea) associated with bulbar or high spinal involvement, 9) intolerance to cold secondary to involvement of the nerve supply to blood vessels, 10) nerve transmission abnormality between nerve fiber and muscle fiber, 11) additional muscle shortening or contracture with deformity or mechanical disadvantage at joints, and 12) new neurological disease.[10]

This chapter will specifically address the issues of contractures, deconditioning, and aging as they relate to the new problems people with poliomyelitis are experiencing. Contractures from muscle shortening cause pain, deformity, and instability. The muscle shortening may be directly related to the acute poliomyelitis,[5] or it may be secondary to gravity, unopposed muscle contraction, or limb discrepancy. We have found that many of the patients coming to our clinic had a very low level of cardiopulmonary conditioning. Some had given up vigorous activity with changing lifestyles and responsibilities. Others were fearful of exercise based on experience or early reports of overuse damage to weakened muscles. Aging contributes to the adverse effects of contractures and deconditioning. Another dimension of aging involves the loss of motor neurons and perhaps a vulnerability to decay of the sprouted compensatory large motor units related to the early recovery from acute infection. Many of the electromyographic studies suggest that a process of denervation and reinnervation goes on constantly. There is the possibility that aging itself potentiates that process. We believe that deconditioning, hypoxygenation, and cold intolerance may also encourage the onset of weakness and muscle fatigue in the compensatory reinnervated units.

CONTRACTURES

Kenny reported her observations of pain and muscle spasm with muscle shortening as the predominant early expression of acute poliomyelitis.[12] Her treatment protocol addressed this issue with hot packs and early mobilization of the patient. She believed that the pain and shortening blocked muscle retraining in the agonist and antagonist muscle groups. The most common muscles involved were the neck and upper back extensors, the low back extensors, hamstrings, and calf muscles. Contractures occurred in the untreated tight muscles, leading to deformity, pain, and mechanical disadvantage for weakened musculature.

Anderson recently summarized the role of pain and tightness in postpolio syndrome.[1] He pointed out that tightening is commonly overlooked and yet represents the most frequent cause of pain and disability in patients entering a postpolio clinic. Tight hamstrings in the presence of weakened knee extension and ankle plantar flexion contribute to a shortened stride, mechanical stress on the back, and buckling of the knee.

Contractures commonly developed in extremities treated by immobilization for extended periods of time. The neutral position of the Toronto splint, once used for positioning during the acute and early convalescent stages of polio, was hip flexion, hip abduction, and knee flexion. Shortening of the iliotibial band and the Achilles tendon occurred in individuals who were kept flat and whose positioning received inadequate attention. Where there is leg length discrepancy, the calf musculature in the short limb is often contracted secondary to adaptation to function. The high arch of pes cavus is associated with contracture in the plantar fascia and shortening of the anterior tibial tendon. Pes cavus deformity causes pain and results in shoe and orthotic problems.

During ambulation, the shortened musculature is vulnerable to overstretch and injury. Destabilization of a joint limited by contracture is particularly noticeable in joints affected by two muscles. The rectus femoris and gastrocnemius are good examples of two joint muscles that affect knee stability. The person with a short rectus femoris may have discomfort and muscle injury at the end of the stance phase with extension of the hip, knee, and ankle. Equinus and cavus deformities of the feet are often quite painful and difficult to treat conservatively.

Treatment is determined by the patient's response to a stretching exercise program. Formal physical therapy using heat or hydrotherapy as a prelude to prolonged gentle stretching is required in those individuals who underwent little or no stretching at the time of their initial acute disease. Many individuals recall their self-managed programs once they are reinitiated. Neck and shoulder range-of-motion exercises often overcome tension and postural pain in those areas. Stretching of the back extensors may relieve back pain if carried out in conjunction with abdominal strengthening or support. Tight hip flexors and anterior thighs frequently cause lower extremity and back pain by stretching the shortened muscle and accentuating lumbar lordosis. Exercise to lengthen these muscles requires careful positioning to avoid further strain on the knee or back during stretch. Contractures of the hamstrings and calf muscles may present a problem in the absence of antagonists because of instability at the involved joints. Shortening and contracture that is attended by joint capsule tightness may require a surgical release. Tenotomy, capsulotomy, or subtalar fusion may be necessary in the case of foot and ankle deformity and pain. Stretching casts and orthoses are not usually tolerated well. An orthosis for function and position may be needed after a full range of motion is achieved, either through exercise or surgery.

DECONDITIONING AND UNDERTRAINING

General and local fatigue are characteristics of postpolio syndrome. In some individuals, the symptom of weakness probably stems from a weakening or localized fatigue in response to sustained repetitive activity. This condition may represent a myoneural junction abnormality associated with blockade of motor end plate stimuli in enlarged compensatory motor units. Underoxygenation and deconditioning may contribute to the blockade and weakening in polio-involved muscles.

We have demonstrated increased muscular endurance and an improved level of cardiopulmonary conditioning in response to an adapted cardiopulmonary conditioning program.[4] I believe that the fatigue experienced in involved extremities occurs in the muscles of ventilation as well. Therefore, hypoxygenation is compounded by poor ventilation and diminished cardiopulmonary conditioning. We found a poor cardiopulmonary conditioning status in most of our early postpolio clinic patients, with level of fitness comparable to cardiac rehabilitation patients after a recent myocardial infarction.[11] An adapted conditioning program was established to increase exercise tolerance while minimizing the risk of overuse and abuse of weakened musculature. An interval training protocol was used in which the subject would exercise three times a week for a period of 20 minutes broken up by rest periods of one to two minutes. A target pulse rate served as a guide to a successful conditioning challenge. Cardiopulmonary status, as measured by VO_2 max, increased 16% over the 13 weeks of the interval training program. Endurance of the quadriceps and hamstring musculature increased between 25% and 36% based on total work capacity in those muscles measured on a Cybex apparatus. A similar study has been completed using an arm ergometer. This adapted program was as successful as that which used a combined arm and leg ergometer.[9] The benefits of the exercise program carried over into daily activities and general endurance.

It is important to note that no one experienced new weakness in response to either protocol, and most experienced a sense of well being.

The benefits of conditioning in nondisabled subjects are well known. The work of Knowlton and colleagues[6,7] had raised concerns that exercise could be damaging to polio-involved musculature. However, our studies demonstrated that carefully structured exercise with attention to rest and the avoidance of fatigue can safely increase endurance and conditioning. We believe that flexibility and stretching exercises and a defined, adapted cardiopulmonary conditioning program can address many of the problems experienced by people who had poliomyelitis years earlier.

AGING

The impact of aging on all individuals has been defined and reviewed by Valbona and Baker,[15] who summarized the benefits of an active program of flexibility exercises and appropriate activities and conditioning. Some of the factors that accentuate disability suggest a premature aging of nerve and muscle tissue in the postpolio state. The possibility of a vulnerability to early decay of the large compensatory motor units has been suggested by Wiechers and Hubbell.[16] Tomlinson and Irving[14] found that about 1% of anterior horn cells were lost per year after age 60; however, this study did not include postpolio subjects. The electromyographic studies of postpolio subjects with and without "postpolio syndrome" are similar and suggest that the processes of denervation and reinnervation are going on in all subjects with polio-involved musculature.[2] Decreased activity, intercurrent health issues, bone and joint disease, underventilation, and a loss of marginal muscle function all would contribute to a sense of loss associated with aging, but at an earlier age than in nonpolio subjects. Reduced pulmonary excursion can occur in individuals who have not been fully expanding their chests with inspiration. This can result in a reduced pulmonary compliance and a vulnerability to respiratory insufficiency in the event of a superimposed infection or increased oxygen demand. Postexercise pulmonary function studies should be carried out to identify those who might be at risk for further breathing disability. Oximetry would be helpful for persons who experience severe generalized fatigue, since those who are hypopneic may respond to supplemental oxygen or ventilator assistance.

Kottke and Stillwell reported on the symptoms and signs associated with increased vasomotor tone in the lower extremities following anterior poliomyelitis.[8] Intolerance to cold with pain, cyanosis, swelling, cold skin, and new weakness is accentuated with aging. In our experience, it can also be related to nocturnal cramping. The additional weakness and discomfort can be quite disabling, even in rooms cooled by air conditioning. Individuals with upper extremity involvement may have difficulty carrying out their usual manual activities in a cold environment. Ambulation may be impaired further by loss of adequate contraction in the cold. Sprouted motor units are vulnerable to jitter and blockade of the motor end plates when the extremity is chilled. The physician should be aware of cold intolerance and advise the postpolio patient to guard against overcooling of the extremities to the extent possible.

SUMMARY

The postpolio syndrome presents a number of problems from the standpoints of research, diagnosis, and management. The disease itself is self-reported. The criteria are having had acute poliomyelitis and experiencing new symptoms of fatigue, weakness, pain, breathlessness, and disability. No satisfactory laboratory procedures exist to define the origin of the process or the intensity of its progression. Electromyographic studies are useful for identifying individuals who actually had poliomyelitis. Cephalophosphokinase studies have been positive in about 20% of the people reporting new problems. Many have contractures or muscle shortening that causes pain and instability at related joints. Many are sedentary, have changed their lifestyles, have gained weight, have abandoned intentional exercise, and have reduced the level of their incidental exercise. Most have not been involved in an active cardiopulmonary conditioning program. Ventilatory limitations have often imposed further restrictions on activity. Aging compounds the problems owing to the vulnerability to decay of the sprouted compensatory motor fibers, as well as natural aging of the spinal cord. Intolerance to cold is accentuated, adding pain, swelling, cyanosis, nocturnal cramps, and cold-induced weakness to the syndrome.

Stretching and flexibility exercises are critical physical hygiene measures for the management of pain, instability, and deformity. These exercises should also precede cardiopulmonary conditioning and other vigorous physical pursuits. An adapted cardiopulmonary conditioning program has been devised to safely provide improved cardiac status without the risk of damage to nerve and muscle from overuse. Harpuder defined the issues of training and fitness in rehabilitation in the Eighth Coulter Memorial Lecture.[3] The management of postpolio syndrome requires the application of traditional physical treatment principles, with specific attention given to the vulnerability of compensatory mechanisms to injury and the need to provide a balanced prescription of rest, activity, support, and judicious accommodation to additional disability.

REFERENCES

1. Anderson TP. The role of pain and tightness in residuals of polio. Lecture delivered at Postpolio International Conference, Jewish Heart and Lung Institute, Louisville, Kentucky, May 1990.

2. Cashman NR, Maselle R, Wollmann RL, Roos R, Simon R, Antel JP. Late denervation in patients with antecedent paralytic poliomyelitis. *N Engl J Med.* 1987;317:7–12.
3. Harpuder K. Training and fitness: concepts and problems in rehabilitation. *Arch Phys Med Rehabil.* 1958;39:751–755.
4. Jones DR, Speier J, Canine K, Owen R, Stull GA. Cardiorespiratory responses to adapted aerobic training by patients with poliomyelitis sequelae. *JAMA.* 1989;261:3255–3258.
5. Knapp ME. The Kenny treatment for infantile paralysis. *Arch Phys Ther.* 1942;23:668–673.
6. Knowlton GC, Bennett RL. Overwork. *Arch Phys Med Rehabil.* 1957;38:18–20.
7. Knowlton GC, Bennett RL, McClure R. Electromyography of fatigue. *Arch Phys Med.* 1951;32:648–652.
8. Kottke FJ, Stillwell GK. Studies on increased vasomotor tone in the lower extremities following anterior poliomyelitis. *Arch Phys Med.* 1951;32:401–407.
9. Kriz JL, Jones DR, Speier J, Canine K, Owen RR, Serfass RC. Cardiorespiratory response to upper extremity aerobic training in postpolio subjects. [In press].
10. Owen RR. Polio residuals clinic and exercise protocol: research implications. In: Halstead LS, Wiechers DO, eds. *Late effects of poliomyelitis.* Miami, Florida: Symposia Foundation; 1985.
11. Owen RR, Jones D. Polio residuals clinic: conditioning exercise program. *Orthopedics.* 1985;8:882–883.
12. Pohl JF, Kenny E. The Kenny concept of infantile paralysis and its treatment. Minneapolis: Bruce Publishing Co; 1943.
13. Speier JL, Owen RR, Knapp ME, Canine K. Occurrence of post polio sequelae in an epidemic population. In: Halstead LS, Wiechers DO, eds. *Research and clinical aspects of the late effects of poliomyelitis.* New York: March of Dimes Birth Defects Foundation; 1987.
14. Tomlinson BE, Irving D. The numbers of limb motor neurons in the human lumbosacral cord throughout life. *J Neurol Sci.* 1977;34:213–219.
15. Valbona C, Baker SB. Physical fitness prospects for the elderly. *Arch Phys Med Rehabil.* 1984;65:194–200.
16. Wiechers DO, Hubbell SL. Late changes in the motor unit after acute poliomyelitis. *Muscle Nerve.* 1981;4:524–528.

Chapter 9

PROGRESS IN THE CLINICAL USES OF EVOKED POTENTIALS

Livio Paolinelli Monti and Gladys del Peso D.

INTRODUCTION

Since the discoveries of Galvani in 1778, measurement of the potentials produced by cellular function has been a prevalent component of experimental studies and of their clinical applications in medicine.

The change in electrical activity in the nervous system in response to an external stimulus is called an "evoked potential." It can be caused in any part of the nervous system (sensory or motor, central or peripheral) as a response to a perceptible stimulus. Nevertheless, the term "evoked potential" is now usually used in reference to studies of recordings of average evoked potentials in the central nervous system.

Dr. Caton, a young assistant in physiology at the Royal School of Medicine, Liverpool, was the first to record electrical activity in the cerebral cortex produced by external stimuli. In his 1875 publication,[13] "The Electric Currents of the Brain," he reported that stimulating a cat's retina with light provoked variations in the currents in certain areas of the brain. He added in an 1877 paper[14] that examination of those currents, which were similar to those seen in peripheral nerves, allowed the functions of the cerebral hemispheres to be studied. Thus, the first evoked potential, which later would be called the visual evoked potential, was described.

Later, in 1913, Pravdich-Neminsky[72,73] reported obtaining in a dog's cortex the first evoked potential produced by stimulating the sciatic nerve. The recording of this response was mixed with an electroencephalogram tracing.

In 1933, Gasser and Grahams[33] recorded potentials in the dorsal region of the spinal medula of a cat for the first time by stimulating the afferent nerve fibers with submaximal threshold intensity.

George Dawson, of the University of London, in 1942 obtained the first somatosensory evoked potentials in man, resulting from tactile stimulation.[18] By 1951 a modification was introduced that would be the precursor of present-day techniques. Dawson stimulated the cubital nerve at the wrist and recorded the response in the cortex; to obtain the latency he employed a photographic superposition of the tracings and thus obtained the first "averaged latency" response. Using the same technique, Magladery and coworkers[58] obtained an intrathecal evoked potential in 1951, with a needle recording the response at level L3, by stimulating the peroneal nerve in normal subjects.

During the 1970s, electronics and computers provided great assistance in detecting evoked potentials, which are difficult to distinguish because of their low amplitude (1 to 5 microvolts) and because they become lost in background electronic noise and intermingled with the brain's spontaneous electrical activity. A high-speed operational averager was developed that accumulated responses to repeated stimuli (from 100 to 1,000 signals), eliminated the electronic noise and other spurious potentials, and provided an amplified evoked potential signal that was easy to read and reproduce. Using these devices, Baran in 1980[7] achieved a superficial recording at lumbar levels L2-L3 and thoracic levels T10-T11 by averaging about 1,600 stimuli. With similar signal techniques, numerous investigators—including Cracco,[17] Happel et al.,[43], Jones,[51] and Dimitrijevic et al.[21]—have used superficial electrodes to record spinal evoked potentials at the cervical, lumbar, and sacral levels.

The evoked potentials so far recorded and of greatest clinical use are those which provide us information from the visual sensory system (visual evoked potentials), auditory sensory system (auditory evoked potentials), and somatesthetic system (somatosensory evoked potentials). Transcranial stimulation of the brain has recently been introduced in the study of evoked potentials as a noninvasive method of examining cerebral motor function. This method consists of using two electrodes to stimulate a cortical motor area and recording the motor evoked potential (MEP), which travels through the pyramidal tract, to the corresponding muscle. Responses obtained as evoked potentials have short (from 1 to 100 milliseconds) and long (from 100 to 500 milliseconds) latencies. The short latencies are most often studied.

In general, evoked potential curves have positive (P) and negative (N) peaks. By international agreement, the peaks below the isoelectric line of the recording are called P and those above it are called N. To define each P and N peak, a number is added to it (e.g., N9, N15, P100) which represents the normal average value in milliseconds of the latency for that peak.

EQUIPMENT

Most electromyographs can be used to study visual, auditory, and somatosensory evoked potentials if they have an averager that can record and separate the evoked responses from all the waves generated around them. The averager improves the signal-to-noise ratio in proportion to the square root of the number of averaged signals. For example, if 100 signals are used, the average amplitude of the electronic noise is reduced by a factor of 10.

Generally speaking, at least 200 signals are needed to distinguish the evoked potentials, but it must be borne in mind that if many signals are averaged the "jitter" factor of each separate signal comes into play; this factor relates to the fact that the peak of the curve is displaced a few microseconds between one signal and another. At least two averagings must be obtained to confirm the reproduction of the responses.

The equipment must have sweep speeds ranging from 1 to 500 milliseconds to be able to record all evoked potentials—both short- and long-latency. The sensitivity used is customarily 20 microvolts/division, but it may be 5 or 50 microvolts or even 100 microvolts if the patient is very restless and electromyographic noise and segmental (hand, foot, eye) movements cannot be eliminated. Equipment may have analog or digital filters. For low frequencies, 10 to 20 cycles/second is used, and for high frequencies, 2,000 to 3,000 cycles/second.

The stimuli for peripheral nerves are pulses of current lasting 0.1 and 0.2 milliseconds. Their frequencies are from 2 to 5 cycles/second, the latter being the most common (in use in our laboratory). With a pulse of 0.1 milliseconds, the intensity needed to obtain a response is from 10 to 15 milliamperes, or from 80 to 120 volts. For visual stimuli, a flash or the reverse checkerboard pattern may be used. The latter is most used because its responses present less variation in latency, amplitude, and wave form than those obtained with a flash in the same subject. For auditory stimuli, short clicks of from 50 to 100 microseconds are used. They are produced by electromechanical transducers introduced directly into the ear or are transmitted through headphones.

STIMULATION, RECORDING, AND GENERATION

Somatesthetic Evoked Potentials

Stimulation

Conventionally, sensory and motor nerve conduction studies have enabled us to evaluate the peripheral nervous system. The advent of somatesthetic evoked potentials (SEPs) has given us an opportunity to explore the afferent conduction of sensory nerves at both the peripheral and central levels.

Electrical stimulation can be done either from pure sensory cutaneous fibers or from mixed nerves containing both afferent cutaneous and muscular fibers. Stimulation of sensory cutaneous fibers does not present great technical difficulty and the response is similar to that obtained with the mixed nerve (currently the most used). However, the amplitude of the response is smaller, and averaging requires two to five times as many responses as when a mixed nerve is stimulated. Even though they are similar in form and amplitude, the latencies of the maximal negative and positive peaks of the responses obtained when sensory cutaneous nerves are stimulated are from 2 to 5 milliseconds longer. It is important for every laboratory to establish its own normal parameters according to the technique used.

In the upper limbs the nerves most often stimulated are the median, ulnar, radial, and musculocutaneous (Figure 1, Table 1). To selectively explore spinal segmental sensory disturbances (radiculopathies, myelopathies), specific segmental stimulation may be added, for example, the thumb (C6), middle finger (C7), and little finger (C8).

In the lower extremities, the peroneal (L5-S1), posterior tibial (L5-S1), internal saphenous (L4), and sural (S1) nerves are customarily stimulated (Figure 2, Table 2). High lumbar (L1 to L3) and dorsal exploration is done through spinal segmental stimulation.

Recording and Generation

The most common technical problem with SEPs is that muscular electrical activity contaminates responses. It is essential that the subject be in a supine position, fully relaxed, and in a comfortable environment.

Two kinds of electrodes may be used for recording: gold-plated surface electrodes 1 cm in diameter and monopolar needles with or without a Teflon coating. Both the recording and ground electrodes should have an impedance of less than 5,000 ohms.

Stimulating any of the nerves chosen for exploration provokes a response that can be detected at any point, from the most peripheral (e.g., the forearm, elbow, arm, and plexus) to the central area (spinal and cortical).

Upper Extremities.   The most used recording sites are the brachial plexus (at Erb's point), spinal at CVII, CV, or CII, and cortical C3' or C4' (10–20 EEG system), depending on the side stimulated.

Many anatomic sites for placing the reference electrode have been described in the literature; depending on the placement, they are called cephalic or noncephalic. The cephalic site is the Fz point (10–20 EEG system), and the noncephalic ones are the shoulder (Sh or Sc), knee (Kn), clavicle (CC or Erb), ear (Ea or A), hand (h), and iliac crest (IC) (Figures 3a and 3b).

The choice of the reference electrode site is important because the polarity of the peaks of the waves recorded changes according to the reference site used. For example, peak N9, which is recorded at Erb's point, becomes P9 when a noncephalic reference is used. The most used reference point today is the cephalic site (Fz), since it decreases the muscular contamination of the response (used in our laboratory.)

Brachial plexus recording: A biphasic response is obtained with the Erb-Fz recording technique, with a first peak of maximum negative amplitude called N9 because the average normal latency from the stimulation site at

Figure 1. Stimulation sites on upper extremities.

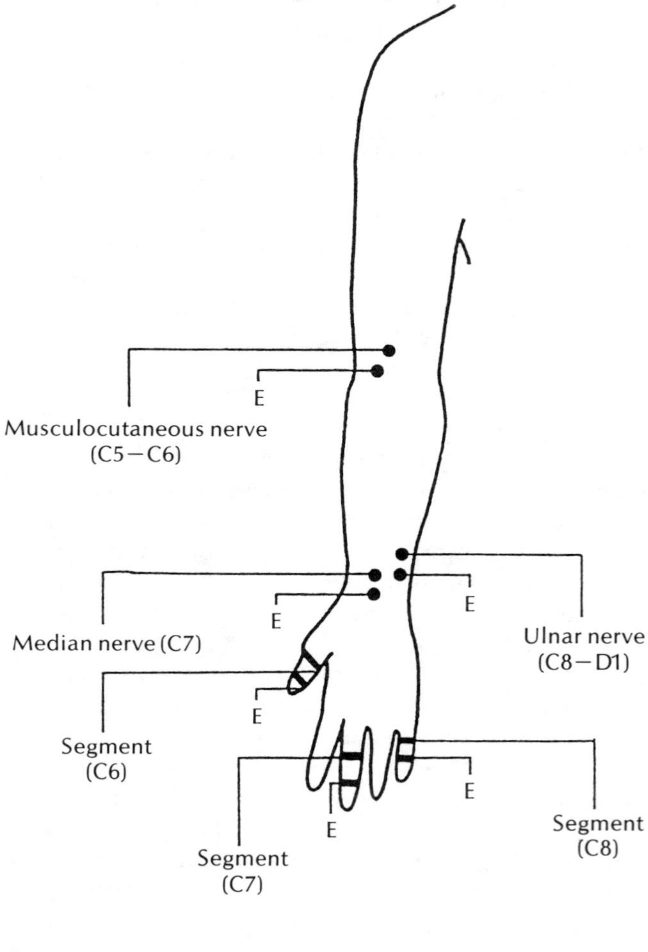

Table 1. Nerve stimulation of upper limbs.

Nerve	Stimulation site	Intensity
Median	Wrist (mixed trunk)	Minimal threshold with minimal contraction of thenar eminence
Ulnar	Wrist (mixed trunk)	Minimal threshold with minimal contraction of hypothenar eminence
Radial	Wrist (sensory trunk)	Minimal threshold, nonpainful
Musculocutaneous	Elbow crease (sensory trunk)	Minimal threshold, nonpainful

Figure 2. Stimulation sites on lower extremities.

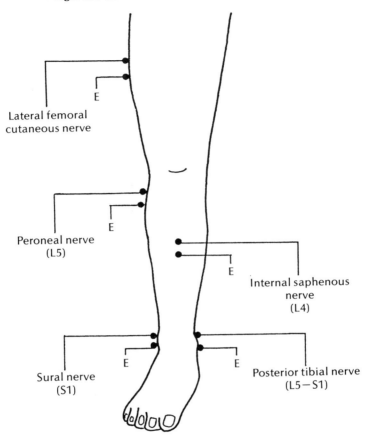

Table 2. Nerve stimulation of lower limbs.

Nerve	Stimulation site	Intensity
Peroneal	Popliteal space (mixed trunk)	Minimal threshold with minimal contraction of lateral peroneal
Posterior tibial	Medial malleolus (mixed trunk)	Minimal threshold with minimal contraction of peroneus brevis
Internal saphenous	1/3 up inner leg (skin)	Minimal threshold, nonpainful
Sural	Lateral malleolus (skin)	Minimal threshold, nonpainful

Figure 3a. Placement of recording electrodes for stimulation of the median nerve.

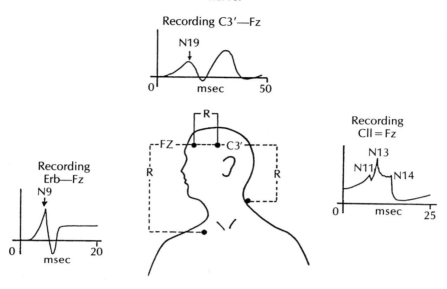

Figure 3b. Placement and identification of recording electrodes on the head.

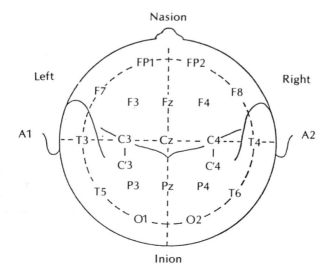

the wrist to Erb's point is 9 milliseconds (median, ulnar, and radial nerves). For the musculocutaneous nerve, the peak for Erb's point has an average latency of 7 milliseconds (N7), since the stimulation site is at the elbow and the stimulus-response distance is thus less.

As for its origin, N9 represents the afferent sensory conductive volume in its course through the distal brachial plexus. This fact has been corroborated in numerous clinical studies, since the response persists when there are high lesions of the brachial plexus with root avulsion.

Spinal recording: With CVII-Fz, CV-Fz, or CII-Fz recording, a response with a maximum negative slope and three recognizable peaks is obtained: N11, N13, and N14; N13 is the peak of maximum amplitude. It is assumed that the N11 peak is generated presynaptically from the entry zone of the dorsal root; it has also been suggested that its origin is the dorsal root or the dorsal column. The N13 peak is thought to be generated postsynaptically in the dorsal spinal column or in the dorsal columns at a high, median cervical, or foramen magnum level. Its origin in the cuneate nucleus has also been suggested. The N14 peak is rarely detected with the Fz reference. With the reference at the ear and cortical recording, this peak becomes P14 and its origin seems to be caudal to the thalamus at the pontine level and related to the leminiscal generator located over the decussation of the so-matesthetic path. Other origins given for P14 are the cervicomedullary junction and the cuneate nucleus.

Cortical recording: This recording is made at points C3' and C4' (EEG 10–20 system), whether the right or left upper extremity is stimulated (C3' is 2 cm behind C3). With the Fz cephalic reference, there are two consistent negative peaks, N19 (N20) and N30 (N32). N19 appears to originate in the ventrolateral nuclei of the thalamus. Other authors suggest that it originates in the thalamocortical or cortical structures. N30 (N32) probably represents the response of the sensory cortex.

Peaks with longer latencies, such as P40, N60, N150, P250, and N350, can also be observed in the cortical response. Peaks N40 and N60 depend on the subject's level of consciousness and cognitive functions; they are affected by sleep, which causes prolongation of their latency and diminution in amplitude. Double stimulation, ipsilateral and contralateral, for each hemisphere is customarily used to obtain these responses. The latest peaks (N150, P250, and N350) appear to be related to nonspecific projections of the thalamocortical system. These latencies have been the object of few studies, but they seem to be related to adaptation, habituation, and attention to the stimulus.

Lower Extremities. *Spinal recording*: The most used spinal recording sites are spaces L4-L5, D12-L1, and CVI-CVII (Figure 4). The reference used for dorsolumbar spinal recordings is the iliac crest (IC), since a bipolar recording (e.g., L1-T10) tends to cancel responses. The reference used with CVII

Figure 4. Placement of recording electrodes for stimulation of the peroneal nerve.

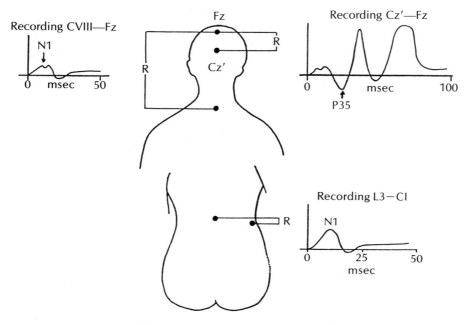

Recording CVIII—Fz

N1

0   msec   50

Fz

R

Cz'

R

Recording Cz'—Fz

0   msec   100

P35

R

Recording L3—Cl

N1

0   25   50
msec

recording is Fz. In thoracodorsal spinal recordings, responses decrease significantly in amplitude.

The spinal response with IC reference has a triphasic form with an initial positive peak of low amplitude followed by a negative peak of maximum amplitude (N1). If the recording is made ventrally, the response reverses polarity and peak N1 becomes P1. This response probably represents postsynaptic activity of the gray matter of the lumbar medulla as a response to the impulses coming from the collateral axons. The response is most recognizable between levels L4 and T9, and the latencies do not vary much among these levels. The greatest amplitude of the response is achieved with T12 and T10 recordings, which indicates that the medullary cone ends between L1 and L2. For the sural and posterior tibial nerves, which are stimulated at the lateral and medial malleolus, respectively, peak N1 has an average normal latency of 22 milliseconds (N22), while for the peroneal and saphenous nerves its latency is 10 milliseconds (N10), since the stimulus-response distance is shorter.

At level CII with reference IC, the N1 peak has an average latency of N29; the response is of very low amplitude and has a long refractory period. Seyal and coworkers[85] suggested that this response reflects the postsynaptic activity of the nucleus gracilis. For purposes of measuring isolated spinal conduction, recordings from D12 and CVII (with reference IC) are commonly used. The conduction time obtained should exclude radicular participation (cauda equina).

More peripheral recordings can be made by stimulating the lower extremities at the popliteal space and in the gluteal region. When the posterior tibial nerve is stimulated, the response obtained is biphasic with an initial negative peak (N1). This response represents the peripheral presynaptic afferent sensory conductive volume.

Cortical recording: The central cortical point Cz (10–20 system) is that which represents the lower extremities in the cerebral homunculi. It is used in active recording of all responses coming from stimuli applied to the lower limbs and the trunk. The most used reference is Fz, but to obtain shorter subcortical components a noncephalic reference (shoulder or lower cervical area) is used. With noncephalic recording and by stimulating the posterior tibial nerve, a response is obtained with an initial positive deflection (P31), followed by a negative phase of very low amplitude (N34) and a positive phase of greater amplitude (P38, P40).

Eisen and Elleker[26] posit that the P31 response may be generated by the afferents caudal to the medial lemniscus. Peak N34 probably reflects subcortical postsynaptic activity in the trunk and/or thalamus. Peak P38 (P40) is probably the primary cortical response, reflecting the localization of the leg in the mesial apex of the postcentral gyrus inside the interhemispheric fissure.

With cephalic reference Fz, the first positive phase of the response (P31) is usually cancelled and the negative phase N34 diminishes in amplitude. The response obtained with the Cz-Fz recording is W-shaped. The positive peak of greatest amplitude, usually called P1, is important; for the posterior tibial nerve it becomes P40, for the sural nerve, P42, and for the peroneal and internal saphenous nerves, P35. These latencies are the best known and most commonly used as reference in clinical studies. Peak P1 is proposed to be generated by one of various structures: as a response of the primary cortex (postcentral gyrus), or as thalamocortical projections. Subsequent peaks N2 P2 are responses generated in the cortical structures.

Factors Influencing SEP Parameters

In 1983, Allison and coworkers[1] studied 130 males and 156 females aged 4 to 95 years to correlate age, weight, and height with SEP characteristics. They analyzed the latencies of cortical and spinal SEPs obtained by stimulating the median nerve. In relation to these three factors, they concluded that in children latencies increase with age together with height and the corresponding increase in the length of the afferent pathway. Height and latencies reach an asymptote around 17 years. There is no significant difference in latencies between the sexes. In adults latencies in males are significantly longer than in females. There is no significant difference between the sexes in peaks. Interpeak distances increase with age except for interpeak N19-N13, which keeps getting shorter in children until reaching its normal length at 17 years. Latencies in the right median nerve were longer than those in the left one in both adults and children.

E. González and coworkers[37] considered that height is a statistically significant factor affecting normal parameters of short latencies and developed a formula that correlated a patient's height with the expected normal latency (Table 3). They performed their study only in the lower extremities, where they thought this factor was most critical. The study was conducted in 33 normal subjects.

A 1989 study by Verroust and coworkers[102] presents an analysis of normal values for the posterior tibial nerve and concludes that age does not have a significant effect on latencies, but that the effect of height is statistically significant for the normal values of latencies, which corroborates González's findings. Verroust et al. developed a regression formula that relates age and height to the predicted latency.

Central Conduction Time

Interpeaks between both spinal and cortical responses are an important factor to look at in SEP studies. The most significant interpeak is between latencies N13 (cuneate nucleus) and N19 (ventrolateral nucleus of the thalamus), which was defined in 1978 by Hume and Cant[47] as "central conduction time." Its average value for nerves in the upper extremities (median, ulnar, and radial) is 5.5 milliseconds. This value remains constant from 10 to 49 years of age, but increases approximately 0.3 milliseconds between the sixth and seventh decades. It is thought that this increase in central conduction time results from slowing of the synapses in the cortex. Central conduction time is independent of height and the distance between nasion and inion.

Clinical Applications of Central Conduction Time. The first successful clinical application of central conduction time was in detecting demyelinating plaques in asymptomatic patients with multiple sclerosis, as demonstrated by Mastaglia and coworkers[59] and later confirmed by other investigators.[4,23,91] Currently, the most frequent applications are (1) early diagnosis of multiple sclerosis, (2) detection of lesions in occult structures, (3) prognosis of coma and central nervous system trauma, and (4) intraoperative monitoring to prevent neurologic complications during surgery.

Because of the different recording levels used by different investigators, calculations of spinal conduction time for the lower extremities vary also.[26,92] Eisen and Elleker[26] obtained a spinal conduction time from the posterior tibial nerve of about 18 milliseconds by measuring the time be-

Table 3. Deviation of latency of P1 from expected normal, in milliseconds, in relation to subject's height from a study by González et al.[37]

Nerve	Expected P1 (Ht = height)	Deviation
Peroneal	P1 = Ht x 0.269	−7.12
Posterior tibial	P1 = Ht x 0.30	−13.3
Sural	P1 = Ht x 0.344	−16.7
Internal saphenous	P1 = Ht x 0.299	+3.18

tween peak N19 in thoracolumbar recording and P40 in cortical recording. If the distance between the recording made at L1 and CII is measured, the spinal conduction velocity can be calculated. Using this method, they calculated a velocity of 59.9 ± 5.7 meters/second for this segment.

In 1984, S. Rapaport[74] made a study of spinal conduction velocity by peroneal nerve stimulation in 35 normal subjects. He used bipolar recordings in spaces D12-L1 and L4-L5 distally and in CII-Fz and CV-Fz proximally. Conduction velocity was calculated by dividing the distance between the recording points by the difference in times between the initial peaks of both responses. Normal values ranged from 49.5 to 86.2 meters/second ($\bar{x}$ = 69.0), with a difference between sides of 5.3 (SD = 4.4 meters/second). The conduction velocity varied significantly with age, sex, and height. This method allows conduction velocity to be compared between the right and left posterior dorsal columns. It can also aid in detecting more rostral demyelinating lesions in the spinal afferent pathway.

The most important diagnostic applications of spinal conduction without intracranial participation are: (1) compressive, demyelinating, traumatic, and/or degenerative myelopathic disturbances; and (2) peripheral disturbances involving the nerve roots (radicular traumatic and compressive lesions, cauda equina and medullary cone syndromes) and Guillain-Barré syndrome and certain axonal neuropathies that compromise long spinal pathways (uremic, toxic, hereditary, demyelinating polyneuropathies).

Visual Evoked Potentials

Visual evoked potentials (VEPs) result from the change in cerebral activity following intermittent light stimuli. The nature of the VEP depends on many parameters: light intensity, level of contrast, type of light stimulus (screen or flash), stimulus size and model, and method and speed of presentation. The reverse checkerboard screen is the most used stimulus because it evokes the longest potentials.

VEPs can be recorded with two electrodes, one placed in the occipital zone (Oz) with reference at the vertex Cz (10–20 system) and the ground placed at Fz. Oz is located 1 to 2 cm above the inion. Another recording used is O1-O2 (10–20 system). The Oz monopolar recording is used preferentially with a reference electrode at the ear, mastoid, or middle frontal region (Figure 5). A triphasic curve is obtained with recording Cz-Oz, with an initial negative wave of very small amplitude, a second positive peak of large amplitude (P100), and a third long negative phase of small amplitude. This response appears 100 milliseconds after the stimulus when the reverse checkerboard model is used and is of greater amplitude when it is recorded at middle point Oz. Normal latency ranges are between 95 and 110 milliseconds.

It is believed that P100 is generated in the striate and peristriate occipital cortex as a result of activation of both primary and, subsequently, thalamocortical pathways. Positron emission tomography of human cerebral metabolism reveals that the reverse checkerboard stimulus activates both primary and association areas of the visual cortex.

Auditory Evoked Potentials

Auditory evoked potentials (AEPs) are sensitive to anatomic changes in the auditory pathway, especially those caused by disruption of the myelin. They are influenced by temperature, but they are little affected by level of consciousness, drugs, or metabolic imbalances. These properties allow the use of AEPs to evaluate many lesions of the posterior fossa. The usual recording site is the vertex (Cz), with a reference electrode on the ear lobe (A) or mastoids (ipsilateral to the stimulus).

The early components (short latencies) composing the AEP are seven waves designated with Roman numerals I to VII (Figure 6). Waves I to V

Figure 5. Placement of recording electrode for visual evoked potentials.

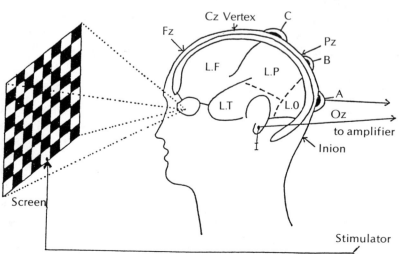

Figure 6. Short latency peaks recorded along the pathway of auditory evoked potentials.

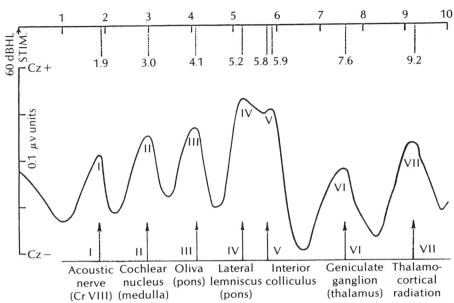

Interpretation of the originating structures of
human auditory evoked potentials

Wave	Proposed origin
I	Distal 8th pair (nerve). Summation of cochlear potentials?
I-II	8th pair and internal auditory meatus.
II	Proximal 8th pair and cochlear activity.
II-III	8th pair (Nz) and internal auditory meatus.
III	Activity of the superior oliva complex. Cochlear nucleus to exit?
IV	Ascending sensory fibers rostral and dorsal in the protuberance.
V	Activity in the area of the inferior colliculus. Activity at the exit of the medial geniculate nucleus.
VI	Activity at the exit of the medial geniculate nucleus. Activity of the inferior colliculus area?
VII	Activity of the distal auditory radiations? Activity of the inferior colliculus area?

correspond to the sequential activation of peripheral, medullary pons, pontine, and mesencephalon pathways. The origin of waves VI and VII is less certain. All these peaks are seen within the 10 milliseconds following the auditory stimulus. This stimulus should have an intensity above the patient's threshold. The threshold of each ear is customarily measured separately, and then stimulation is given monaurally 60 to 70 decibels higher. The most used stimulation frequency is around 10 clicks per second. Normal interpeak latencies of AEPs are: I-V, less than 4.59 milliseconds; I-III, less than 2.63 milliseconds; and III-IV, less than 2.31 milliseconds. The difference in interpeak latencies between the ears should be less than 0.5 milliseconds.

Peaks I to V are the most constant on Cz-A1 or A2 recording. Peaks VI and VII may not appear with this recording in some normal subjects; recordings at the cerebral median line are suggested in such cases.

CLINICAL APPLICATIONS OF EVOKED POTENTIALS

Evoked potentials are of great importance to the physical medicine and rehabilitation specialist as an aid in diagnosis and particularly prognosis of both acute and chronic disabling processes.

Somatosensory Evoked Potentials in Peripheral Lesions

Plexopathies

Although it is possible to use SEPs to show distal peripheral axonal lesions after stimulating an upper or lower extremity nerve, it is easier to use the classical method of measuring the antidromic segmentary sensory conduction speed at the wrist, elbow, and axilla for upper extremities and at the ankle, popliteal space, and gluteus for lower extremities. These responses are usually free from muscular contamination, which is not the case if an attempt is made to record these responses superficially along the nerve by SEP techniques. Only when such conventional methods cannot be performed should SEP be used to verify the most peripheral axonal continuity after a trauma to a nerve trunk.

In contrast, at the level of the brachial plexus, given the difficulty of measuring the trajectory of the nerve between axilla and plexus, recording the SEP at Erb's point is quite useful since it provides precise information about brachial plexopathies. In recent traumas of the plexus, comparative serial study of the Erb's response (N9) during the first 10 days allows the topographic extent of the lesion and the degree of compromise of each nerve to be determined and a prognosis to be established. If the N9-N13 interpeak is also studied, the more proximal compromise of some of the cervical roots, including their avulsion, can be shown.[51]

Thoracic outlet syndrome is one of the pathologies in which an SEP study at the level of Erb's point and cervical spine CVII can pinpoint the dynamic sensory neuropathic compromise, which preferentially affects the inferior primary trunk of the brachial plexus (C8-T1). This syndrome is secondary to transient vascular compression at Erb's point, which is produced by different anatomic structures: anterior scalene muscle, cervical rib, or pectoralis minor. Glover and coworkers[36] in 1981 were the first to suggest that

SEP changes in the supraclavicular fossa (Erb's point) could reflect the neuropathic lesion of thoracic outlet syndrome.

In 1984, Chodoroff and coworkers[16] performed a functional study of sensory evoked potentials at the brachial plexus (N9) and at spinal level CVII (N13) in patients with thoracic outlet syndrome. While stimulating the ulnar and median nerves, they recorded the two responses in two positions: (1) supine with arm at side and (2) supine with arm abducted 90° and rotated externally. The absolute latencies of N9 and N13 as well as the N9-N13 interpeak were measured in the 14 patients in whom thoracic outlet syndrome was suspected based on clinical findings. Six patients showed disappearance of spinal response N13 in the dynamic position; this response was normal in the resting position. Significant variations were not found in any of the cases at the Erb's point level (N9).

Our laboratory has used this technique with positive results since its appearance. We have introduced a change in the method of recording at Erb's point by using Teflon monopolar needles to preclude the displacement that superficial electrodes undergo when Adson's maneuver is applied.

A variation of less than a millisecond between the values obtained for N13 in the normal versus the Adson position may be considered in the normal range.

Radiculopathies in Upper Extremities

Spinal recording (N13) and selective nerve stimulation allows exploration of the sensory component of a root when compromise is suspected clinically. Although this stimulation explores two to three radicular segments simultaneously, electrophysiologic evaluation is important, especially in traumatic compromises.

In practice and according to our experience, there are roots that predominate in their conduction of nerve fibers from the peripheral nerve:

Median nerve	Preferentially	Rootlet:	C7
Ulnar nerve	Preferentially		C8
Radial nerve	Preferentially		C7
Musculocutaneous nerve	Components		C5–C6

In the musculocutaneous nerve the peak N13 corresponds to N10 since the stimulus-recording distance (elbow-spinal CV) is less than when the median, ulnar, or radial nerve (wrist-spinal CVII) is stimulated.

In cervical radiculopathies, spinal segmental stimulation will clearly provide more objective information about the compromise. A comparative study has now been implemented in our laboratory to correlate stimulation of nerve trunks and spinal segments with radiologic and clinical findings. In rehabilitation, such studies permit both diagnosis and monitoring of patients with these pathologies, which are often difficult to pinpoint, especially in disabling cases.

As for cases in which such compromises exceed peripheral participation, El Negamy and Sedgwick[29] in 1979 published a study of SEPs in the median nerve with recordings in the brachial (N9) and spinal (N13) plexus in 14 patients with cervical spondylosis and radiculopathy. The results were as follows: four patients had SEP with normal N11 and N13 spinal latencies; five patients had prolongation of the N11 and N13 latencies; five did not present recognizable responses at the spinal level; and all the patients had normal N9 (plexus) latencies. Since the postulated origin of peak N11 is spinal, it would be the first to be altered in compromises involving the dorsal roots, and changes in N13 would show participation of the fibers in the ascending dorsal columns; thus, the latter's compromise would be logical when a myelopathic disturbance presents conductive slowing. The authors posit that the increase in this N9-N11 or N9-N13 interpeak is the most important SEP finding for differentiating a cervical compromise with myelopathic participation from demyelinating pathologies that also affect the SEPs in intramedullary conduction. Rubio Esteban and coworkers[79] recently found similar changes in 30 patients with cervical spondylosis.

In patients who presented doubtful pyramidal compromise based on clinical signs and only slight radiologic alterations, Iwasaki and coworkers[49] performed a dynamic myelography study during extension and flexion. During flexion, myelography showed a marked narrowing of the spinal canal between C4 and C7, as though the canal were pinched between the posterior margin of the vertebrae and the posterior portion of the dura mater. In light of these radiologic findings, we thought it very important to develop a new dynamic method of electrophysiologic evaluation in our laboratory through SEPs recorded during flexion of the neck in patients with radiologic signs of spondylosis or spondyloarthrosis and cases of posttraumatic column instability, many of whom presented clinically doubtful signs of myelopathic compromise.

In 1989 we presented the experience of 11 patients, of whom 6 had severe spondyloarthrosis (four with spinal stenosis), three had posttraumatic instability of the cervical column, and two had listhesis in C4-C5 and C5-C6. All the patients had undergone computed tomography and/or myelography. Only five of these patients presented clinical pyramidal signs.

The study of SEPs in the normal position showed a prolonged N13 or N10 short latency in nine of these patients. When the neck was flexed, the latencies were significantly prolonged or, in some cases, were totally blocked. In the two remaining patients, the spinal response was normal in the resting position, but it was significantly prolonged during flexion, with frank diminution of the amplitude of the response. Six of these patients reverted to normal after surgery (cervical arthrodesis), demonstrating the extent of regression of the spinomedullary compromise.

We believe that this dynamic method of studying cervical SEPs, developed in our laboratory, illuminates the physiology of the dynamic peripheral compromise of the root (foramen and interapophyseal articulations) and at the medullary level (spinostenosis due to spondylotic bars, listhesis, post-traumatic columnar instability), where it reveals the medullary deficit during postural changes of the cervical column. In cases of clinically doubtful compromise this noninvasive method can help clarify the patient's symptomatology, which aids the treating physician in selecting the appropriate radiologic studies and, subsequently, surgical intervention.

Lower Extremity Radiculopathies

Cassvan,[12] in 1981, was one of the first authors to study the correlation between the distortion of the short latency (P35) of the peroneal nerve SEP and radicular compression of the fifth lumbar root. He found that all patients with nucleus pulposis protrusion at L4-L5 had significant prolongation, even to the point of abolition, depending on the extent of the lesion. He established a latency of 37 milliseconds as a normal limiting value. In 50 patients in whom other laboratory studies showed L5 radiculopathy, he found an average latency of 40 milliseconds in the affected side, with considerable diminution in the amplitude. On the basis of this study, we added the cortical SEP from the peroneal nerve to the fifth lumbar root to our routine electrodiagnostic exploration in radiculopathies (EMG, H reflex, F wave). In 1983 we studied 58 patients aged 25 to 65 years who had lumbo-sciatic syndrome. Five patients had no changes; of the 53 remaining patients, 33 showed fifth lumbar root compromise and 20 showed compromise of the first sacral root. The 33 patients with compromise of the fifth lumbar root had altered Cz-Fz (P35) cortical SEPs; 19 had a P35 prolonged beyond 37 milliseconds, and in the other 14 a P35 short latency was absent (Figure 7). These findings were not related to how long the clinical picture had persisted but only to its intensity.

Of the 53 patients studied, 13 underwent surgery, which corroborated the level of the lesion as determined by the SEP. In three of them, intraoperative monitoring of the cortical SEP of the peroneal nerve was performed during diskectomy of the fourth lumbar disk. During surgery there was a complete blockage of the Cz-Fz cortical response. A serial study during the first 10 postoperative days showed that some of the phases of the cortical response appeared between 48 and 72 hours in two patients. Gradual improvement followed, until on the tenth day there was 80% recovery of SEP amplitude, with a normal P35 short latency (Figure 8).

A third patient who was monitored postoperatively continued to have an altered Cz-Fz cortical response, and some preoperative clinical signs and symptoms became accentuated during the next month. He underwent surgery again and a periradicular fibrosis was found. We believe that SEP study

Figure 7. Prolongation or absence of Cz-Fz (P35) cortical sensory evoked potential resulting from compromise of the fifth lumbar nerve root.

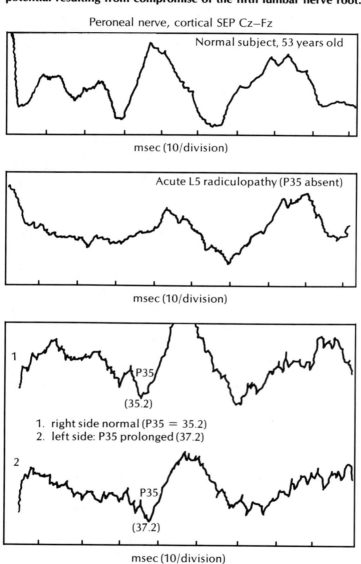

Peroneal nerve, cortical SEP Cz–Fz

Normal subject, 53 years old

msec (10/division)

Acute L5 radiculopathy (P35 absent)

msec (10/division)

1

P35
(35.2)

1. right side normal (P35 = 35.2)
2. left side: P35 prolonged (37.2)

2

P35
(37.2)

msec (10/division)

Figure 8. Serial recordings of the cortical sensory evoked potential response to peroneal nerve stimulation, from complete blockage of Cz-Fz response during surgery (L4 disk protrusion removed) to recovery of normal P35 on the seventh postoperative day.

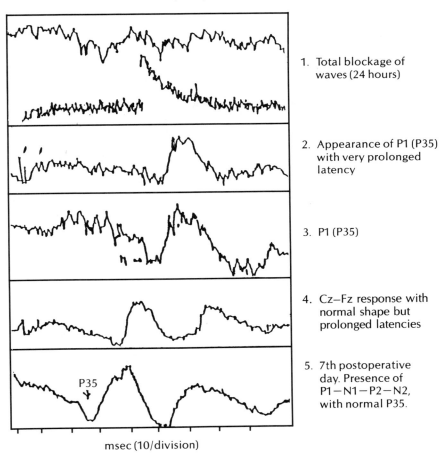

1. Total blockage of waves (24 hours)

2. Appearance of P1 (P35) with very prolonged latency

3. P1 (P35)

4. Cz–Fz response with normal shape but prolonged latencies

5. 7th postoperative day. Presence of P1 – N1 – P2 – N2, with normal P35.

msec (10/division)

in lumbar radiculopathies is an excellent noninvasive aid in quantifying and localizing the level of the compromised root from the inception of the lesion, and additionally provides a method for identifying postoperative sequelae.

A serial study from the start of a clinical picture of L5 radiculitis shows a direct relationship with the extent of compression this root undergoes. Gradual alteration of the SEP may follow this sequence:

1. P35 with normal latency bilaterally and only diminution in amplitude on the compromised side.

2. P35 latency prolonged beyond 37 milliseconds or with a difference greater than 2 milliseconds between the compromised side and the normal, healthy side.

3. P35 absent on the compromised side and within normal limits on the healthy side.

4. P35 latency prolonged bilaterally.

5. P35 latency absent on the compromised side and prolonged on the other.

6. P35 wave absent bilaterally.

7. Cortical response absent.

In 1985, Aminoff et al.[3] published a very contradictory study on the diagnostic value of somatosensory evoked potentials in L5 and S1 radiculopathies. They studied the spinal and cortical SEPs of the peroneal nerve and the L5 and S1 distal segments. Their results showed no alteration in the cortical SEPs obtained from the peroneal nerve, even in patients in whom radiologic examinations and electromyography showed L5 compromises, many of which were corroborated surgically. The cortical SEP obtained by stimulation of L5 and S1 dermatomes was altered in only seven of 28 patients, showing the correct radicular level of the lesion.

The explanation given by the authors to justify the normality of the cortical response of the peroneal nerve is that it possesses multiradicular L4-L5 and S1 innervation. They do not give any explanation for the normality of the cortical response of segments L5 and S1 found in 75% of the patients studied by this method, especially when 10 of them had only sensory clinical alterations.

This study contrasts completely with our findings and with those of Scarff et al.,[82] Cassvan,[12] and Notermans and Vlek,[65] among others. The common denominator in these studies has been the excellent correlation (70% to 100%) between the level of the lesion identified by the Cz-Fz SEP, clinical and radiologic findings, and surgical confirmation of the compromised root. In these cases, we have no doubt as to the precocity with which the cortical Cz-Fz SEP of the peroneal nerve is altered in L5 radiculopathies, which enables the extent of compression of these sensory fibers and their regressive evolution to be revealed from the start of the picture, without considering functional factors that usually occur with such pictures.

In long-term postoperative monitoring, cortical SEPs can demonstrate fibrosis and in some instances secondary spinostenosis. In the latter case, the evoked potentials present good form and amplitude, but latencies are prolonged symmetrically at more than one metameric level (usually L4 and L5).

Polyneuropathies

In 1980, Jones and coworkers[52] correlated the alterations in peripheral conduction and central neuroconduction that occur in Friedreich's ataxia.

Eisen et al.[27,28] had also reported desynchronization and delay in the cortical SEPs of patients with hereditary sensory neuropathy.

In 1981, Arezzo et al.[5] conducted experimental studies in monkeys intoxicated with acrylamide and proved that this neurotoxin not only caused degeneration of the distal portion of the long peripheral axons but also degeneration of the terminal and preterminal portions of the axons in the fasciculus gracilis. Since study of the sensory fibers of the upper extremities going to the cuneate nucleus did not find alterations, it is assumed that, owing to its great length, the fasciculus gracilis is more vulnerable to toxic, metabolic, and genetic factors that produce distal axonal degeneration.

Metabolic. *Diabetes*: Grupta and Dorfman[41] reported similar findings in 1981 regarding alterations that occur in diabetics with moderate or asymptomatic neuropathy. It is believed that the site of the primary neural defect is in the ganglion of the dorsal root, from whence conduction is altered to both distal peripheral sites and central projections. Nevertheless, this mechanism does not give a clear explanation when transmission of the afferent pathway is slowed at the intracranial level. In our laboratory we have studied SEPs in diabetic patients since 1986 by analyzing only cortical responses from the lower extremities and central conduction time from the upper extremities (N13-N19). We have found spinal conduction compromise only in patients with severe mixed distal peripheral neuropathies. It might be necessary to add a specific calculation of "spinal conduction time" or "spinal conduction velocity" to show such compromise early.

Renal: In 27 patients with chronic renal insufficiency treated with diet and dialysis, Rossini et al.[76] studied spinal conduction from the median and peroneal nerves. Eleven patients presented spinal conduction slowing from the lower extremities and only one from the upper extremities. The authors suggest that this study enables early states of central-distal peripheral axonopathy to be confirmed. In 1985, Paradiso and coworkers[67] made similar findings in nine patients undergoing hemodialysis and two successful renal transplant patients. In eight of the nine dialyzed patients, spinal conduction was prolonged, while it was normal in the two transplanted patients. The authors postulate that the metabolic factor that produces this prolongation in spinal conduction is rapidly reversible after transplant and is not a structural compromise.

Toxic. Arezzo's findings have been confirmed in several later studies.[44,63] The toxicity caused by organic solvents in subjects with chronic alcoholism produces central-distal peripheral axonopathy. In the case of patients with thallium intoxication, spinal SEP studies allow evaluation of the level of compromise, which at times is limited to only the peripheral part or radicular spine, or, in the most severe cases, includes participation of the trunk, mesencephalon, and cortex. In our laboratory, such study enabled us in

1988 to serially quantify the effect of treating these patients with Prussian blue.[19] It can also identify the toxic side-effects of vincristine on spinal conduction.

Hereditary.   There are numerous publications relating to SEP alternations in these pathologies.[4,17,25,52] Noteworthy is the work of Jones et al.,[52] in which peripheral neuroconduction and intracranial conduction were studied in persons with Charcot-Marie-Tooth disease and Friedreich's ataxia. Of 14 patients with Charcot-Marie-Tooth, six had prolonged central conduction times (6.41 to 8 milliseconds), which reveals the atypical symptoms of CNS participation in these pictures. Of 22 patients with Friedreich's ataxia, 11 presented major prolongation of central conduction times (15.4 to 16.5 milliseconds), which was expected since the greater compromise is due to degeneration of the long spinal tract.

In a recent work published by Triantafyllou and coworkers,[98] visual and auditory evoked potentials were analyzed in nine patients with Charcot-Marie-Tooth disease. Three patients showed anomalies in visual evoked potentials (prolongation of the P100). Eight presented abnormal auditory evoked potentials: one had I-III prolongation, two had prolonged latencies in wave I, and six had repeated responses that were not comparable unilaterally or bilaterally. These findings prove that the II and VIII pairs of cranial nerves are involved in the demyelinating process of Charcot-Marie-Tooth.

In patients with hereditary sensorimotor neuropathies and Kulgelberg-Welander spinal muscular atrophy, Egerhazi et al.[25] have reported prolongation of the central conduction time. In patients with Type I hereditary sensorimotor neuropathies there was prolongation of both spinal (N13) and cortical (N19) short latencies and central conduction time (N13-N19). In contrast, in patients with Type II hereditary sensorimotor neuropathies spinal (N13) and cortical (N19) short latencies were prolonged, but central conduction time was normal.

Idiopathic.   Regarding Guillain-Barré syndrome, in 1980 Eisen and Elleker[26] reported a case of tetraparesis with absence of the P40 short latency in the cortical SEP of the peroneal nerve (obtained by stimulating the lateral malleolus, sensory branch).

Since 1982 we have been conducting, together with the neurology service in our hospital, a serial pre-/postplasmapheresis study in patients with Guillain-Barré syndrome.[101] Our laboratory and the clinical neurologic examination are the starting point for diagnosis and prognosis regarding entry into treatment.

To the classic sensorimotor neuroconduction examinations used in Guillain-Barré syndrome (segmentary motor conduction velocity, distal sensory latency, F wave, H reflex, blink reflex) we have added spinal and cortical SEP studies in both the lower extremities (peroneal nerve) and the upper extremities (median and ulnar nerves) with plexal recording (Erb's point). The pudendal nerve has sometimes been studied in cases of transient bladder dysfunction.

In 22 Guillain-Barré patients, nine of whom were treated with plasmapheresis during the first 15 days of the syndrome's evolution, we found that the SEP study elucidated the initial clinical sensory symptomatology and, together with the classic axonal neuroconduction examinations, enabled us to choose the patients to be started on plasmapheresis. The complete blockage of the spinal response from both upper and lower extremities coincides with motor blockage of the F wave in the proximal segment. These findings demonstrate the degree of proximal segmentary demyelinization, both motor and sensory, and the risk of severe neuropathic compromise, which may result in respiratory insufficiency and risk of death for the patient. One of the nine patients went into shock upon entering plasmapheresis therapy and could not continue it. This patient, who died 22 days later, had initially presented complete blockage of the spinal SEPs in the median, ulnar, peroneal, sural, and pudendal nerves.

In a 1988 study, Granji and Frazier[31] analyzed the SEPs in 13 patients with Guillain-Barré syndrome and found prolongation of all upper extremity interpeaks—N13-N19, Erb-N19, and Erb-N13.

SOMATOSENSORY EVOKED POTENTIALS IN SPINAL COMPROMISE

Factors Affecting Spinal Conduction

The kind of recording used is an important factor in spinal conduction. Invasive recording techniques with subdural electrodes[58] or epidural electrodes[11,18] were initially used. The superficial recording technique was first employed by Liberson[56] and Cracco.[17] Today the latter is the most used recording method.

In 1974, Happel[43] carried out an experimental study in cats to determine how the level of recording and kind of spinal lesion affect spinal conduction. He stimulated the sciatic nerve in 20 cats and recorded the spinal SEPs at the lumbar, thoracic, and cervical levels directly from the medullary surface. At the lumbar level an initial negative wave was obtained, followed by a variable wave; when the electrode was moved rostrally, the initial large negative peak decreased in amplitude and the duration and latency of the response increased. At the cervical level the response was polyphasic with an increase in latency and low amplitude.

When a posterior rhizotomy was performed on the lumbar and sacral roots ipsilateral to the sciatic stimulus, the response was completely blocked. A thoracic medullary section also blocked the response on the cervical medulla.

In 1983, Schramm et al.[84] also published a study in cats in which they performed a chronic spinal compression and compared the change in spinal and cortical SEPs and motor alterations. They found that the spinal SEPs were first altered when 36% of total medullary compression was reached, before clinical neurologic signs appeared. In contrast, the cortical SEPs were only altered after the appearance of neurologic signs and on reaching 91% of total compression.

In summary, it can be concluded that:

- Spinal responses differ in their form, duration, amplitude, and latency according to the kind of recording (extradural, intradural, or superficial) and placement of the electrodes (lumbar, dorsal, or cervical).
- For clinical use in medullary lesions, a spinal SEP recording is preferable to a cortical SEP recording, since the former is the first to change.
- In compressive medullary lesions due to extrinsic mechanisms, the spinal SEP generally changes in amplitude and latency; complete blockage appears only if the compression is quite accentuated.[7]
- In inflammatory medullary lesions, the spinal SEP is completely blocked above the level of the lesion.

Prognostic Value

The literature is contradictory in regard to the prognostic value of SEPs in medullary lesions, whether the recording is spinal or cortical.

Rowed and coworkers[78] studied patients who had suffered medullary damage more than six weeks earlier and demonstrated a probable correlation between the reappearance of spinal SEPs and a prognosis of recovery.

Perot and Vera[70] studied 55 patients with incomplete cervical medullary damage and found that early return to normal ranges of the SEPs from the median and posterior tibial nerves indicated a good prognosis. In patients with incomplete, progressive damage, the SEPs presented progressive alterations in amplitude and latency.

McGarry et al.[61] studied walking capacity and the cortical SEP from the peroneal nerve in 25 patients with old, incomplete medullary damage. The results were quite contradictory since patients who presented a good cortical response did not have good walking capacity. Of the nine patients who had a normal cortical SEP, four did not have useful activity in the lower extremities. The other 16 patients had a cortical SEP with prolonged latencies; eight of them could walk functionally. The patients who had normal cortical SEP but could not walk functionally probably presented damage in the anterior and lateral columns of the spinal medulla but relatively little in the dorsal columns. In contrast, the injury in patients able to walk functionally but who had an altered cortical SEP was probably in a central area of fusiform necrosis which involved the ventral portion, dorsal columns, and gray matter adjacent to the posterior horn. Such damage may abolish or delay the cortical SEP while having little effect on motor function. These findings led McGarry to conclude that recording the cortical SEP of the peroneal nerve does not predict motor function nor, consequently, ambulatory capacity after a medullary trauma.

In the area of evaluating proprioception after medullary lesions, Dimitrijevic et al.[22] conducted a study in 1983 in 66 patients with old medullary lesions and found that alterations in the cortical SEP of the posterior tibial nerve correlated with the proprioception damage.

To identify the optimal kind of SEP study to be used in medullary lesions, Shiff and coworkers[87] determined the conduction velocities of the medullary and cortical afferent pathways in three groups: normal controls, patients with medullary lesions of varied etiology and severity, and patients with peripheral nerve pathology. The peroneal nerve was stimulated at the popliteal space and superficial spinal recordings were made at levels L3, T12, T6, and Cz-Fz. The normal spinal conduction velocity values found are shown in Table 4.

In the patients with medullary compromise, no absolute correlation was found between proprioceptive alteration and slowing of the spinal conduction velocity. Nevertheless, there was a good correlation between the nature of the lesion and the associated abnormality of the SEP. Focal lesions of the medulla, especially local epidural compressions, cause a slowing of the medullary conduction velocity; this shows that such local lesions selectively damage the fastest conduction fibers. Patients with severe diffuse pathology, including demyelinating diseases, more often have absent rostral and cortical spinal responses than slowing of the spinal conduction velocity; this can be explained on the basis of blockage of conduction in some axons and asynchronic central conduction in others. In summary, focal compressive medullary lesions cause slowing of the spine-to-spine and spinocortical medullary conduction velocity. Multifocal lesions of the medulla generally inhibit cortical response. There is a clear correlation between the SEP findings and clinical prognosis of these lesions.

Table 4. **Normal spinal conduction values found in the study by Shiff et al.[87] (1984).**

Site of stimulation	Site of recording electrode	Conduction velocity (msec)	Standard deviation
Popliteal space	L3	70.9	4.5
L3	CZ	32.8	2.3
T12	CZ	30.7	2.8
T6	CZ	26.7	2.8
L3	T12	58.6	7.0
T12	T6	53.8	5.6

Small and Matthews[92] used spinal conduction time instead of conduction velocity to reveal medullary lesions. They called this time the medullary transit time, and it was measured between interpeaks N21 (lumbar L1), N27 (CVII), N29 (CV), and P33 (CII). The authors believe that in this way the responses are not contaminated with intracranial central conduction time and thus "lesioned spinal segments" are being explored.

Conclusions from the use of somatosensory evoked potentials as a diagnostic tool in medullary lesions are as follows:

- The presence of a cortical or spinal response above the lesion rules out complete medullary anatomic section.
- The presence of cortical or spinal response above a lesion indicates a hopeful prognosis for the future.
- The presence of cortical or spinal response above a lesion does not predict functional ambulation.
- Slowing of the spinal conduction time may be caused by various pathologies.
- Alteration of the cortical SEP may be correlated with proprioception disturbances.
- To determine the level of a spinal lesion, segmentary medullary studies should be carried out.
- Immediate, appropriate study of SEPs in medullary lesions enables decisions to be made regarding emergency surgery in some cases.

EVOKED POTENTIALS IN INTRAOPERATIVE MONITORING

Preventing damage to the central nervous system during surgery close to it is quite important since such damage is often irreversible. Nervous system monitoring can identify complications early enough to allow them to be treated or corrected before they become permanent.

Evoked potentials provide a method for intraoperative monitoring of the CNS in major surgery on the spinal column or aorta and neurosurgery in the posterior fossa. Here both auditory and somatosensory evoked potentials are used.

Somatosensory evoked potentials enable monitoring of the pathways of the posterior columns and their rostral connections up to the central region of the cortex. In this way, somesthetic monitoring provides information on medullary function and on substantial parts of the trunk and central region of the hemispheres. Different recording techniques are used: direct dural recording in each corner near the conus medullaris, or superficial spinal and/or cortical recording. Superficial spinal recording has the disadvantage of providing responses of very low amplitude at the thoracic and cervical levels.

The stimuli used may be invasive in the extradural space at the high thoracic level or at the peripheral (superficial) level in nerve trunks (posterior tibial, peroneal, internal saphenous, or sural).

Intraoperative SEP monitoring is used most often during the insertion of Harrington instrumentation or similar devices to stabilize the column in patients with scoliosis. In such cases, SEP monitoring is a procedure without risk to the patient which allows medullary function to be evaluated continuously. This monitoring should take several factors into account: (a) the recording and stimulation techniques to be used; (b) the organization of the operative suite; (c) the instrumentation in use; (d) the methods of anesthesia; and (e) interpretation of the results and costs of the procedure.

With respect to technique, the most satisfactory recording is Cz-Fz superficial cortical and/or spinal, with stimulus at the posterior tibial nerve. Electrosurgery generally interferes with recording.

A nitrous oxide/O_2 mixture, thiopental, succinylcholine, and D-tubocurarine are the anesthetic agents of choice. Meperidine and fenanyl citrate may improve SEP recording. Halogenated agents are incompatible with monitoring since they alter SEPs, but their use in minimal proportion and in combination with nitrous oxide/O_2 decreases alterations. Halothane and estrane are incompatible with SEP monitoring.

Bolus injection of any medicine may change the monitoring. Controlled hypotension decreases the amplitude of the SEP by 50%, and thus should be avoided during monitoring.

Monitoring should be performed during the following phases of surgical intervention: preincision, hypotension phase, instrumentation, postinstrumentation, and skin closure. As for the costs, González et al.[39] posits that they are approximately 300% less than the cost of treating paraplegia secondary to a surgical process.

The effectiveness of monitoring is clearly seen in the spinal stenosis operation. González et al.[38] found a frank improvement in P1 and N1 (cortical) amplitude and latency after decompression. This demonstrates that stenosis of the spinal canal produces a compression of the nerve root and consequently an ischemia that primarily affects the larger-diameter myelin fibers. Their decompression improves their axoplasmic flow.

In surgery with Luque instrumentation for cervical column instability, the cortical SEP from the median nerve is used for monitoring.

Ischemia causes diminution in the amplitude of the cortical SEP when the cortical flow falls below 20 ml/100 g/minute. The SEP is lost with a flow of 15 ml/100 g/minute. Recordings of subcortical and spinal evoked potentials are more resistant to ischemia. This trait makes them useful in monitoring carotid endarterectomy and aneurysm surgery.

Evoked potential monitoring in cardiopulmonary bypass has been used only recently. Visual, auditory, and somatosensory evoked potentials are used. The N19 (N20) peak is probably the most resistant to the effects of hypothermia, an additional factor always present in this type of surgery.

In posterior fossa surgery, auditory evoked potential monitoring of the brain stem is most used. The use of AEPs is noteworthy in procedures at the cerebellopontile angle (acoustic neuron resection, microvascular decompression of cranial nerves, retrolabyrinthine vestibular neurectomy, and other tumor resections) and other posterior fossa procedures (basilar artery aneurysm, arteriovenous malformation of the posterior fossa, intrinsic tumors of the trunk).

EVOKED POTENTIALS IN DIAGNOSIS OF MULTIPLE SCLEROSIS

Many investigators have studied evoked potential alterations in this pathology. Most agree in their conclusions regarding the changes found, and especially regarding the great usefulness of this examination in diagnosis.

Baker and coworkers, in 1968,[6] recognized the utility of SEPs in detecting subclinical lesions in multiple sclerosis.

Mastaglia et al.[59] wrote that alterations in the cervical SEP (N13) were found in 58% of multiple sclerosis patients. He also reported that it is possible to detect SEP alterations in patients who did not have sensory signs or symptoms. The abnormal SEPs in such patients indicate silent plaques and may aid in documenting multiple lesions.

In 1982, Chiappa and Ropper[15] reported comparisons of three methods of stimulating evoked potentials (visual, somesthetic, and auditory) in multiple sclerosis patients. They found that visual and somesthetic evoked potentials are equally good in revealing clinically unsuspected lesions. The AEP had the least sensitivity (between 30% and 50%). The three types of studies are complementary.

Chiappa and Ropper found that the SEPs in the upper extremity were normal in about 75% of all patients with multiple sclerosis (confirmed, probable, or possible) and in close to half of multiple sclerosis patients who did not have sensory symptoms or signs. SEPs in the lower extremities, in contrast, were altered more often, presumably because of the greater distance from the spinal medulla and consequently through the white matter being studied. Approximately one-third of the SEP abnormalities were unilateral. The bilateral abnormalities presented various degrees of compromise on each side.

The demyelinating plaques in multiple sclerosis are distributed in multiple locations in the CNS, and therefore the diagnosis is "confirmed" only if such multifocal changes are evidenced by the evoked potentials. A combined study by visual, auditory, and somatosensory evoked potentials (preferably from the posterior tibial nerve) can aid in demonstrating the multiple localizations of the disease. This evoked potential combination is called the "multimodality test."

Many authors—Green and Walcoff,[40] Phillips et al.,[71] and Aminoff et al.[2]—have combined visual, auditory, and somatosensory evoked potentials in the study of multiple sclerosis. Some have found VEPs more sensitive, others SEPs. All agree that AEPs have very low sensitivity.

Recently, Giesser and coworkers[34] compared trimodal evoked potentials with magnetic resonance imaging (MRI) for diagnosing multiple sclerosis. They found the following sensitivities: visual evoked potentials, 71.4%; auditory evoked potentials, 51.6%; somatesthetic evoked potentials, 36.8%; trimodal evoked potentials, 90.5%; magnetic resonance imaging, 71.4%. This study concluded that VEPs and MRI have similar sensitivity, but the sensitivity of trimodal evoked potentials is higher.

In our laboratory, the SEPs from both lower extremities (cortical, peroneal nerve) and upper extremities (spinal and cortical, median nerve) are used for routine study. The comparative bilateral central conduction time includes the median nerve since in suspected multiple sclerosis this factor has been found to be the first to change, showing a statistically significant prolongation (comparative bilateral study). In addition, the P35 of the cortical response of the peroneal nerve is prolonged, unilaterally or bilaterally, and in most cases the altered side in the upper extremities is not the same as in the lower extremities.

EVOKED POTENTIALS IN CENTRAL LESIONS

Somatosensory Evoked Potentials in Cerebral Ischemia

It is important to have another tool for diagnosing cerebral ischemia, and one that will indicate the lesion early, since it has been confirmed in animals (cats) that the cerebral cells surviving after an ischemia and subsequent recovery depend not only on the independent effects of the residual flow and duration of the ischemia but on the combined influence of these two factors.[46]

Meyer and coworkers[62] provoked an experimental cerebral ischemia in animals and compared the SEP changes to ischemic lesions. They studied 17 cats whose right medial cerebral arteries they occluded. The SEP was measured before the occlusion (24 hours and 1 hour) and after it (immediately, 6 hours, and 24 hours). They found that before the occlusion the SEPs were identical in the right and left cortical recordings. Postocclusion: (a) interpeak N1-P1 latency slowed in the right hemisphere (3.53 milliseconds before ischemia versus 3.99 after); (b) P2 component and greater negative peaks showed prolonged latencies and diminution of their amplitude immediately after occlusion; (c) P1 latency became more prolonged if the ischemia extended to the thalamus (4.38 milliseconds); and (d) components of greater negativity were more prolonged in severe infarcts in the medial suprasylvian and posterior ectosylvian area when compared with less severe infarcts in the same area (20.6 versus 16.4 milliseconds).

Through this experimental study, the authors demonstrated that SEP measurement is a sensitive method that can indicate the beginning and extension of cerebral ischemia.

Symon and coworkers[96] conducted studies from which they concluded that a close correlation exists between cerebral ischemia, diminution in the amplitude of the cortical SEP, and prolongation of the central conduction time, even if central conduction time changes occur before the clinical compromise. This finding is quite important in diagnosis and for the initiation of treatment while the lesions are still reversible.

In 1984, Robinson and coworkers[75] compared the results obtained from SEPs, computed tomography (CT), and clinical findings in patients with purely sensory apoplexy and sensorimotor apoplexy. All 11 patients with sensory apoplexy presented sensory alterations that affected all modalities on the compromised side of the body, but none presented complete hemianesthesia. All had normal SEPs and CT scans. The three patients with sensorimotor apoplexy presented a motor and sensory deficit with absence of defects in the visual field, aphasia, or behavioral changes. All presented unilateral changes in the SEPs. In two, the thalamic or thalamocortical wave was absent, and one had marked diminution in the amplitude of the N20 response.

The SEP alterations were detected immediately after the vascular accident, and were present in one patient before CT changes were found. In subsequent CT scans, the three patients showed a defined lesion of low density that compromised the thalamus and/or posterior limbus of the internal capsule.

From this study it was concluded that only sensorimotor apoplexies present changes in the cortical SEPs. Since these changes occur early, they can aid in a patient's initial diagnosis.

In 1983, Stohr and coworkers[94] presented a study of the cortical SEP from the median nerve and computed tomography in 30 patients with unilateral lesions and kinesthetic alterations. Their findings were as follows:

- Abnormal P15 with normal P13 and P14 (using noncephalic references) correlated with lesions of the thalamus, internal capsule, and putamen.
- Low-amplitude or blocked N20 and altered late latencies indicated lesions of the postcentral gyrus.
- Blocked N20 and normal later components signaled lesions of cortical area 3b.
- Normal N20 and altered later components indicated lesions of the cortical parietal association area.
- Altered N55 and later components showed ischemia in cortical area 39.
- Loss of P13, P14, and P15 correlated with a lesion between the thalamus and putamen.

Most published studies state that a compromise at the thalamic level changes component P15 (noncephalic reference) or N14 (cephalic reference), but in 1984 Tsuji and coworkers[99] found an N16 peak in a study of Parkinsonian patients using direct recording over the thalamus (cortical recording with noncephalic reference) during stereotactic surgery, which suggests that it is probably generated in the thalamus. The peaks with shorter latencies probably originate caudal to the thalamus and peak N18 rostrally to it.

Somatosensory Evoked Potentials in Other Central Nervous System Compromises

Somatosensory evoked potentials provide evidence of tumors of the brain stem or medial lemniscus and pontine infarct (claustral syndrome).

In patients with vascular or neoplastic lesions of the thalamus, the SEPs may be abnormal if the patient shows a clinically significant sensory deficit. In lesions located primarily in the ventroposterior area of the thalamus, the SEPs of both upper and lower extremities are consistently changed or are lost. When the lesion is located laterally the SEP of the lower extremity (posterior tibial nerve) is preferentially affected, whereas if the lesion is located more medially it will affect the SEP of the median nerve.

Infarcts that compromise the corona radiata cause changes in the SEP similar to those found with ventroposterior thalamic lesions, except that in this case the SEP is never lost. With subcortical infarcts there is a relative preservation of the short latencies compared to the medium and late components of the response.

Tumors that affect the thalamus change the SEPs in different ways, depending on whether they are extrinsic or intrinsic. Parietal lesions secondary to vascular pathologies produce abolition of the cortical response of the median nerve in the affected hemisphere. Mauguiere and coworkers[60] found that a complete parietal lesion produced a contralateral hemianesthesia with pyramidal signs, eliminating the N19-P27-P45 components in the SEP response without affecting the prerolandic peaks (P22-N30).

In tumors of the posterior fossa, such as acoustic neuromas, tumors of the cerebellopontine angle, and trunk gliomas, auditory evoked potentials have high sensitivity (even greater than that of computed tomography), though perhaps not exceeding that of magnetic resonance imaging. In such cases interpeak III-V increases when the opposite ear is stimulated.

In toxicometabolic encephalopathies, the auditory evoked potential is extraordinarily resistant; in some cases, interpeak I-V is prolonged.

In Alzheimer's disease the late AEP and SEP peaks are prolonged, indicating anomalies of the associative parieto-occipital cortex. In dementia caused by multiple infarcts the late components of auditory evoked potentials are the most prolonged, which may reflect the pathology of the temporal lobe.

Evoked Potentials as Prognostic Aids in Hemiplegia

In 1982, LaJoie et al.[55] studied the cortical SEPs of the median nerve in 68 patients with right-side hemiplegia in order to determine the correlation between the SEP and functional changes in the right upper extremity.

They found the following alterations:

- SEP was absent in 42 patients; only one of them had minimal function in the right upper extremity on discharge.
- SEP had diminished amplitude in 14 patients; five (36%) had some function in the right upper extremity on discharge.
- SEP was normal in eight patients; three (38%) had good function on discharge.

Sixty-four patients did not have function in the right upper extremity on admission, and those with absent SEP showed no functional recovery in 98% of cases. Four patients had normal SEP and some function in the right upper extremity on admission, which increased by discharge.

This study suggests that cortical SEP of the median nerve may be useful in prognosis of right hand function in hemiplegic patients, so that these patients can be started early on a rehabilitation plan.

On the basis of the LaJoie study, Jacobs et al.[50] conducted a study of spinal (N13) and cortical (N19) SEP from the median nerve and central conduction time (N19-N13) in 55 selected patients with hemiplegia. SEPs and central conduction times were analyzed in relation to activities of daily living, hand function, and functional recovery. A significant correlation was found between both the SEP response and central conduction time at the start of hemiplegia and ability for activities of daily living. The results were as follows at discharge:

- Patients who did not have cortical SEPs could not perform activities of daily living or did so only minimally.
- The amplitude of the cortical response was always diminished in patients with hemiplegia.
- If the diminution in the amplitude is greater than 50% between the right and left sides, a patient had scant hand function.
- If there was a marked difference in N19 latency and central conduction time between right and left, the patient was dependent on discharge.
- The SEP from the median nerve did not have prognostic value regarding the extent of a hemiplegic patient's recovery. A combined study of the upper and lower extremities might provide clearer data since the SEP from the upper extremity was only able to evaluate hand function.

In summary, the difference in latencies is an indirect indicator of functioning in activities of daily living, while amplitude alterations are a good predictor of hand function. However, none of the three variables is a good predictor of motor recovery.

Evoked Potentials in Coma

Evoked potentials have been useful in reaching prognoses about patients with cerebral injury severe enough to cause coma. One of the most complete studies is that of Hume et al.,[48] who through studying SEPs correctly predicted recovery from coma in 38 of 49 patients evaluated within three days of the start of their coma. The loss of median nerve (N19) cortical responses in both hemispheres was viewed as an indicator of fatal coma, while responses that were reduced or absent on one side or displayed a prolonged latency on the other almost always implied the development of a severe neurologic deficit such as hemiplegia.

The persistence of spinal response N13 in such cases indicated preservation of the lower medullary components, even among comatose patients in whom evidence suggested pontine and upper medullary necrosis. The preservation of these components is probably related to the fact that the cervicomedullary junction receives less injury associated with an increase in intracranial pressure than structures that are completely confined in the cranium. In contrast with these findings, the auditory evoked potential of the brain stem in most brain-dead patients shows an absence of response of the VIII nerves; however, the medullary mechanisms described are present in such patients.

A quantitative correlation does not always exist between evoked potential findings and prognosis, since in some cases the serial SEPs showed significant variations in the same patient. For example, 44 patients in coma with poor SEP responses died or were left with a severe residual deficit. Thus, although somatosensory evoked potentials have provided good prognostic information about coma in some cases, more studies are needed before they can be used as a prognostic guide in patients.

In 1983, Rumpl and coworkers[80] studied cortical and cervical SEPs and central conduction time from the median nerve in 44 comatose patients. Thirty-four patients were studied in acute coma (one or two days). Twenty-three were studied in prolonged coma (three to 12 days), six of whom were diagnosed as brain dead. Ten patients could be studied only after recovery but before the 30th day posttrauma.

The pontine compromise was classified clinically and by computed tomography as (a) lesions secondary to displacement of the supratentorial mass, or (b) lesions due to trauma directly over the pons.

A correlation was made in the study between outcome and the central conduction time (N13-N19) and N19/N13 amplitude ratio. Those with supratentorial lesions and central conduction time as well as N13 and N19 amplitudes close to normal had a good evolution. Those with increased central conduction time or a decrease in the N13 and N19 amplitudes, in both acute and prolonged coma, had a very poor evolution.

Asymmetry of the SEP indicated moderate to severe final disability. There is a close relationship among the degree of cerebral ischemia, decrease in cortical SEP amplitude, and increase in central conduction time. The SEP may aid in diagnosis as to the extent and location of the cerebral ischemia.

"Trimodality" of evoked potentials was used in patients with coma in a 1984 study by Newlon and Greenberg.[64] Clinical signs, evoked potentials, computed tomography, and the Glasgow coma scale were compared. These authors found that trimodal evoked potentials (SEP, VEP, and AEP) provided 100% prediction in coma. The clinical signs plus sensory evoked potentials yielded 96%, the Glasgow scale 96%, clinical signs alone and clinical signs plus CT 91%, and CT 71%.

Recently (1989), Shin and coworkers[89] conducted a study of auditory and somatosensory evoked potentials in 29 patients from 1 to 67 months after a closed head injury, comparing the trimodality of evoked potentials with the Rancho Los Amigos scale and other clinical parameters to evaluate the discharge prognosis in these patients. The Rancho Los Amigos scale had a predictive value of 60% at discharge. When age and SEPs were taken into account, the predictive value of the Rancho Los Amigos scale increased to 72%. Trimodality does not appear very sensitive in discharge prognosis in relation to the Rancho Los Amigos scale. This could be because the SEPs do not reflect adaptation to chronic processes in patients with high cognitive function.

We have conducted some examinations on comatose patients but without the frequency necessary to draw conclusions. But in one patient who suffered cerebral trauma in 1988 and in whom a serial study was conducted between the third and fourteenth days of coma, we found complete blockage of both cortical responses (N19) on the fourth day and in later examinations. We predicted a vegetative state, which has persisted until today (1990).

In cases of coma due to anoxic ischemia, a study of 30 patients conducted by Brink[8] showed that none of the 30 patients in whom cortical SEPs were absent recovered consciousness. The presence of cortical SEPs for several hours after cardiac arrest was associated with recovery of consciousness in some patients and persistence of coma or development of vegetative state in others.

With regard to the use of organs for transplantation from "brain-dead" donors, Fotiou and coworkers[30] have used brachial plexus (N9) and spinal (N13) recordings to certify the preserved peripheral functional status in a patient who might be a good donor. The persistence of a good N13 spinal response (spinogram) indicates maintenance of spinomedullary function, which in some instances would explain the partial maintenance of respiratory function in patients who meet other criteria for cerebral death. In Fotiou's study, seven patients with cerebral death who had a normal spinogram were kidney donors, and the transplants were successful.

Recently, Shaw[86] conducted an experimental SEP study in rats that had been subjected to experimental cerebral concussion by acceleration. He recorded the short cervical (N13) and cortical (N19) latencies during the immediate postconcussion period. The thalamic and primary cortical responses were abolished, but the spinal response was preserved. This loss of the cortical response is presumably due to the rapid acceleration (or deceleration) of the head on the axis of the neck; in this case it is understandable to find a dysfunction of the brain stem. Within the 60 seconds following concussion, the potentials that had been lost began to reappear.

Shaw concludes that the site of action of the concussion lies in the cervicomedullary junction and thalamus. The brain stem and lemniscal pathway may therefore be almost as vulnerable during the acute period following a closed cerebral contusion as the collateral reticular formation.

Drechsler[24] studied a group of 32 patients two years after cerebral concussion. None of the patients showed neurologic anomalies. Their only noteworthy symptoms were headache and neurasthenic syndrome. The most significant finding in these patients was prolongation of central conduction time (N13-N19), which was significantly longer in comparison to an age-matched control group.

Our experience has been similar to that of Drechsler. In patients with cerebral concussion who do not have clinical neurologic alterations we recommend conducting a follow-up study of serial SEPs from the median nerve and central conduction time to verify regression of the subclinical cerebral compromise.

SPECIAL SOMATOSENSORY EVOKED POTENTIAL TECHNIQUES

Pudendal Nerve

In 1970 Bradley and Fletcher[9] studied the distribution of the somatic innervation of the external urethral sphincter in the spinal medulla in cats. Later, in 1982, Haldeman and coworkers[42] studied the cortical response of the SEP coming from the pudendal nerve by stimulating the dorsal nerve of the penis in men and clitoris in women (both sensory branches). These responses were compared in morphology, latency, and peripheral and central conduction time with those obtained at the spinal and cortical level when the posterior tibial nerve was stimulated.

The latency parameters Haldeman et al. found were the following: in men, 35.2 ± 3.0 milliseconds for the N34 peak (initial) and 42.3 ± 1.9 milliseconds for P1 (P40); in women, 32.9 ± 2.9 milliseconds for N34 and 39.8 ± 1.8 milliseconds for P40. These values were similar to those found in the same subjects' posterior tibial nerve.

The findings led to the following conclusions:

- The cortical latencies of the pudendal nerve are quite similar to those of the posterior tibial nerve.
- The spinal response in L1 had very low amplitude and at times was difficult to define. The latency to L1 from the pudendal nerve is 12

milliseconds shorter than from the posterior tibial nerve (stimulated at the ankle).

- The spinal conduction of the pudendal nerve from the conus terminalis proximally is therefore 12 milliseconds slower than that of the posterior tibial nerve.
- The greatest amplitude of the cortical response was obtained at the medial line of the sensory cortex (interhemispheric fissure line). This unsuspected finding may be explained by: (a) a difference in the route followed by the afferent pathway of the pudendal nerve in the spinal medulla and pons; (b) the spectrum of conduction velocities of the various fibers in the central afferent pathway; (c) a difference in the fibers that were stimulated: in the case of the posterior tibial nerve, pure sensory cutaneous and sensory fibers from the neuromuscular spindle, and in the case of the pudendal nerve, pure sensory cutaneous fibers which probably conduct more slowly, both peripherally and centrally.

In 1983, Kaplan[53] studied the SEP of the pudendal nerve in patients with cord lesions at both the cervical and thoracolumbar levels. He studied 10 patients with a complete cervical lesion (quadriplegia), 15 with an incomplete cervical lesion, and 10 with a complete thoracolumbar lesion (paraplegia). In patients with complete lesions, the cortical SEP of the pudendal nerve was absent. In those with incomplete cord lesions, vesical function does not return very soon after the trauma. Conducting this study is thus quite useful to predict probable return of this function.

Sarica and Karacan[81] recently presented a new method for exploring vesical function through cortical SEP by stimulating the ureterovesical junction. In 22 normal subjects, a Foley catheter containing a pair of electrodes 7 mm apart was inserted into the bladder; when the balloon was inflated, it was oriented so that the electrodes touched the ureterovesical junction. The cortical response at Cz-Fz had an average latency of 91.4 ± 11.1 milliseconds at the first negative peak. This peak was preceded by a small positive deflection with an average latency of 64.3 ± 11.9 milliseconds. Because of the great difference in latency, the authors postulate that axons other than those coming from the pudendal nerve are carrying the afferent impulses to the cortex.

Up to 1987 we conducted the classic electrophysiologic studies of the pudendal nerve (cortical somatosensory evoked potential and bulbocavernosis reflex from the dorsal nerve of the penis) in our laboratory in patients with urinary, anal, and/or sexual dysfunction. Exploration of the dorsal nerve of the penis does not provide good correlation in the area of sexual dysfunction. Owing to this fact and motivated by the concern of urologist Dr. E. Pino, we developed a new technique for exploring the nerves of the corpus cavernosum (pelvic splanchnic nerve) to correlate the Cz-Fz cortical

SEP and the bulbocavernous reflex from the pelvic splanchnic nerve with sexual dysfunction in males. In 1987 we presented the first results from a normal control group of 20 subjects. These values are shown in Table 5.

In 1988 we reported on this new technique at the International Congress on Impotence in Boston as applied in 32 patients who had undergone prostatectomy (transurethral resection). We obtained an effective correlation of 100% of abnormality among patients who were impotent postoperatively and positivity of SEPs and bulbocavernous reflexes in the pelvic splanchnic nerve.

In 1989 we presented a study of 64 impotent patients, of whom 20 were diabetics and 15 had undergone prostatectomy; in the remaining 29 the impotence was associated with various factors (alcohol, premature ejaculation, ingestion of antihypertensive drugs). The cortical SEP from the pelvic splanchnic nerve was altered in 98% of these patients, while SEPs from the dorsal nerve of the penis and the superficial perineal nerve (pudendal branch) were altered in only 48% and 60%, respectively. All of the diabetic and prostatectomized patients had altered cortical SEP from the splanchnic nerve. When the Mac-Nemar test was applied both to the nerves explored and the type of examination conducted, only the pelvic splanchnic nerve was found to be significantly compromised, and the examination that revealed the alterations earliest was the Cz-Fz cortical SEP.

From this study, we conclude that study of the SEP and bulbocavernous reflex through the new technique developed in our laboratory—by stimulating the pelvic splanchnic nerve—enables exploration of the neurovegetative pathway involved in erection.[69] The preliminary findings point to this level as a probable site of autonomic neuropathy since, because of its anatomic constitution as described by Lue,[57] the pelvic splanchnic nerve is probably responsible for controlling blood supply to the corpus cavernosus. We believe that this research indicates the greater significance of study of the pelvic splanchnic nerve instead of the pudendal nerve in impotent pa-

Table 5. Normal values of latencies of the bulbocavernous reflex and somatosensory evoked potential (n = 20, age 25–66 years).

	Dorsal nerve of penis	Superficial perineal nerve	Pelvic splanchnic nerve
Bulbocavernous reflex	28.5–39.4	39.2–38.3	27.0–37.5
Somatosensory evoked potential (P40)	36.2–42.2	37.0–42.3	37.8–42.5

Note: Other values for bulbocavernous reflex (BR) and somatosensory evoked potential (SEP) from dorsal nerve of penis:
Haldeman et al., 1982—35.9 ± 9.0 (BR), 42.3 ± 1.9 (SEP)[42]
Opsomer et al., 1986—43.4 ± 2.95 (SEP)[66]
Dick et al., 1974—27-40 (BR)[20]
Siroky et al., 1979—28-42 (BR).[90]

tients, since the former probably exercises the principal neurologic control of erection. Thus, SEP carried out in the pelvic splanchnic nerve would be the examination of greatest sensitivity in detecting impotence of neuropathic origin.

Trigeminal Nerve

Stohr and Petruch[95] studied the SEPs of the trigeminal nerve through electrical stimulation of the medial inferior branch. Later work standardized the parameters of the responses and noted their clinical importance in various groups of patients.[10]

More than 200 subjects were included in the latter study, among them healthy volunteers, patients with CNS compromise, patients with a possible diagnosis of multiple sclerosis (46 with confirmed multiple sclerosis), 20 patients with trigeminal neuralgia, 7 with ischemia of the pons (Wallenberg's syndrome), and 11 with tumors of the cerebellopontile angle. The technique used was stimulation of the upper and lower lips at the angle of the mouth. The intensity of the stimulus provokes a small contraction of the lips. The recording electrode was placed in the T3 or T4 cortical zone, according to the side to be explored, with an Fz reference.

The response is a wave with two negative and two positive peaks within 50 milliseconds. The first positive peak (P19) has an average latency of 18.5 milliseconds, with a limiting value of 22.3 milliseconds. A difference of more than 1.9 milliseconds between the sides was considered pathologic. In the patients with trigeminal neuralgia average latency was 21.1 ± 1.9 milliseconds. Separate stimulation of each branch may be made when a single branch of the trigeminal nerve is compromised. In the patients with multiple sclerosis, 61% had an altered P19 short latency. Ischemic lesions of the lateral medulla oblongata produced alterations in six of seven cases.

In 1985, de la Parra and Bertotti[68] of the Physical Medicine and Rehabilitation Service of the Costa Buero Institute of Neurosurgery in Argentina studied 35 patients affected by essential trigeminal neuralgia who underwent surgery with Sweet's technique. The preoperative SEPs of the trigeminal nerve were normal, which is congruent with the functional integrity characteristic of essential neuralgia. Only one patient showed definite alteration in latencies, but he also demonstrated clear clinical signs of multiple sclerosis, with a sensory deficit in the area affected.

On the basis of these findings, the authors drew the following conclusions:

- The SEP from the trigeminal nerve is normal in patients affected by trigeminal neuralgia.
- As far as can be determined, this normality represents overall anatomic integrity, which would justify the label "essential."
- Abnormality in any branch might correspond to a compressive process

or demyelinating plaque in that branch, which would call for more specific studies.

- Postoperative study of the SEP from the trigeminal nerve after Sweet's technique (used as integral treatment of essential neuralgia) would confirm the protection of the tactile pathways, together with hypalgesia of the affected area.
- SEP studies in the trigeminal nerve could contribute valuable information on the physiopathology of the trigeminal system and its diseases.

This study contradicts the results of one conducted earlier by Buettner and coworkers[10] in 200 patients with possible trigeminal pathology of varied etiology, including 20 with "trigeminal neuralgia." Overall, they found a significant difference in the P19 short latency between the healthy side and the compromised side.

We have little experience with this technique in our laboratory owing to the great difficulty associated with the recording, which includes a major artifact of the stimulation technique. This may be due to either perspiration, which increases skin resistance, or the proximity of the recording and stimulation electrodes.

EVOKED POTENTIALS IN PEDIATRICS

The literature on evoked potentials in pediatric medicine is quite limited. Since evoked potentials provide a noninvasive method of studying the somatosensory system from the periphery to the central area, they can be of great utility in infants and children, in whom at times no other method is suitable.

Somatosensory Evoked Potentials

Several changes occur as the somatosensory system matures: the pathway lengthens, average myelinization of portions of the pathway varies, and the number of synapses in the pathway increases. In the most peripheral part, nerve conduction velocity reaches its maximum between 18 and 27 months of age. At the cerebral level, not all the components of the SEP are present in a term infant; N19 is consistent after 6 to 12 weeks of life. The thalamus contains myelin in 87% of term newborns. Subcortical radiations may appear as P37 (P40) responses around three months of age (posterior tibial nerve).

Non-REM sleep affects cortical peak P22 (median nerve), but not N19 or P37 (posterior tibial nerve). REM sleep does not affect peak P22. The effect of non-REM sleep is greater in infants than in children. It is preferable not to sedate children before three months of age. Gilmore[35] found that when children are sedated, peaks N19 (median nerve) and P35 (posterior tibial nerve) are attenuated. The latencies may also be prolonged, which may lead to the false conclusion that a pathology exists.

Willis et al.[103] conducted a study of SEPs in 61 normal children up to one year of age, establishing normal parameters and clarifying the optimal technique. Both median nerves were stimulated at the wrist with the same technique used in adults, and the recording was at cortical levels C4' and C3', spinal CII-Fz, and brachial plexus Erb-Fz. None of the children was sedated. All were term infants without neurologic alterations.

The children tolerated the procedure quite well. They cried when the electrodes were put in place and at the beginning of the stimulation, but after a short time they calmed down and slept during the recording. The normal latency values (in milliseconds) are shown in Table 6.

Several premature children who survived intraventricular intracranial hemorrhages had SEP anomalies that reflected the clinical situation. This suggests the utility of SEP study in following the progress of such infants.

In degenerative compromises of the nervous system, SEP anomalies have been described in polioencephalopathies (affecting primarily the gray matter) and leukodystrophies. In most of these compromises the peripheral components are normal, except in the case of metachromatic leukodystrophy. Tobimatsu et al.[97] demonstrated that the SEPs of the median nerve are of great value in differentiating between adrenomyeloneuropathy and adrenoleukodystrophy. The central conduction time is prolonged in both cases, but in adrenomyeloneuropathy the latencies are also prolonged. Gary and coworkers[32] suggest that the somatosensory evoked potential is more sensitive than the auditory evoked potential in showing anomalies associated with the adrenoleukodystrophy gene.

Rossini and associates[77] reported alteration of the SEPs in other neurodegenerative compromises: Friedreich's ataxia, hereditary sensorimotor neuropathy, familial spastic paraplegia, olivopontocerebellar atrophy, and ataxia-telangiectasia.

Obstetric compromise of the brachial plexus is a common peripheral lesion. We have conducted a few prognostic examinations in cases of this

Table 6. Normal latency values for SEPs from the median nerve in children under 1 year of age, from a study by Willis et al.[61]

Age	N9	N13	N19	Central conduction time
Newborn	6.2 ± 0.7	9.4 ± 0.4	24.3 ± 2.1	15.5
2 months	5.6 ± 0.5	8.7 ± 0.7	20.2 ± 1.5	11.5
4 months	5.6 ± 0.3	8.3 ± 0.7	19.1 ± 1.3	10.6
6 months	5.6 ± 0.6	8.1 ± 0.4	17.4 ± 0.9	9.1
8 months	5.3 ± 0.6	8.1 ± 0.6	17.2 ± 1.7	9.1
10 months	5.5 ± 0.7	11.3 ± 1.4	17.7 ± 0.9	6.4

pathology in the ulnar, median, and musculocutaneous nerves, depending on which plexal trunk has the greatest compromise. We began recording at three upper extremity levels: brachial plexus (N9), spinal (N13), and cortical (N19). Given that the more peripheral Erb's point and spinal levels proved difficult and provided little precise information, we have routinely used cortical recording as the follow-up technique, since it is easier and more reliable in young infants. Prolongation of the cortical response has a direct correlation with the degree of compromise of the brachial plexus (primary and/or secondary trunks) and can be used for prognosis.

Auditory Evoked Potentials

Schulman-Galambos studied 373 infants treated in an intensive care unit who had severe auditory sensorineural deficits revealed by auditory evoked potentials. These deficits were later confirmed by conventional audiometric techniques. The authors recommend that AEP testing be used routinely in all pediatric intensive care units.

In a study of 41 infants and children who had bacterial meningitis, 26 had normal AEPs (Group 1), 10 had a prolonged wave I (Group 2), and 5 had no response (Group 3). There was no correlation of these results with age, bacterial organism involved, antibiotic therapy, spinal fluid electrolytes, or spinal fluid proteins. Five children in Group 2 were tested again after nine months, and four of them had normal responses. The five children in Group 3 had auditory evoked potential abnormalities in subsequent tests.

It has been reported that the auditory evoked potentials were normal in victims of sudden infant death syndrome. Stockard and Hecox[93] studied 47 children with other apnea syndromes and found abnormal AEPs in 15 (32%); among these children the incidence of respiratory arrest was high (5 of 15) compared to those who had normal AEPs. None of the children died from respiratory arrest during follow-up period of 3 to 36 months.

Prolongation of interpeaks has been reported in children with metabolic disorders (hyperglycemia and phenylketonuria).

Abnormal auditory evoked potentials have been found in gliomas of the brain stem in all 21 cases reported in the literature.

Hecox et al.[45] studied 126 children who had experienced a significant period of asphyxia. Twenty-one of them had a marked anomaly in the amplitude of waves I-V; all had severe neurologic deficits. Nevertheless, amplitude of waves I and V within the normal range does not always indicate normality on discharge since 10 children continued to have severe disability.

Visual Evoked Potentials

Visual evoked potentials have been recorded in children of all ages, including neonates, since they have been used to follow the development of the visual system and to monitor the efficacy of treatment of amblyopia and corneal opacity.

Kurtzberg[54] reported the results of flash VEP in 79 high-risk children. Fifty-one percent had normal responses; the remaining 49% displayed anomalies, with asymmetry of amplitude in the responses between the hemispheres. Ninety-two percent of the children with normal VEPs continued to have good responses in follow-up during their first six months of life. Those with VEP anomalies continued to have them.

Multimodality

Multimodality is indicated in children with severe hypoxia. It is believed that auditory evoked potentials and the somatosensory evoked potential of the median nerve are better predictors of a chronic vegetative status than EEG and clinical examination.

In 18 pediatric patients with AIDS, Udani and coworkers[100] investigated development using clinical findings, AEPs, SEPs, and MRI. Results were as follows: 33% had microcephaly, 56% had motor alterations, 18% had changes in the AEP and central conduction time (N19-N13), 25% had peripheral anomalies of the AEP, 79% had abnormal median nerve SEPs, and a little over 20% of the MRI studies showed specific alteration. The authors conclude that an SEP anomaly is common in early stages of this disease and can be useful in its follow-up.

REFERENCES

1. Allison T, Wood C, Goff W. Brain stem auditory, pattern-reversal visual, and short-latency somatosensory evoked potentials: latencies in relation to age, sex, and brain and body size. *Electroencephalogr Clin Neurophysiol.* 1983;55:619–636.
2. Aminoff MJ, Davis SL, Pantich HS. Serial evoked potential studies in patients with definite multiple sclerosis: clinical relevance. *Arch Neurol.* 1984;41:1197–1202.
3. Aminoff MJ, Goodin DS, Barbaro NM, et al. Dermatomal somatosensory evoked potentials in unilateral lumbosacral radiculopathy. *Ann Neurol.* 1985;17:171–176.
4. Anziska B, Cracco RQ, Cook AW, Feld EW. Somatosensory far field potentials: studies in normal subjects and patients with multiple sclerosis. *Electroencephalogr Clin Neurophysiol.* 1978;45:602–610.
5. Arezzo J, Schaumburg H, Vaugh H, Spencer P, Barna J. Hind limb somatosensory evoked potentials in the monkey: the effects of distal axonapathy. *Ann Neurol.* 1982;12:24–32.
6. Baker JB, et al. Evoked potentials as an aid to the diagnosis of multiple sclerosis. *Neurology (Minneapolis).* 1968;18:286.
7. Baran EM. Spinal cord responses to peripheral nerve stimulation in man. *Arch Phys Med Rehabil.* 1980;61:10–17.
8. Barber C, Blum T. *Evoked potentials III.* Stoneham, MA: Butterworth's; 1987.
9. Bradley O, Fletcher W. Spinal cord distribution of somatic innervation of the external urethral sphincter of the cat. *J Neurol Sci.* 1970;10:11–23.
10. Buettner U, Petruch F, Scheglemann K, Stohr M. Diagnostic significance of cortical somatosensory evoked potentials following trigeminal nerve stimulation. In: Courjon J, Mauguiere F, Revol M, eds. *Clinical applications of evoked potentials in neurology.* New York: Raven Press; 1982:339–345.
11. Caccia MR, Ubiali E, Andreussi L. Spinal evoked responses recorded from the epidural

space in normal and diseased humans. *J Neurol Neurosurg Psychiatry.* 1976;39:962–972.

12. Cassvan A. Cortical somatosensory evoked potentials following peroneal nerve stimulation in lumbo-sacral radiculopathies [abstract]. *Arch Phys Med Rehabil.* 1981;62:508.
13. Caton R. The electric currents of the brain. *Br Med J.* 1975b;2:278.
14. Caton R. Interim report on investigation of the electric currents of the brain. *Br Med J.* 1977(Suppl);1:62–63.
15. Chiappa K, Ropper A. Evoked potentials in clinical medicine (second of two parts). *N Engl J Med.* 1982;306(20):1205–1210.
16. Chodoroff G, Lee DW, Honet JC. Dynamic approach in the diagnosis of thoracic outlet syndrome using somatosensory evoked responses. *Arch Phys Med Rehabil.* 1985;66:3–6.
17. Cracco RQ. Spinal evoked response: peripheral nerve stimulation in man. *Electroencephalogr Clin Neurophysiol.* 1973;35:379–386.
18. Dawson GD. Cerebral responses to electrical stimulation of peripheral nerve in man. *J Neurol Neurosurg Psychiatry.* 1947;10:134–140.
19. Díaz V, Tapia R, Brink G, Gutiérrez M, Hurtado C, del Peso G. Intoxicación por talio: tratamiento con azul de Prusia en 4 casos. *Rev Med Chile.* 1990;118:183–185.
20. Dick HD, Bradley WE, Scott FF, Timm GW. Pudendal sexual reflexes: electrophysiologic investigations. *Urology.* 1974;3:376.
21. Dimitrijevic MR, Larson L, Lehmkuhl D, Sherwood A. Evoked spinal cord and nerve root potentials in humans using a non-invasive recording technique. *Electroencephalogr Clin Neurophysiol.* 1978;45:331–340.
22. Dimitrijevic MR, Prevec MTS, Sherwood A. Somatosensory perception and cortical evoked potentials in established paraplegia. *J Neurol Sci.* 1983;60:253–256.
23. Dorfman LJ, Bosley TM. Age-related changes in peripheral and central nerve conduction in man. *Neurology (Minneapolis).* 1979;29:38–44.
24. Drechsler F. Short latency SEP to median nerve stimulation: recording methods, origin of components and clinical application. *Electromyogr Clin Neurophysiol.* 1985;25:115–134.
25. Egerhazi A, Dioszeghy P, Mechler F. Somatosensory evoked potentials in spinal muscular atrophies and hereditary motor sensory neuropathies. *Electromyogr Clin Neurophysiol.* 1988;28:285–288.
26. Eisen AM, Elleker G. Sensory nerve stimulation and cerebral potentials. *Neurology.* 1980;30:1097–1105.
27. Eisen A, Stewart J, Nudleman K. Cord to cortex conduction in multiple sclerosis. *Neurology (Minneapolis).* 1979;29:189–193.
28. Eisen AM, Stewart J, Nudleman K. Abnormalities of early-latency somatosensory potentials in multiple sclerosis. *Neurology.* 1979;29:104.
29. El Negamy E, Sedgwick EM. Delayed cervical somatosensory potentials in cervical spondylosis. *J Neurol Neurosurg Psychiatry.* 1979;42:238–241.
30. Fotiou F, Tsisopoulos P, et al. Evaluation of the somatosensory evoked potentials in brain death. *Electromyogr Clin Neurophysiol.* 1987;27:55–60.
31. Ganji S, Frazier E. Somatosensory evoked potentials studies in acute Guillain-Barré syndrome. *Electromyogr Clin Neurophysiol.* 1988;28:313–317.
32. Gary BP, et al. Evoked response studies in patients with adenoleukodystrophy and heterozygous relatives. *Arch Neurol.* 1983;40:355–359.
33. Gasser HS, Graham HT. Potentials produced in spinal cord by stimulation of dorsal roots. *Am J Physiol.* 1933;103:303–320.
34. Giesser BS, Kurtzberg SD, Vaughan JHG, et al. Trimodal evoked potentials compared with magnetic resonance imaging in the diagnosis of multiple sclerosis. *Arch Neurol.* 1987;44:281–284.
35. Gilmore RL. Effects of sleep on central conduction time in infants and children. Paper presented at International EEG Congress Scientific Session. London; August 1983.
36. Glover JL, Worth RM, Bendick PJ, Hall PV, Markand OM. Evoked responses in the diagnosis of thoracic outlet syndrome. *Surgery.* 1981;88:86–89.
37. González EG, Berman WS, Hajdu M. Influence of height and type of lower extremity nerve tested on P1 somatosensory evoked potential [abstract]. *Arch Phys Med Rehabil.* 1983;64:502.

38. González E, Hajdu M, Keim R, Brand L. Lumbar spinal stenosis: analysis of pre- and postoperative somatosensory evoked potentials. *Arch Phys Med Rehabil.* 1985;66:11–15.
39. González E, Hajdu M, Roye D, Brand L. Intraoperative somatosensory evoked potential monitoring. *Orthop Rev.* 1984;13:573–578.
40. Green JB, Walcoff MR. Evoked potentials in multiple sclerosis. *Arch Neurol.* 1982;39:696–697.
41. Grupta PR, Dorfmann LT. Spinal somatosensory conduction in diabetes. *Neurology (Minneapolis).* 1981;31:841–845.
42. Haldeman S, Bradley WE, Bhatia N, et al. Pudendal evoked responses. *Arch Neurol.* 1982;39:280–284.
43. Happel LT, Leblanc HJ, Kline DG. Spinal cord potentials evoked by peripheral nerve stimulation. *Electroencephalogr Clin Neurophysiol.* 1975;38:349–354.
44. Hazemann P, Jeftic M, Lille F. Somatosensory evoked potentials in alcoholics and patients occupationally exposed to solvents and lead. *Electromyogr Clin Neurophysiol.* 1987;27:183–187.
45. Hecox KE, Cone B, Blaw ME. Brainstem auditory response in the diagnosis of pediatric neurologic disease. *Neurology.* 1981;31:832.
46. Heiss WD, Rosner G. Functional recovery of cortical neurons as related to degree and duration of ischemia. *Ann Neurol.* 1983;14:294–301.
47. Hume A, Cant B. Conduction time in central somatosensory pathways in man. *Electroencephalogr Clin Neurophysiol.* 1978;45:361–375.
48. Hume A, Cant B, Shaw N, Cowan J. Central somatosensory conduction time from 10 to 79 years. *Electroencephalogr Clin Neurophysiol.* 1982;54:49–54.
49. Iwasaki Y, Tashiro K, et al. Cervical flexion myelopathy: a "tight dural canal mechanism." *J Neurosurg.* 1987;66:935–937.
50. Jacobs H, Vanderstragten G, et al. SEPS and central somatosensory conduction time in hemiplegics. *Electromyogr Clin Neurophysiol.* 1988;28:355–360.
51. Jones SJ. Short latency potentials recorded from the neck and scalp following median nerve stimulation in man. *Electroencephalogr Clin Neurophysiol.* 1977;43:853–863.
52. Jones S, Carrol W, Halliday A. Peripheral and central sensory nerve conduction in Charcot-Marie-Tooth disease and comparison with Friedreich's ataxia. *J Neurol Sci.* 1983;61:135–148.
53. Kaplan P. Somatosensory evoked responses obtained after stimulation of the pelvic and pudendal nerves. *Electromyogr Clin Neurophysiol.* 1983;23:99–102.
54. Kurtzberg SD, Vaughan JHG Jr. Electrophysiologic assessment of auditory and visual function in the newborn. *Clin Perinatol.* 1985;12(10):277–299.
55. LaJoie WJ, Reddy NM, Melvin J. Somatosensory evoked potentials: their predictive value in right hemiplegia. *Arch Phys Med Rehabil.* 1982;63:223–226.
56. Liberson W. Scalp distribution of somatosensory evoked potentials and aging. *Electromyogr Clin Neurophysiol.* 1976;16:221–224.
57. Lue T, Salim J, et al. Neuroanatomy of penile erection: its relevance to iatrogenic impotence. *J Urol.* 1984;131:273–280.
58. Magladery JW, Porter WE, Park AM, Teasdall RD. Electrophysiological studies of nerve and reflex activity in normal man; IV, two-neurone reflex and identification of certain action potentials from spinal roots and cord. *Bull Johns Hopkins Hosp.* 1951;88:499–519.
59. Mastaglia FL, Black JL, Collins DWK. Visual and spinal evoked potentials in diagnosis of multiple sclerosis. *Br Med J.* 1976;3:732.
60. Mauguiere F, Desmedt J, Courjon J. Neural generator of N18 and far-field somatosensory evoked potentials; studies in patients with lesion of thalamus or thalamo-cortical radiations. *Electroencephalogr Clin Neurophysiol.* 1983;56:292–293.
61. McGarry J, Friedgood DL, Woolsey R, Horenstein S, Johnson C. Somatosensory evoked potentials in spinal cord injuries. *Surg Neurol.* 1984;22:341–343.
62. Meyer KL, Dempsey RL, Roy MW, Donaldson DL. Somatosensory evoked potentials as a measure of experimental cerebral ischemia. *J Neurosurg.* 1985;62:269–275.
63. Mutti A, Ferr F, Lommi G, Lotta S, Lucertini S, Franchini I. Solvent induced changes in nerve conduction velocities and somatosensory evoked potentials. *Int Arch Occup Environ Health.* 1982;51:45–54.

64. Newlon PG, Greenberg RP. Evoked potentials in severe head injury. *J Trauma.* 1984;24:61–66.
65. Notermans SL, Vlek NM. Cortical and spinal somatosensory evoked potentials in patients suffering from lumbosacral disc prolapse. *Electromyogr Clin Neurophysiol.* 1988;28:33–37.
66. Opsomer RJ, Guerit Wese FX, Van Cangh PJ. Pudendal cortical somatosensory evoked potentials. *J Urol.* 1986;135:1216–1218.
67. Paradiso G, Fernández M. Potenciales evocados somatosensitivos espinales y corticales de los nervios tibial y mediano en pacientes con insuficiencia renal crónica y transplante renal. *Rev Neurol Argent.* 1985;11(3):152.
68. Parra SA de la, Bertotti AC. Neuralgia esencial trigeminal. *Rev Neurol Argent.* 1985;11:127–132.
69. Peso G del, Paolinelli L. Neuroconducción en las disfunciones sexuales masculinas. *Rev Sanidad Def Nac (Chile).* 1991;8:38–47.
70. Perot PL, Vera CL. Scalp recorded somatosensory evoked potentials to stimulation of nerves in the lower extremities and evaluation of patients with spinal cord trauma. *Ann NY Acad Sci.* 1982;388:359–368.
71. Phillips KR, Potvin AR, et al. Multimodality evoked potentials and neurophysiological tests in multiple sclerosis. *Arch Neurol.* 1983;40:159–164.
72. Pravdich-Neminsky VV. Ein Versuch der Registrierung der elektrischen Gehirnerscheinungen [Experiments on the registration of the electrical phenomena of the mammalian brain]. *Zentralbl Physiol.* 1913;27:951–960.
73. Pravdich-Neminsky VV. Einige elektrische Erscheinungen in Zentralnervensystem bei *Rana temporaria. Arch Anat Physiol.* 1913:321–324.
74. Rapaport S. Spinal conduction velocities determined with peroneal nerve stimulation in man. *Neurology.* 1984;34(suppl 1):134.
75. Robinson RK, Richey ET, Kase CSM, Mohe JP. Somatosensory evoked potentials in pure sensory stroke and allied conditions. *Neurology.* 1984;34:231.
76. Rossini P, Treviso M, Di Steffano E, Di Paolo B. Nervous impulse propagation along peripheral and central fibers in patients with chronic renal failure. *Electroencephalogr Clin Neurophysiol.* 1983;56:293–303.
77. Rossini PM, Zarola F, Di Capu M, et al. Somatosensory evoked potentials in neurodegenerative system disorders. In: Gallai, ed. *Maturation of the CNS and evoked potentials.* Amsterdam: Elsevier; 1986.
78. Rowed DW, McLean JA, Tator CM. Somatosensory evoked potentials in acute spinal cord injury: prognostic value. *Surg Neurol.* 1978;9:203–210.
79. Rubio Esteban G, Remartinez Lagranja A, Cid López MA, Marin Redondo M, Asiron Yribarren P. Delayed short-latency somatosensory evoked potentials in premature diagnosis of medullar disturbances in cervical spondylosis. *Electromyogr Clin Neurophysiol.* 1988;28:361–368.
80. Rumpl E. Prugger M, Gersterbrand F, Hackl JM. Central somatosensory conduction time and short latency somatosensory evoked potentials in post-traumatic coma. *Electroencephalogr Clin Neurophysiol.* 1983;56:583–596.
81. Sarica Y, Karacan I. Bulbocavernosus reflex to somatic and visceral nerve stimulation in normal subjects and in diabetics with erectile impotence. *J Urol.* 1987;138:55–58.
82. Scarff TB, Dallmann DE, Toleikis JR, Bunch WH. Dermatomal somatosensory evoked potentials in the diagnosis of lumbar root entrapment. *Surg Forum.* 1981;32:489–491.
83. Scarff TB, Toleikis JR, Bunch WH, Parrish S. Dermatomal somatosensory evoked potentials in children with myelomeningocele. *Z Kinderchir.* 1979;28:384–387.
84. Schramm J, Shigeno T, Brock M. Clinical signs and evoked response alterations associated with chronic experimental cord compression. *J Neurosurg.* 1983;58:734–741.
85. Seyal M, Emmerson RG, Pedley TA. Spinal and early scalp recorded components of the somatosensory evoked potential following stimulation of posterior tibial nerve. *Electroencephalogr Clin Neurophysiol.* 1983;55:320–330.
86. Shaw NA. The effects of experimental concussion on cervical and thalamic somatosensory evoked potentials. *Electromyogr Clin Neurophysiol.* 1988;28:67–73.
87. Shiff JA, Cracco RQ, Rossini PM, Cracco JB. Spine and scalp somatosensory evoked potentials in normal subjects and patients with spinal cord disease: evaluation of afferent transmission. *Electroencephalogr Clin Neurophysiol.* 1984;59:374–384.

88. Shimoji K, Kano T, Higashi H, Morioka T, Herschel EO. Evoked spinal electrograms recorded from epidural space in man. *J Appl Physiol.* 1972;33:468–471.
89. Shin DY, Ehrenberg B, Whyte J, Bach J, DeLisa JA. Evoked potential assessment: utility in prognosis of chronic head injury. *Arch Phys Med Rehabil.* 1989;70:189–193.
90. Siroky M, Sax D, Krane R. Sacral signal tracing; the electrophysiology of the bulbocavernosus reflex. *J Urol.* 1979;122:661–664.
91. Small DG, Beauchamp M, Matthews WB. Spinal evoked potentials in multiple sclerosis. *Electroencephalogr Clin Neurophysiol.* 1977;42:141.
92. Small M, Matthews WB. A method of calculating spinal cord transit time from potentials evoked by tibial nerve stimulation in normal subjects and patients with spinal cord disease. *Electroencephalogr Clin Neurophysiol.* 1984;59:156–164.
93. Stockard JJ, Hecox K. Brainstem auditory evoked potentials in sudden infant death syndrome (SIDS), near-miss for SIDS and infant apnea syndromes [abstract]. *Electroencephalogr Clin Neurophysiol.* 1981;51:43P.
94. Stohr M, Dichgans J, Voigt K, Buettner U. The significance of somatosensory evoked potentials for localization of unilateral lesions within the cerebral hemisphere. *J Neurol Sci.* 1983;61:49–63.
95. Stohr M, Petruch F. Somatosensory evoked potentials following stimulation of the trigeminal nerve in man. *J Neurol.* 1979;220:95–98.
96. Symon L, Hargdine J, Zawirski M, Branston N. Central conduction time as an index of ischaemia in subarachnoid hemorrhage. *J Neurol Sci.* 1979;44:95–103.
97. Tobimatsu S, Fukui R, Kato M, et al. Multimodality evoked potentials in patients and carriers with adrenoleukodystrophy and adrenomyeloneuropathy. *Electroencephalogr Clin Neurophysiol.* 1985;62:18–24.
98. Triantafyllou N, Rombos A, Athanasopoulou H, Siafakas A, Loulakaki SM. Electrophysiological study (EEG, VEPS, BAEPS) in patients with Charcot-Marie-Tooth (Type H, MSN 1) disease. *Electromyogr Clin Neurophysiol.* 1989;29:259–263.
99. Tsuji S, Shibasaki H, Kato M, Kuroiwa Y, Shima F. Subcortical, thalamic and cortical somatosensory evoked potentials to median nerve stimulation. *Electroencephalogr Clin Neurophysiol.* 1984;59:465–476.
100. Udani V, Cracco JB, Hittelman J, et al. Clinical and developmental evaluation, evoked potentials and MRI in pediatric AIDS. American EEG Society Scientific Session, St. Louis, 18 September 1987.
101. Urra X, del Peso G, Gutiérrez A, Díaz V. Estudio precoz de electrodiagnóstico neuromuscular comparativo en pacientes con síndrome de Guillain-Barré con tratamiento de plasmaferesis o sin él. *Rev Hosp Clin Univ Chile.* 1990;1(2):52–59.
102. Verroust J, Blinowska A, Vilfrit R, Couperie D, Malapert D, Perrier M. Somatosensory evoked potentials from posterior tibial nerve; normative data. *Electromyogr Clin Neurophysiol.* 1989;29:299–303.
103. Willis J, Seales D, Frazier E. Short-latency somatosensory evoked potentials in infants. *Electroencephalogr Clin Neurophysiol.* 1984;59:366–373.

Chapter 10

INSTITUTION OF REHABILITATION DURING INTENSIVE CARE

Murray M. Freed

The advances in diagnostic and therapeutic skills let many patients survive diseases and trauma which would have doomed them in decades past. The price of survival, however, may be a permanent or temporary disability which may include long periods of immobilization. The morbidity of a long term illness or surgery is often in part caused by the immobilization that circumstances have imposed on the patient.

F.U. Steinberg, 1980[5]

ENVIRONMENTAL MANIPULATION

The measures needed for environmental manipulation during intensive care are as important to consider as those carried out during the entire rehabilitation process and during independent living after treatment in an institution. These measures are mainly for prevention of psychological and physical complications and for maintenance of neuromusculoskeletal function.

In many instances, when the patient is isolated in a poorly lighted area without external stimulation except for the incessant drone and pulsing of monitoring devices, this lack of stimulation leads to anxiety and, not infrequently, visual and auditory hallucinations.[7] In the elderly patient, the problem is compounded by the pre-existing deterioration of vision—one of the most frequent changes that occur with senescence—and commonly by conductive hearing loss as well.

Stimulation includes acceptable lighting as a vision enhancer, clocks and calendars in the field of vision to provide time orientation, and provision of prism spectacles for improved environmental vision when the individual must be kept supine. Also included is the placement near the patient of familiar pictures and objects brought from home.

STRESS MANAGEMENT

Occupational therapy programs during the period of intensive care include relaxation techniques to decrease the stress imposed by isolation and sensory deprivation. The following are common techniques for the reduction of stress:[1]

Breathing.   Rapid and/or shallow breathing is one component of a physiological awareness and controlled response to stress. By learning to control breathing, individuals can begin to reverse their own "fight or flight" response and alter their experience of stress.

Imagination.   Visualization, or the active focusing of attention on healing images, successful treatment, or a healthy state, can be used to reduce tension and anxiety and to mobilize inner resources toward recovery. Guided imagery is a more passive resting of attention and a self-directing as one listens to music or a voice and imagines a particular "haven" from a stressful experience.

Autogenic training.   Based on the work of Oskar Vogt,[6] this systematic program is designed to teach the body and mind to respond quickly and effectively to self-given commands to relax.

Progressive relaxation.   This technique uses the voluntary tensing and releasing of muscle groups to identify muscles and muscle groups holding tension in the body. Individuals are taught to distinguish between tension and deep relaxation and to begin to control the level of muscle tension they experience.

Relaxation music.   Peaceful, soothing music that contains no lyrics and does not evoke an emotional response can be used alone or in tandem with other techniques to reduce stress.

Meditation.   As practiced independently of any religious or philosophical orientation, meditation is an experiential exercise involving the resting of an individual's attention and focus on one object, thought, or word for a period of time.

PULMONARY THERAPY

Surgical and medical conditions, compounded by enforced bed rest, interfere with adequate pulmonary function. In the upright position motion of the ribs contributes to tidal volume; in recumbency the costal movements are reduced, resulting in decreased tidal volume. Muscle weakness resulting from immobilization reduces vital capacity. Poor ventilation of the dependent segments of the lungs results in hypoxemia, since perfusion is not altered.

Bronchioles are made susceptible to infection by prolonged bed rest. The recumbent position interferes with normal ciliary function; mucus pools on the underside of the bronchioles, causing the uppermost surfaces of the bronchioles to lose this protective layer.

The indications for consideration of chest physical therapy are the following:

Medical Patients

- patients with increased sputum production (or increased pooling of secretions, whether in large airways or in lungs, discovered by chest x-ray showing an infiltrate);
- patients with increased intrapulmonary shunting secondary to atelactasis or pulmonary edema;
- patients having a history of chronic obstructive lung disease;
- patients with restrictive lung disease;
- patients with occupational lung disease;
- elderly, semi-immobile, or obese patients;
- patients with diagnosed pulmonary conditions such as cystic fibrosis, lung abscess, interstitial lung disease, etc.;
- patients with neuromuscular conditions such as spinal cord injury, Guillain-Barré syndrome, myesthenia gravis, amyotropic lateral sclerosis, cerebral vascular accident, and others that may involve or have potential to compromise respiratory muscle function;
- patients with single or multiple rib fractures and consequent interference with normal respiration;
- patients after drug overdose;
- patients with restrictive burns to thoracic cage or inhalation burns;
- patients with aspiration pneumonia.

Surgical Patients

- all open heart surgical patients (they are seen preoperatively for evaluation and teaching and are followed postoperatively for pulmonary management, mobility, and exercise);
- surgical patients with a history of or predisposition to respiratory complications (these patients should be seen preoperatively for training in breathing techniques);
- any surgical patient who has or develops recurring bronchitis, asthma, chronic obstructive pulmonary disease, or pneumonia; a known heavy smoker or obese patient;
- all postoperative thoracotomy patients;
- all upper abdominal surgical patients;

- lower abdominal surgical patients with respiratory problems;
- patients requiring prolonged ventilator support after surgery.

Precautions in Chest Physical Therapy

The following are guidelines to contraindications or precautionary measures in giving chest physical therapy when certain invasive procedures have been used in patient management or in the face of certain diagnoses.

Invasive Procedures

Transvenous pacemaker.   Patient must be kept as still as possible. Aggressive percussion and vibration could dislodge pacing wires. Precautions to avoid vigorous treatments should be taken, especially during the first 48 to 72 hours.

Intra-aortic balloon pump.   Presence of the pump should alert the therapist to patient's poor left ventricular function. Treatment, including percussion and vibration is *not* contraindicated. It is important to note that patient should not flex hip or knee of the lower extremity through which the balloon is inserted. Caution should also be taken not to percuss or vibrate over the cardiac monitor leads.

Left ventricular assist device.   Treatment is delayed for the first 24 to 48 hours. After this period of time, based on patient stability and need, treatment can be initiated.

Chest tubes.   There is no contraindication to treatment. Percussion and vibration over the site of insertion should be avoided. It is important to encourage chest expansion on the side of the chest tube.

Peritoneal dialysis.   Deep breathing and coughing and use of incentive spirometry are good prophylactic measures. If percussion or vibration is required, it should be avoided during swelling or infusion of liquid.

Hemodialysis.   Therapy can be done, with caution, while patient is on hemodialysis unit. Positions are modified to accommodate tubing length.

Diagnoses

Acute spinal cord injuries.   Patients with cervical cord injury can be treated vigorously with percussion and vibration. When placed in skeletal traction, patients with cervical cord injury are not tipped for postural drainage. It is very important to know the level of injury and the stability of the fracture site before treating.

Low platelets.   The normal range is 200,000 to 500,000 per cu. mm. Percussion should be avoided on patients with a platelet count of 50,000 or less; deep breathing should be stressed, and vibration may be continued in spite of low platelet counts.

Rib fractures.   If fracture site is unstable or there is flail chest, percussion and vigorous vibration are to be avoided. Deep breathing and coughing are very advantageous in treatment of fractured ribs. Binders may be used for patient comfort when the patient is encouraged to cough or inspire deeply. The binder should *not* be kept on constantly as it may impede adequate breathing.

Abscess.   In the case of lung abscess, careful positioning of patients is imperative to avoid spread of the abscess to other lung segments. Techniques including percussion and vibration are often very important treatments in conjunction with specific drug management.

BASIC GUIDELINES: PERCUSSION, VIBRATION (SHAKING), POSTURAL DRAINAGE

Postural Drainage

Indications

1. Secretions—infiltrate present in the lung
2. Atelectasis
3. Splinting with decreased breath sounds in an area
4. Collapse of a lung segment

Contraindications

1. Unstable cardiac conditions
2. Unstable fluid balance resulting in:
   a. Congestive heart failure
   b. Pulmonary edema
   c. Unstable blood pressure
3. Unstable neurologic conditions
   a. Cerebral aneurysm
   b. Increasing intercranial pressure
   c. Coma or loss of consciousness with unestablished etiology
4. Increased abdominal girth
   a. Obesity
   b. Distention
5. Nausea
6. Shortness of breath

Percussion

Indications

1. Excess secretions
2. Aspiration
3. Atelectasis
4. Collapse of a lobe
5. Collapse of a lung—after chest tube insertion

Contraindications

1. Rib fracture—flail chest
2. Degenerative bone disease
3. Excessive pain
4. Obesity over rib cage
5. High-dose anticoagulant drugs
6. Unstable cardiac conditions
7. Hemoptysis

Vigorous Shaking

Indications

1. Excess secretions
2. Aspiration
3. Atelectasis
4. Collapse of a lobe
5. Collapse of a lung—after chest tube insertion

Contraindications

1. Rib fracture—flail chest
2. Degenerative bone disease
3. Excessive pain
4. High-dose anticoagulant drugs
5. Unstable cardiac conditions
6. Hemoptysis
7. Presence of a Greenfield filter.

Moderate Shaking

Indications

1. Excess secretions
2. Aspiration

3. Atelectasis
4. Collapse of a lobe
5. Collapse of a lung—after chest tube insertion

Contraindications

1. Rib fracture—flail chest
2. Unstable cardiac conditions
3. Hemoptysis
4. Presence of a Greenfield filter.

Vibration

Indications

To be used whenever shaking is contraindicated; use in conjunction with relaxation breathing exercises.

Contraindications

None.

Postural Drainage Positions

Left upper lobe, posterior segment: One quarter turn to left from prone lying position with right arm outstretched posteriorly; three pillows used to raise head and shoulders.

Right upper lobe, posterior segment: One quarter turn to right from prone lying position with left arm outstretched posteriorly; one pillow supporting right arm.

Upper lobes, anterior segments: Supine position with pillow under knees to aid relaxation.

Left upper lobe, lingula: One quarter turn from supine position with left side uppermost; knees are flexed, foot of bed raised 12 inches, a pillow supports back.

Right middle lobe: One quarter turn from supine position, with right side uppermost; knees are flexed, foot of bed raised 12 inches, a pillow supports back.

Lower lobes, apical segments: Lying prone with pillow under abdomen to flatten back and another pillow under ankles.

Left lower lobe, lateral basal segment: Lying on right side. Pillow at waistline to keep spine straight, foot of bed raised 18 to 20 inches, or hips on three pillows.

Right lower lobe, lateral basal segment: Lying on left side. Pillow at waistline to keep spine straight, foot of bed raised 18 to 20 inches, or hips on three pillows.

Lower lobes, anterior basal segments: Supine position with pillow under knees to aid relaxation, foot of bed raised 18 to 20 inches.

Lower lobes, posterior basal segments: Lying prone with two pillows under abdomen, foot of bed raised 18 to 20 inches. If patient can tolerate, he tips over side of bed with forearms resting on a pillow on the floor, trunk at a 45° angle to floor.

THERAPY DURING IMMOBILIZATION

Immobilization leads to deconditioning, a result of weakness, atrophy, and poor endurance.[3] This problem is compounded by loss of range of motion of joints resulting from persistent faulty positioning and lack of active joint motion. These adverse effects are frequently neglected in the seriously ill or injured patient while more manifest problems are being treated.

Body Positioning

Prevention of contracture due to the inherent illness or injury or persistent faulty positioning requires specific postural measures.

Lower extremity positioning includes maintaining the ankle at the neutral position by use of either a footboard or bilateral ankle-foot orthosis (AFO), the latter fabricated from well-padded available materials. The knees are maintained in extension and the hips in the neutral position, held by a trochanter roll to avoid hip flexion.

The upper extremities are positioned with the shoulders in abduction to 90° if possible. The elbow is placed to form a right angle, the wrist at 20° dorsiflexion (maintained by a cloth roll or splint), the digits in partial flexion, and the thumb in the opposed position. To avoid edema of the dorsum of the hands, they should be positioned above heart level.

For the intubated patient, the ventilator should be moved from right to left once daily, since the patient has a tendency to turn to the side of the ventilator.

Attention must be directed to prevention of pressure ulceration by providing periods of relief of pressure over the sacrum, trochanters, ischial tuberosities, and malleoli.

Therapeutic Exercise

All joints, when accessible and when conditions permit, should be moved through their full range of motion two to three times daily. Particular attention should be directed to the shoulders, wrists, hands, hips, and ankles.

Under the condition of complete bed rest and immobilization, a muscle will lose 1% to 3% of its strength per day, 10% to 15% per week, and 50% during a three to five week period.[2,4] It is recommended that muscle contractions at 20% to 30% of maximum tension for several seconds be performed at least four to six times daily. When the situation precludes joint motion, isometric exercises are appropriate. There is no general agreement on the use of electrical stimulation to retard muscle atrophy or strengthen individual muscles.[5] However, this technique is in use as an accepted form of muscle reeducation or training.

In some situations, overwork from treating weakness may prove to be injurious. Evidence exists that overuse or overwork of recovering muscles may result in an increase in weakness, often to the point of no recovery.[5] This phenomenon has been observed in poliomyelitis, Guillain-Barré syndrome, and other peripheral neuropathies, as well as in Duchenne muscular dystrophy. However, long-duration, low-intensity activity may not have adverse effects.[4]

In summary, there are appropriate, well-recognized rehabilitation measures available for use during intensive care to prevent the adverse consequences of isolation and immobilization. When followed, the likelihood of complications that require correction during the ongoing rehabilitation process is reduced.

REFERENCES

1. Affleck AT, Lieberman S, Polon J, Rohrkemper K. Providing occupational therapy in an intensive care unit. *Am J Occup Ther.* 1986;40:323–332.
2. Halar EM, Bell KR. Rehabilitation's relationship to inactivity. In: Kottke FJ, Lehmann JF, eds. *Krusen's handbook of physical medicine and rehabilitation.* 4th ed. Philadelphia: WB Saunders; 1990:1113–1133.
3. Herbison GJ, Jaweed MM, Ditunno Jr JF. Exercise therapies in peripheral neuropathies. *Arch Phys Med Rehabil.* 1983;64:201–205.
4. Jaweed MM, Herbison GJ, Ditunno Jr JF. Effect of swimming on compensatory hypertrophy of reinnervating soleus and plantaris muscles. *Am J Phys Med.* 1974;53:35–40.
5. Steinberg FU. *The immobilized patient.* New York: Plenum; 1980.
6. Vogt O, cited by Mason GL. *Guide to stress reduction.* Berkeley, CA: Peace Press; 1980.
7. Zubek JP, MacNeill M. Effects of immobilization: behavioral and EEG changes. *Can J Psychol.* 1966;20:316–334.

Chapter 11

QUANTITATIVE EVALUATION OF PHYSICAL DISABILITY AND RESTORATION FOR RETURN TO WORK

Richard F. Harvey, Norman A. Aliga, Jeffrey S. Cameron, and Burton J. Silverstein

INTRODUCTION

The practice of physiatry encompasses care of persons with impairments and disabilities during various segments of their continuum of health care. Since impairments and disabilities are usually secondarily contracted, there is a need for accurate quantitative measurement to describe the impairment or disability at first contact and to identify the effect of physiatric management and outcomes. In order to categorize quantitative measures, it is important to define an organizational concept of the continuum served by the physiatrist. The World Health Organization has assisted in this process with descriptions of the terms impairment, disability, and handicap. Recently, H. Livneh has provided a descriptive operational context of the continuum in rehabilitation.[18] This continuum describes a four-level system divided into biophysical, mental, and affective categories. The four-level system represents what he refers to as a person-environment congruence model (Table 1). Each of the levels are components of the continuum of health care which often require physiatric quantification.

The first level, or sub-body system, deals with cellular or molecular activities or, specifically, disease and injury elements. Quantitative measures of these elements are generally part of the acute care system and include our extensive laboratory, radiological, anatomical, and physiological measures. These are generally well quantified and are usually described with interval measures such as weight, length, degrees, etc. This quantification is readily available to the physiatrist when consulting on a given patient.

The second level, or body system, refers to organ systems, where deficiencies are called impairments. For such impairments as muscle weakness, decreased range of motion, and others, expanded quantifiable measures are needed to identify the entry points and the effect of physiatric care. Typically, observational measures using ordinal or estimated interval scales are employed by physiatrists. These include ordinal scales for strength or sensation and interval scales for measures of actual force of muscle contraction. Other body system or organ impairments involve the sensory, mental, and affective areas. Quantification of these impairments often utilizes psychometric testing methods.

The third level, or self system, involves person-integrated activities, more commonly called activities of daily living. An impairment affecting this system interferes with a person's ability to perform a specific activity and can be described as a disability. Functional assessment systems have been developed in many centers to describe these limitations or disabilities, and they most often use a nominal or ordinal scale.[26] True interval scales or measures are only recently appearing in the literature and are an important aspect of quantification of the entry level of disability, the effect of management, and outcome.

The final level, according to Livneh, is the extero-self system. At this level, a person's disability interferes with the capacity to function in the community in which he or she is active. Such interferences are referred to as handicaps. Key to the quantification of a handicap are quantifiable measures of impairment, disability, *and* environment. Quantifiable measures of environment are still being researched, and only a few operational methodologies have been published. Outcome measures, such as the ability to return to home, school, or work, are gross quantifiable measures of handicap.

In this chapter, quantifiable measurement of neuromuscular and musculoskeletal impairments will be discussed, as will quantifiable measures of disability. In order to interrelate these scales, it is important to utilize interval level measures whenever possible. Interval measures allow for comparisons and correlations of the impaired, disabled, or handicapped functions. These comparisons should make it possible to differentiate individuals, benefits of physiatric care, and rehabilitation outcomes. Such comparisons and correlations will then assist physiatric care in restoring persons towards

Table 1. Four-level "person-environment congruence model," adapted from H. Livneh.[18]

Levels	Health care problem	Quantifiable measures
Sub-body system	Disease, injury	Anatomical, physiological, laboratory, radiological
Body system	Impairment	Strength, flexibility, sensation, cognition, affect
Self system	Disability	Activities of daily living, functional performance
Extero-self system	Handicap	Environment-disability interaction

a specific goal and, it is hoped, with further research, toward predictable outcomes.

CENTRAL NERVOUS SYSTEM IMPAIRMENTS

Physiatric care is commonly provided to those persons with central nervous system impairments and disabilities. Significant advances have been made in the quantification of key impairments and disabilities, such as spasticity, loss of balance, and pain. Some of the methods to measure these impairments will be discussed.

Spasticity Quantification

Spasticity, which is present in a wide variety of neurological impairments with upper motor neuron dysfunction, can have both tonic and phasic components. The tendon tapping typically performed in the bedside examination tests the phasic component of the muscle stretch reflex. The tonic phase may be measured utilizing Ashworth's method.[2] In this method, spasticity is assessed manually by estimating resistance to passive range of motion, and the result is recorded with the Ashworth scale, an ordinal scale of values from one to four. One equals no tone, two equals considerable increase in tone with passive motion easily accomplished, three equals marked increase in tone with passive motion difficult, and four equals rigid limb positioning in flexion and in extension.

Numerous physiological methods have been devised to measure spasticity more quantitatively. EMG studies can demonstrate the latency, threshold, and magnitude of muscle response to tendon tapping, using a mechanical tapper that triggers the EMG sweep. Another measure utilizes the H reflex, since facilitation of H reflex recovery is enhanced in spasticity as compared to normals and the peak amplitude of the recovery curve is higher. Other recovery curve features may differentiate spasticity from various rigidity states. Pharmacological and mechanical intervention effects have been noted by comparing the H reflex response curves in treated and untreated spastic patients. Recorded EMG responses to tonic stretch reflex stimulation by angular velocity changes allow differentiation of spastic from normal limbs. Summated EMG responses vary in time of onset and magnitude with increasing angular velocity change. Studies utilizing the tonic stretch reflex measures have been shown to differentiate pharmacological and mechanical methods of intervention for the treatment of spasticity.[11]

In all quantitative measurements of spasticity, it is important to realize that wide variability in spasticity is seen in a given patient at different times of the day and with different levels of arousal or activity. This variability can obscure any changes seen as a result of modifications of medication or other treatments.

Balance Impairments

Many central nervous system disorders can result in impairments of balance. With recent advances in the field of posturography, we are now able to quantify what was previously a purely qualitative assessment. In the typical physical examination, balance is assessed by observing the patient's stance, gait, and tandem gait and by the Romberg Test. Sometimes, balance reactions are tested by the examiner perturbing the patient's balance. The results of these observations are generally recorded in qualitative, subjective terms (such as "very unsteady") because there is no standardized and accepted quantitative scale.

Fregly and Graybiel described a test for ataxia which challenges the patient to maintain balance for 30 seconds standing on the floor or on a foam cushion. The patient is asked to accomplish five consecutive trials of balancing for 30 seconds on each of the two surfaces utilizing three strategies: eyes open, eyes closed, and eyes open wearing a visual dome to obstruct vision. Displacement of the feet or the dropping of an arm is a failure in the test. Summation of time without failure for each of the challenges tested is totaled, with 900 seconds being the maximum score.[13]

Other authors have described ordinal scales to assess the response to a destabilizing strategy or perturbation of the patient in the situations described by Fregly and Graybiel. These measures are quantifiable, but depend upon human observation and scoring using an ordinal or interval scale.

With the advent of posturography, balance can be quantified in terms of amount of sway relative to the limits of stability, and quantitative information can be obtained about the motor and various sensory contributions to balance. In posturography, the patient stands on a force plate that is capable of perturbing balance by rapid horizontal translation forward or backward or by rotation about the ankle axis. By measuring a person's stability with a stable base of support and stable visual field, and then by presenting different sensory conditions (see below), the differential contributions of the somatosensory, visual, and vestibular systems to balance can be assessed.[29] Balance can be quantified under different sensory conditions, and the strength, symmetry, and latency of motor responses to perturbations of balance can be determined; all of these measurements can also be compared to standardized normal values. This system can characterize and quantify a balance disorder, identify malingerers, and help direct treatment approaches.

In the sensory organization subtest of posturography, the differential contributions of the somatosensory, visual, and vestibular inputs to balance are tested by measuring the degree of spontaneous sway under six different sensory conditions. The subject stands on a force plate and is surrounded by a visual screen that has horizontal fixation points. Both the force plate and the visual screen are independently capable of rotating about the ankle axis in response to the subject's spontaneous sway, in such a way as to render useless the somatosensory and/or visual information (this is called sway referencing). Balance is tested under six different sensory conditions. In condition 1, the eyes are open, the force plate is fixed, and the visual screen is fixed. In condition 2, the force plate is fixed and the eyes are closed. In condition 3, the force plate is fixed, the eyes are open, but the visual screen is sway-referenced. In condition 4, the force plate is sway-referenced, the eyes are open, and the visual screen is fixed. In condition 5, the force plate is sway-referenced and the eyes are closed. In condition 6, both the force plate and the visual screen are sway-referenced and the eyes are open. Impairments of the vestibular, somatosensory, or visual systems produce different patterns of performance under these sensory conditions. For example, a person with both visual and vestibular impairments will be very reliant on somatosensory systems and will, therefore, do well in conditions 1, 2, and 3, but poorly in conditions 4, 5, and 6. A person with a purely vestibular disorder will do well in conditions 1 through 4, but poorly in both conditions 5 and 6, because the force plate is sway-referenced and the eyes are closed in condition 5, and the visual field is sway-referenced in condition 6, making the visual information useless; thus, the only useful information is coming from the vestibular system. In a similar fashion, other patterns of performance under the different conditions are seen with other sensory deficits.

In the movement coordination subtest, a subject's balance is perturbed by either horizontally translating the force plate or rotating the force plate about the ankle axis. The strength, symmetry, and latency of the motor response is then measured. Different strength perturbations are used to assess the appropriateness of the magnitude of the patient's response, and repetitive identical perturbations are given to evaluate the patient's adaptation to the same stimulus. Normal values are also available for this subtest.

In addition to helping to localize the problem in a balance disorder, posturography can also help direct the treatment approach and can be useful in measuring treatment outcome. For example, patients who do worse in conditions 3 and 6 than in conditions 2 and 5 have what is referred to as visual preference pattern of deficit. They do better with their eyes closed than when their eyes are open and they are presented with inappropriate visual stimuli, which indicates an inability to suppress inaccurate visual information. This type of patient may have difficulty in a visually complex environment such as a shopping mall. Patients with a visual preference pattern may benefit from wearing a visual conflict dome on the head to help them learn to suppress the inaccurate visual information and to rely on their intact vestibular systems. On the other hand, patients who do well in conditions 1 through 4, but very poorly in conditions 5 and 6 have a vestibular disorder, and these patients should be counseled that they may experience balancing difficulties on uneven surfaces in conditions of poor lighting. These patients would have difficulty walking outdoors at night, for example, and may even need to use a cane in that environment to expand the base of support. Patients with vestibular disorders may also benefit from therapy in which repetitive challenges to balance are given in conditions requiring gradually more and more reliance on the vestibular system, with the aim of enhancing the patient's use of vestibular information.

Pain Quantification

To date no method has been found to accurately quantify pain. Subjective instruments, such as the McGill Pain Questionnaire, Dallas Pain Questionnaire, and Pain Drawing, are often used for assessment.

Pain threshold for a pressure stimulus and the degree of tenderness of accessible nonvisceral soft tissues may be measured with a pressure threshold meter (or algometer, also called dolorimeter). There is as yet no standardized instrument. An algometer is essentially a handheld dynamometer modified to pick up resistance in a localized area. Pressure is progressively increased by one kilogram per second, and the level at which the subject reports pain is recorded. Using an instrument resembling a dial-type tire-pressure gauge with a 1 cm^2 round metal tip, a pain threshold of less than 3 kg/cm^2 or a left/right difference in the pain thresholds of greater than 2 kg/cm^2 is considered significant.[7]

Another algometer is essentially a pinch dynamometer with a 2 cm^2 rubber tip meant to resemble an examining thumb. There is apparently good reliability among tests done by the same examiner and also between different examiners, except in tests on the trapezius and gastrocnemius muscles.[34] Stress and fear of pain decrease the threshold of pressure-induced pain. The algometer has been useful in documenting decrease in trigger point sensitivity following passive stretch. Correlation between the pressure threshold meter and thermography is claimed.

Thermography depicts surface temperature distribution. Telethermography picks up infrared radiation that is transduced to a cathode ray screen. Contact thermography, on the other hand, depends on the changes in liquid crystals coated on a framed flexible sheet that is gently pressed on the body surface being examined. A side-to-side difference of 1°C is considered clinically significant, although these instruments may be sensitive to 0.1°C.[12]

Any condition that alters blood flow or otherwise results in changes in body surface temperature, such as ischemia or inflammation, would be detected by thermography. It may be used to document vasomotor activity that may be induced by pain. While localized "hot spots" may mark myofascial trigger points, correlation may be less reliable for cutaneous thermal changes related to radiculopathy because of the poor dermatomal congruence of superficial and deep somatic and autonomic nerves. Nevertheless, there have been claims that thermography is more sensitive than electromyography or myelography for the diagnosis of disc disease and radiculopathy.[12]

A neurometer (or vibrometer) finds the pain threshold to a vibratory stimulus of graduated intensity by relying on the subject's report, in a manner very similar to an audiographic test. Normative data have been compiled. This technique may be useful for differentiating neuropathy from spurious complaints in patients with suspected carpal tunnel syndrome.

MUSCULOSKELETAL IMPAIRMENT

Strength Measurement

Although several methods of manual muscle testing have been described, the most practical system remains that of determining a patient's ability to initiate movement of a given muscle against gravity or against resistance provided by the examiner in the direction opposite the movement.[25] An attempt must be made to isolate muscles being tested and to differentiate them from substitutions. A six-level grading system may be used; 0 for no perceptible contraction, 1 for trace contraction, 2 for full-range joint motion without gravity, 3 for full-range joint motion against gravity, 5 for the ability to counter completely the examiner's maximum resistance, and 4 for ability falling between grades 3 and 5.[5] The reliability of this approach is compromised by the likelihood that examiners with varying muscle strength will report different responses in the same patient.

The use of a handheld dynamometer, or strain gauge, minimizes the subjective nature of manual muscle testing. Discrete values for isometric strength can be recorded as read from the dynamometer dial. More refined models of such devices come with digital readouts that can register peak resistance or average peaks over a set period (e.g., three seconds). With the use of precision instruments, variability can be minimized if standards such as placement of the sensor, positioning of the subject, and the direction of application of resistance are observed. Strength testing with the portable dynamometer has been shown to be reliable for upper extremity testing with an intra- and interobserver coefficient of variation of 5% to 8%. Variation is twice as high in lower extremity strength testing with this device.[1]

Dynamic strength may be divided into kinetic or isokinetic categories. In measuring kinetic strength (frequently called isotonic strength erroneously), the torque or internal tension of a muscle is mistakenly presumed to be the same throughout an arc of motion, although this is not the case. This capacity is often expressed in terms of "one repetition maximum" or "ten repetition maximum," i.e., the most weight that a subject can lift through the full range of motion once or ten times.

Isokinetic strength is the peak torque that can be exerted at a preset rate or angular velocity against a device that offers resistance that is proportional to the instantaneous effort exerted. There are a variety of devices that are suited to measurement of different extremities, muscle groups and joints, and positions, as well as to measurement of trunk muscle strength. The kinetic communicator exercise device, similar to Cybex, records and graphs eccentric and concentric torques produced by the muscles. Normative values for extremity strength by age group have been developed utilizing these kinetic communicator devices (Table 2).[3]

Several investigators have used computerized machines for quantifying trunk strength in extension/flexion and rotation. Isometric and isokinetic strengths at various speeds can be measured and a torque curve in relation to the angular position can be obtained, as well as data on peak torque, work performed, and power consumed. Trunk strength is decreased in patients with long-standing lower back impairment, compared to normal subjects of the same sex and approximate body weight. Trunk strength may also vary with sex and age, as noted in Table 3[29] and Figure 1.[16]

Devices are now available to measure multiplanar spinal strength and range of motion. Used primarily in research and industrial clinic settings, they are computerized and can display, record, and print out results, and can compare all data gathered to normative values.

Table 2. Isometric knee flexor and extensor muscle strength.

Age group (years)	No.	Flexor strength in 3 knee-joint positions (kg-cm)			Extensor strength in 3 knee-joint positions (kg-cm)		
		$30^{oa,b}$	$45^{oa,b}$	$60^{oa,b,c}$	30^{oa}	$45^{oa,b,c}$	$60^{oa,b,c}$
20–35	24	719 ± 37	792 ± 38	792 ± 36	1,188 ± 58	1,728 ± 83	1,797 ± 69
42–61	24	682 ± 38	721 ± 40	676 ± 39	1,056 ± 58	1,444 ± 69	1,402 ± 69
70–86	24	502 ± 33	510 ± 32	505 ± 31	903 ± 45	1,110 ± 68	1,124 ± 56

Note: Data expressed as mean ± SE$_M$ and adapted from Murray et al. (personal communication, 1984).
[a]Youngest different from oldest (p < .01).
[b]Middle-aged different from oldest (p < .01).
[c]Youngest different from middle-aged (p < .01).

Table 3. Percentage of people 55–74 years of age who have worked since age 45 with difficulty or inability to lift or carry 25 pounds.

Sample	Age (years)			
	55–59	60–64	65–69	70–74
Men				
Difficulty	11.6	15.4	16.8	23.1
Unable	3.5	3.8	5.6	7.5
Women				
Difficulty	22.9	31.0	33.8	40.8
Unable	9.1	8.7	9.3	10.7

Note: From "Exercise, Fitness, and Aging," by E.R. Buskirk, in *Exercise, Fitness, and Health: A Consensus of Current Knowledge*, Claude Bouchard et al., eds. (Champaign, IL: Human Kinetics, 1990), p. 692. Copyright 1990 by Human Kinetics Publishers. Reprinted by permission.

Figure 1. Difference in strength of back extension between male and female industrial workers.

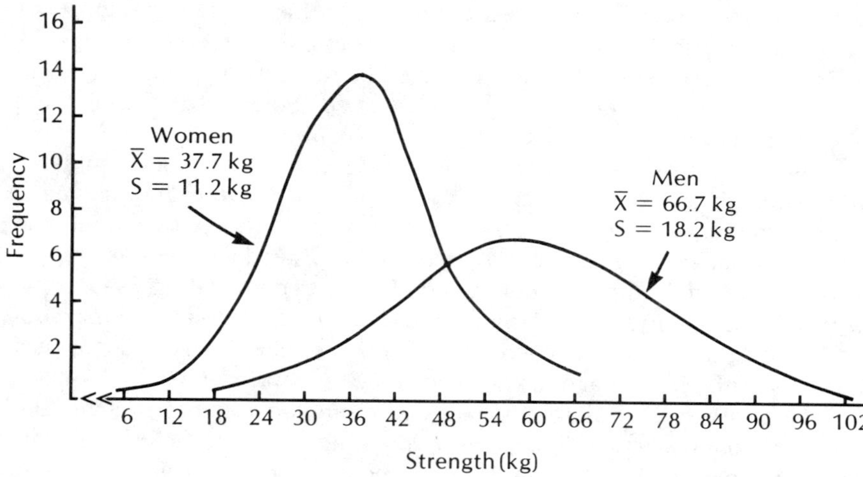

Reprinted from Kamon, E., and A. J. Goldfuss, "In-Plant Evaluation of the Muscle Strength of Workers," *Am Ind Hyg Assoc J* 39: 801–807, 1978, by permission of the American Industrial Hygiene Association.

Quantification of Range of Motion

Because of its simplicity, manual goniometry is the most practical way of measuring joint range of motion. Different methods of recording are used, most notably the "neutral zero" or the 360-degree method. For most joints, the 360-degree method uses the position of the proximal bone as the 0-degree baseline and records the angle on flexion or abduction side. Shoulder external rotation corresponds to the 0-degree baseline. Thumb carpo-metacarpal measurements are based on the position on the palm (third or second metacarpal for abduction or opposition, respectively).[7]

Orthopedists prefer using the neutral anatomic position as the 0-degree baseline. Thus, measurements readily represent deviations from the baseline or normal anatomic position. Normal ranges of motion are available in other texts. In one study, no significant differences in range of motion were attributable to age or sex.[35]

Goniometers must be durable, versatile (preferably with a reversible dial), easily readable, and rigid in the plane being measured. No significant difference in reliability exists between small and large goniometers in experienced hands. For bigger joints, a longer-armed goniometer is easier to line up with the members of the joint in question. A fairly narrow (four degrees) range of variation has been found in repeated measurements under controlled conditions within or between experienced observers.[24]

A carpenter's inclinometer, readily available in hardware stores, is a cheap and practical way of determining spine range of motion. The 1988 edition of the American Medical Association's *Guide to the Evaluation of Permanent Impairment* recommends that all spine range measurements be done with this device.[11] Basically, the range of movement of the more caudal level is subtracted from that of the more cephalad level in relation to the part being measured. The procedure can be done simultaneously with two inclinometers or serially with one. For example, to measure lumbar spine flexion, readings are taken over T12 and over the sacral midpoint when the subject is erect and when he is fully flexed. Then the sacral arc is subtracted from the T12 arc. This method eliminates the contribution of hip flexion.[19]

Electronic digital inclinometers are commercially available. They offer the ease of calculating arcs at the press of a button, but the actual procedure and placement of the sensors are the same.

Other tests of lumbar spine motion have been described. The modified Schober's test measures skin distraction between two midline points 10 cm above and 5 cm below the top of S1 in the patient while erect and again while bent forward. It has less variability in flexion testing than inclinometry (although intertester variability is less than 10% in both). Moll's lateral flexion test measures skin distraction on the sides of the trunk. Moll's extension test uses a plumbline from a point on the side of the thorax and measures the horizontal excursion of the plumbline at the level of the pelvic crest. It is more consistent than inclinometry. A common office test of spine flexion is performed by visually estimating or actually measuring the fingertip-to-floor distance; however, this method has up to 80% variability.[27]

Technical and mechanized refinements in goniometry have been developed to make measurement more precise and accurate. These are used in gait and motion analysis laboratories or in multifunction extremity and spine testing machines.

THE AMA GUIDE TO THE EVALUATION OF PERMANENT IMPAIRMENT

The American Medical Association's *Guide to the Evaluation of Permanent Impairment* is a system of standard clinical tests and ratings based on the principle that "all impairments affect the whole person, and therefore, all impairment ratings should be combined to be expressed as impairment of the whole person."[10] It covers all organ systems and describes how the assigned values for each impairment could be summated in relation to the whole person. It is useful in documenting residual impairment after a sufficient period of treatment.

The musculoskeletal system is divided into the upper and lower extremities and the spine. Upper extremity evaluation was developed and approved for international application by the International Federation of Societies for

Surgery of the Hand. It takes into consideration impairments due to amputation, sensory loss, abnormal motion and ankylosis, and peripheral nerve and plexus injuries. It reduces impairment ratings 5% to 10% for the non-preferred extremity. Sensory loss is tested by two-point discrimination using a paper clip that is opened and bent into a caliper. Range of motion is measured by goniometry using the neutral zero system. Peripheral neurogenic impairment is quantified in terms of decreased sensation with or without pain in relation to activity, and muscle power is graded on a six-level scale. Impairment from vascular conditions is graded based on the presence of claudication, edema, evidence of tissue damage, or Raynaud's phenomenon.

Lower extremity rating is on amputation level, range of motion and ankylosis, peripheral nerve impairment (using the same principles as for the upper extremity), and vascular impairment based on different grades of claudication, edema, or evidence of tissue damage.

Rating of the spine is based on impairments due to specific disorders of the spine and range of motion abnormalities using the inclinometer method. Pain is not a major factor in the rating and is considered only in relation to specific disorders.

RESTORATION FOR RETURN TO WORK

Functional Capacity Evaluation Methods

Job-related physical requirements can prevent workers who have recovered from acute injuries from immediately resuming work. Therefore, functional capacity evaluations are necessary to assess the worker's capability to return to work. Several protocols have been developed to guide these evaluations. Most protocols include a functional assessment which describes a person's activities of daily living. In order to develop a worker's treatment plan, information is also obtained about the worker's education, vocational history, aptitudes, goals, and realistic options, and a job analysis is prepared with descriptions of the work place. A psychological profile, including pain assessment questionnaires, may also be used to assess symptom magnification and whether the worker is capable of giving a valid effort during the evaluation of physical capacity. Physical impairments are then evaluated by the physician and documented with quantifying data for each impairment.

Next, the worker's ability to do activities pertinent to the job is assessed. Static lift strength testing in relevant positions may be administered following protocols, and comparisons made with normative data such as those in Tables 2 and 3 and Figure 1.[30] Computerized equipment has been designed for assisting in this method of evaluation. Chaffin reported an increased risk of back or musculoskeletal injury when a worker's strength in the simulated job position is exceeded by the actual lifting the job requires.[6] To protect against this risk, the worker should receive dynamic strength tests and endurance tests that follow appropriate protocols and are designed to resemble the motions that a worker is expected to perform on the job. The Progressive Isoinertial Lifting Test evaluates dynamic lifting, with the limit being the subject's perception of a safe maximum.[21] Functional capacity evaluations may be compact and administered by one trained person, or they can be expanded as necessary and carried out by a specialized team of health professionals. Ideally, a physician trained or experienced in occupational rehabilitation heads such a team and integrates the data in order to produce a comprehensive report on the worker's functional capacities, tolerances, and restrictions. If these capabilities exceed the demands stated in the job analysis, then the worker is ready for work. A worker who does not meet the job's physical requirements, but who has good potential, may go through a physical restoration and work conditioning program during which job modifications may be recommended. Snook found that "designing the job to fit the worker can reduce up to one-third of industrial back injuries."[33]

Lifting Guidelines and Quantification

The United States Department of Health and Human Services' National Institute for Occupational Safety and Health (NIOSH) has established guidelines for safe lifting based on research.[30] They list two levels of lifting tasks: the acceptable lifting level or action limit (AL), above which some workers will be at risk of injury, and the maximum permissible limit (MPL), which is the upper limit considered safe for workers to lift. The variables to be considered in calculating these limits include: 1) the weight of the object lifted (L); 2) the horizontal distance factor, or the distance from the center of the weight to the body, using a line through the ankles (H); 3) the vertical location or height at which the load is picked up (V); 4) the vertical distance from the origin to the destination of the load (D); 5) the frequency of lifting (lifts per minute) averaged over a period of time (F); and 6) the duration of the period during which the lifting takes place (P).

Certain basic assumptions are associated with the descriptions of these two levels of lifting. At the action limit level, assumptions include the following: 1) a lift will produce 750 pounds (350 kg) of compressive force on the L5-S1 disk; 2) the metabolic rate will be 3.5 kcal per minute; 3) more than 75% of women and 99% of men can perform the task. Assumptions for the lifting task at the maximum permissible limit are that: 1) a lift will produce 1,430 pounds (650 kg) of compressive force on the L5-S1 disk; 2) the metabolic rate will be above 5 kcal per minute; 3) only 25% of men and 1% of women have the strength to perform the task.

In calculating the "perfect" lift, NIOSH has identified an action limit of 90 pounds (40 kg) if a person stands erect holding the weight close to the body and lifts from the waist level no more than 12 inches or 30 centimeters. Figure 2 provides nomograms for calculating the action limit based on the

Figure 2. Individual nomograms of the proportional reduction of tolerance to the stress of lifting as each of four critical factors deviates from optimal.

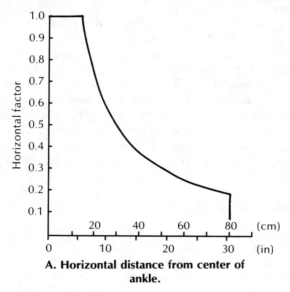

A. Horizontal distance from center of ankle.

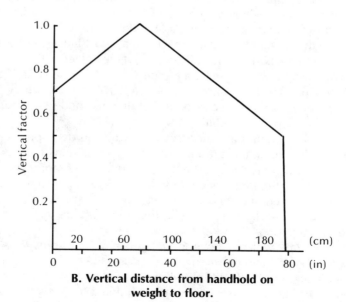

B. Vertical distance from handhold on weight to floor.

Figure 2 (cont.).

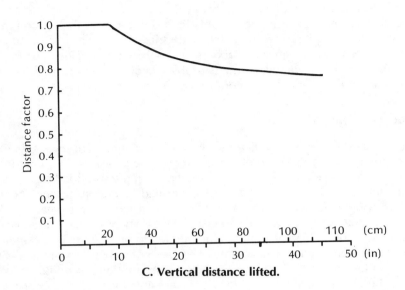

C. Vertical distance lifted.

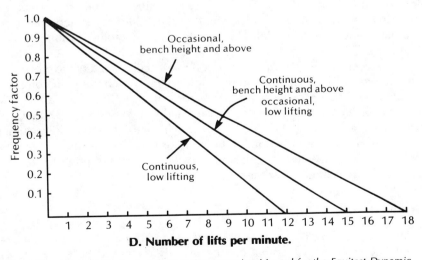

D. Number of lifts per minute.

Reprinted from Nashner, L. M., *Data Interpretation Manual for the Equitest Dynamic Posturography System*, 1–47 (Clackamas, OR: NeuroCom International, 1989), by permission of the publisher.

variables horizontal (H) and vertical (V) distances from the center of gravity of the body, distance lifted (D), and rate of lifting (F). Therefore, as the horizontal distance from the body, the lift distance, or the frequency of lifts per minute increases, the total weight of the object to be lifted (L) will need to be decreased in order to fall below this action limit. In all of these calculations, the maximum permissible limit is three times the action limit.

Safe limits for lifting can be calculated utilizing formulas such as those in the NIOSH method described above, unless there is a specific impairment that needs to be considered. Normative tables for age and sex can be referred to in the NIOSH manuals for more specific comparative data.

Endurance Quantification

Endurance is generally related to the aerobic capacity of the individual performing a task or job. Aerobic capacity can be measured by monitoring the oxygen uptake and heart rate while increasing the workload on a treadmill, stationary bicycle, or steps in a controlled laboratory setting. Actual task measurement can be accomplished through recording oxygen uptake and heart rate during the specific task. Measurement of aerobic capacity and task or job demands is often too complex to be utilized in a standard clinical or work setting. The volume of oxygen consumed per minute (VO_2) for each task divided by the basal oxygen consumption per minute equals a metabolic unit value (MET). Kilocalorie per minute values have been used for comparative data because of the complexities of obtaining the oxygen consumption values for each specific task. Each liter of oxygen uptake per minute is equal to 4.92 kcal/min, which for many tables is rounded off to 5 kcal/min.

Most recently, three dimensional portable accelerometers have been developed to record activities and their intensities, which are then correlated with known energy values. These instruments, such as the Caltrac (Hemokinetics, Inc., 1923 Osmudsen Road, Madison, Wisconsin 53706, USA), are available for about US$75-$100. Through reliability and validity studies, these instruments are continually being improved and seem to have good potential for convenient quantification of energy consumption for tasks in clinical settings and at job sites.[27]

Work Hardening

Work hardening is a psychophysical reconditioning program that uses simulated work activities that can be directly translated by the worker in the job environment. One study of 66 chronic back-pain patients who underwent such a program and 38 who did not, found that 85% of the treatment group had returned to work at one year follow-up, versus 40% of the control group.[22] In a two-year follow-up study, 80% of those who underwent work hardening were working, compared to 45% of those who did not.[23]

Work hardening can either be job-specific or general. The latter, also called work conditioning, is used for patients who lack specific vocational or job goals, but who are incapable of returning to their last employment for various reasons. Activities for these patients are "generic" for their general job classification (e.g., laborer, assembly line, clerical). It is most cost-effective to have a specific job goal so that work hardening activities can focus on the demands of that job. Vocational counseling is very helpful toward this end.[20]

Program attendance is daily, simulating actual employment. However, the time input and the loads, repetitions, or rates of tasks are increased gradually as tolerated. The patient is supervised and taught proper body mechanics in the tasks, pacing, proper responses to discomfort, exercises, relaxation techniques, and other useful habits. Job site analysis helps identify potential barriers to a successful return to work. The program is discontinued when the functional goal is reached and the patient is released to work, or when a plateau in improvement is reached. In the latter case, residual functional incapacities or restrictions are documented, which is useful in matching a worker to a potential job. Such information is also helpful in assessing compensation.[20]

Work conditioning or hardening can also be useful for persons with disabilities from causes other than musculoskeletal impairments. Multidisciplinary goal setting and intervention is more important in these instances. An example of the need for multidiscipinary involvement is the case of a 42-year-old mental health center security officer with a cauda equina syndrome. Vocational assessment and counseling, including employer interviews, were initiated during his paraplegia rehabilitation. A potential job as a telephone operator was identified. The counselor and the social worker analyzed the site to learn how many structural accommodations the employer was willing to make. In the same trip, they scouted accessible dwelling areas close to the job site. In the last week of the patient's stay, as a form of work hardening, he helped handle the telephones at a busy nurse's station at set times compatible with his therapy schedule and his progressive tolerance for sitting; tasks included taking notes, reaching over, and at times standing with braces, with decreasing supervision by the therapist and the nurses.[20] Two weeks after discharge, to allow time to settle into his new apartment and install adaptations in his car, the patient commenced working part-time for one week and full-time thereafter. He was happy doing the same job at follow-up three years later.

FUNCTIONAL ASSESSMENT FOR QUANTIFYING REHABILITATION STATUS AND PROGRESS

Rehabilitation's primary objective is to restore patients' functional performance. Therefore, it is vital that rehabilitation providers measure patients' functional status and use these measures in planning, implementing, and monitoring rehabilitation interventions. Specifically, functional assessment measures the impact of physical or cognitive impairment on a person's ability to perform necessary daily tasks and operations.

This section briefly presents five aspects of functional assessment's role in rehabilitation: 1) characteristics of functional assessment scales; 2) caveats to consider in interpreting functional assessment data; 3) patient screening for rehabilitation appropriateness at the time of admission; 4) documentation of patient improvement and justification for continued treatment; and 5) functional assessment data in formative program evaluation.

Functional Assessment Characteristics

Most functional assessments share a common approach to measuring patient status. First, a specific rehabilitation focus is targeted (e.g., physical mobility, dressing, feeding, expressive language). Second, tasks are graded into hierarchical levels of behavioral competence. In practice, a rater (physician, nurse, or therapist) observes a patient's competence in certain functions, associates that competence with the appropriate category on the rating scale, and assigns that number to the patient as a score.

Assessments, however, vary widely in terms of the number of hierarchical categories used, the degree of behavioral objectivity and detail in the categories' descriptions, and the number of rehabilitation targets measured. The Patient Evaluation and Conference System (PECS), for example, uses seven categories in the assessment of 79 function areas.[15] The PECS scales consistently use category 1 to indicate total dependence and category 7 to denote total independence, or functioning within normal limits. In each PECS scale there is a break between categories 4 and 5, demarcating the critical transition between dependent and independent functioning. Tables 4 and 5 show examples of this continuum from the PECS.

Other widely used instruments, such as the Functional Independence Measure (FIM)[15] and the Levels of Rehabilitation Scale (LORS),[32] use variations of this model, employing seven category scales to rate patient competence. Other measuring systems use fewer, more broadly defined categories. The Barthel Index, for example, assesses patient functioning in 10 areas: feeding, wheelchair transfers, personal hygiene, toilet transfers, bathing, level surface walking, ascending and descending stairs, dressing, and bowel and bladder control. Each item is scored as to whether it is performed independently, with help, or with complete dependence.

Functional Assessment Scale Applications and Caveats

Functional assessment scales offer rehabilitation practitioners several advantages. First, they provide a common framework that the interdisciplinary rehabilitation team can use to describe patients' functioning at admission

Table 4. Scale for ability to comprehend verbal language, from the Patient Evaluation and Conference System (PECS).

1 = No purposeful response to auditory stimuli.

2 = Maximum cuing required to attend to environmental and concrete single-step auditory stimuli; inconsistent responses characterized by latency and variable accuracy.

3 = Responses indicate comprehension of brief personal and contextually based stimuli; reliability decreases for comprehension of abstract stimuli, which requires increased structure and repetition; inconsistent carry-over from minute to minute.

4 = Relies upon the speaker to provide necessary repetition and clarification for comprehension of noncontextually bound stimuli such as multi-step commands, conversation on familiar topics.

5 = Patient comprehends auditory stimuli associated with activities of daily living. Patient demonstrates emerging responsibility for clarification and repetition to enhance auditory comprehension. Breakdown may occur with decreased structure and increased length and complexity.

6 = Patient is independent in utilizing compensatory techniques to maximize recall and new learning for comprehension in his premorbid environments. Sustained concentration to auditory stimuli may be affected by distractions and/or mental fatigue.

7 = Comprehension of verbal language is functional for all situations at the patient's premorbid level of functioning.

Table 5. Ambulation scale from the Patient Evaluation and Conference System (PECS).

1 = Patient attempts to participate or provide some physical assistance in carrying out the activity, but requires significant physical and verbal assistance to complete the activity. Patient is able to assist with up to 25% of the activity.

2 = Patient attempts to participate or provide some physical assistance in carrying out the activity, but requires physical and verbal assistance to complete the activity. Patient is able to assist with 25%–75% of the activity.

3 = Patient is able to participate fully in the activity, but requires intermittent physical assistance and/or contact guard. Patient is able to assist with 75% or more of the activity.

4 = Patient performs the activity without physical/hands-on assistance. May require verbal cuing, prior demonstration, a special physical setting, or supervision to complete the activity for safety purposes.

5 = Patient is independent in the activity, but requires an assistive device or environmental modification.

6 = Patient is independent in the activity but demonstrates an altered quality of movement or requires beyond a reasonable amount of time.

7 = Patient is independent in the activity, with reaction time and quality of movement appropriate for age.

and establish rehabilitation goals. Second, they summarize clinicians' observations into concise, hierarchically defined categories and, as such, facilitate measurement of progress and outcome. While all functional assessment scales have been developed to assist the treatment team in monitoring status and progress, they attempt to do so in different ways. One common method is to assign numerical values to each scale's categories and use the category numbers in arithmetic operations (as in the case of the Barthel, LORS, and FIM). For example, the Barthel Index and the FIM both yield a sum of the individual item scores, which is interpreted as the patient's general level of functioning. The Barthel Index assigns scores of 0, 5, and 10 to item responses, depending on whether the task is performed with total assistance, some assistance, or no assistance. The 10 categories are weighted so as to yield a total score ranging from 0 (totally dependent) to 100 (no need for an attendant). The FIM matches a score from 1 through 7 to an item according to which of seven categories the patient is assigned to. The sum of all item scores from an array of diverse abilities, including feeding, grooming, bathing, bladder and bowel management, walking, language comprehension, problem solving, and memory, is used to compare functional status among patients. In this method, patients with equal item totals are assumed to have equivalent levels of functioning, and the arithmetic difference between admission and discharge scores is represented as the magnitude of patient progress.

Recently, questions have arisen concerning the validity of combining item scores addressing diverse aspects of functional independence to represent general functional status.[26,32] What follows is a brief discussion of unidimensionality and additivity—two measurement characteristics required before items can be combined to produce a total scale score.

Unidimensionality pertains to the extent to which items in a scale measure a unitary underlying trait or construct along a common hierarchical continuum. For example, one would argue that unidimensionality is present in a "gross motor scale" composed of items such as sitting up, crawling, standing, walking, and running. Each task posed to patients must represent a relatively constant difficulty (i.e., easy tasks are relatively easy for all patients and difficult tasks are relatively difficult for all patients). If this requirement is not met, identical scores will have different meanings in different patients.

An example of the problems encountered in interpreting total scale scores in the absence of unidimensionality is displayed in Figure 3. Although the two functional assessment profiles have the same total raw score (57), they depict patients with very different sets of strengths and deficits. The patient represented by the dashed line is at least two levels lower than the patient represented by the solid line in the areas of speech production, feeding, bladder control, and resocialization. Conversely, the dashed line is high relative to the solid line in problem solving, car transfers, and negotiating environmental barriers. Because these items lack unidimensionality (that is, do not retain constant difficulties across patients), the total raw scores belie significant differences between patients and cannot be interpreted meaningfully. It is clear that problem solving and bladder control represent different dimensions of functional independence and their sum has little utility.

The second criterion for combining individual item scores to yield a valid total score is *additivity*: a constant interval unit of measurement. Referring

Figure 3. Functional independence profiles of two patients with identical assessment score totals.

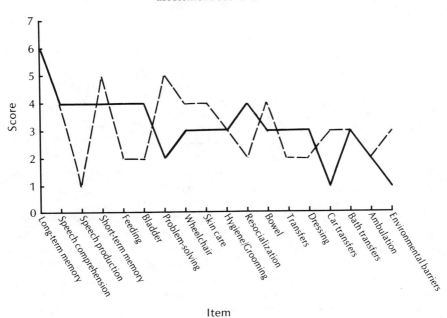

back to Tables 4 and 5 for a moment, in adding individual item scores one assumes that the distance between level 2 and level 4 is the same as between level 4 and level 6 (i.e., it is equally difficult to move the two levels between 2 and 4 as it is to move between levels 4 and 6). Similarly, one assumes that these distances are constant from item to item.

In each scale, however, the item score indicates only the ordinal relationship among the categories. In other words, 1 is less than 2, 2 is less than 3, and so on; but 1 is not necessarily half of 2. The patient receives a score of 2 because the definition of category 2 best describes the patient's level of competence. The patient has not achieved, nor does he/she possess, "2" of anything. Patients in category 2 are more independent than patients in category 1 (but not necessarily twice as competent) and less independent than patients in category 3 (but not necessarily 33% less independent). Measurement of the difference between the abilities of persons who are assigned to different categories is ordinal in nature: the magnitude of difference does not necessarily correspond to the arithmetic differences between the categories' "number names." Consider the respective difficulties represented in the five category items depicted in Figure 4. It shows that achieving a rating of 3 on expressive language might be as difficult as achieving a 4 on ambulation. Raw category scores are therefore not nec-

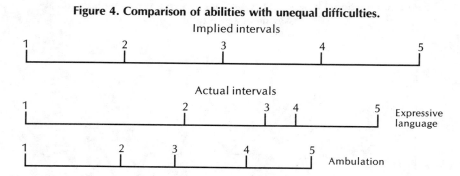

Figure 4. Comparison of abilities with unequal difficulties.

essarily additive across items or within items. An average outcome measure of 2.5 raw score units on "Expressive Language" is not necessarily comparable to an average measure of 2.5 on "Ambulation."

Figure 4 depicts another additivity-related problem in using functional assessments to measure progress arithmetically: the varying distances between scale steps. Consider two patients, one rated a 3 in expressive language and the other rated a 1 in that domain. Because of the respective difficulties involved in moving from 1 to 2 and from 3 to 4, all other things being equal, the category 3 patient will probably progress to the next level sooner than the category 1 patient. Further, the difficulty involved in moving from level 3 to level 5 is much less than in moving from level 1 to level 3. Thus, the patient moving one expressive language level from 1 to 2 has progressed a distance comparable to (or even greater than) the patient moving two levels from 3 to 5. It is clear that these ordinal category scores do not represent equal intervals.

In summary, before combining ordinal items to produce intervally related total scale scores, one must examine the data for evidence of unidimensionality and additivity. A more in-depth presentation of technical issues pertaining to the use of functional assessment data in measuring progress is beyond the scope of this chapter (see Silverstein et al.[32] for a more complete treatment of measurement in rehabilitation and methods of scaling ordinal items to produce interval data). The point of this discussion is that casual use of ordinal functional assessment category numbers in arithmetic operations can easily produce misleading results.

Having cautioned potential users about some misuses of ordinal functional assessment data, let us present some straightforward applications of these data to individual patient management and program evaluation. As stated earlier, the PECS items have seven categories, labeled from 1 to 7. Level 1 denotes maximum dependence/minimal function and level 7 denotes maximum independence and function. The transition between level 4 and level 5 on each item marks the transition between minimal dependence on another person (level 4) and minimal independence (level 5).

Although, as outlined above, the indeterminate distances between ordinal item categories preclude arithmetic operations on the category numbers, *appropriate* use of these ratings can yield valid information. For example, three characteristics of the PECS anchor these functional assessment scales along a dimension of increasing functional independence and provide a basis for comparison with set criteria and across time: 1) the qualitative descriptions associated with each category (see Tables 4 and 5), 2) the consistent use of "1" and "7" as the extreme ends of the continuum, and 3) the consistent use of "4" and "5" as the boundaries of transition between dependence and independence. Some examples of the appropriate use of ordinal functional assessment data follow.

Admissions Screening

A patient appropriate for inpatient rehabilitation displays functional deficits in mobility and major activities of daily living *and* demonstrates the likelihood of progress toward independence. Functional assessment data offer a useful, concise summary of narrative information related to a patient's disabilities and rehabilitation goals. This profile also functions as an effective screening device. A reviewer can determine at a glance whether a particular admission requires more in-depth examination to assure appropriate utilization of treatment resources.

Consider Figure 5: It reveals the profile of a patient's admission status, the progress made during the first two weeks, progress during the next two weeks, and the discharge profile. The rehabilitation goals (shown by the dashed line) provide an individual standard against which to compare the patient's status and progress, and the horizontal dotted line demarcates the transition between dependence and independence (level 4 and level 5). The white portion of Figure 5 represents the profile of an appropriate rehabilitation inpatient. The patient manifests a low level of dependence in the most important self care, ADL, and mobility areas. Further, the interdisciplinary team has placed the rehabilitation goals in the independent range, denoting its judgment that the patient has the potential to regain independence in those areas.

Figure 6, conversely, illustrates the profile of a questionable rehabilitation admission. The rehabilitation team does not believe the patient will regain functional independence during this stay. Patient status is consistently low across the major skill areas, and many of the team's goals are also in the dependent range. This profile raises questions about the patient's ability to profit from rehabilitation. Will this patient be able to follow commands and participate in therapy? What medical complications might limit the patient's involvement? No decisions should be made directly from this profile— except the decision to investigate further and closely monitor the patient's future progress. Although an admissions screener could glean the same

Figure 5. Profile of patient status at admission and discharge from a rehabilitation program, showing progress at two-week intervals.

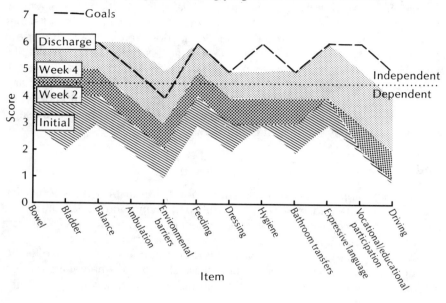

Figure 6. Patient status profile for judging appropriateness for admission to a rehabilitation program.

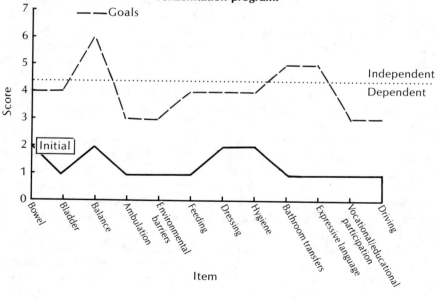

information from a thorough examination of the patient's chart, the profile summarizes a large amount of narrative information for quick, accessible study.

Monitoring of Patient Progress

Beyond screening for admission appropriateness, functional assessment profiles can also assist in scrutinizing patients' status and determining if patients require continued inpatient care. Figure 7 represents a patient who has achieved or exceeded most rehabilitation goals. Although the patient has yet to achieve goals (and functional independence) in the areas of expressive language, vocational planning, and driving, treatment in these areas alone clearly does not justify inpatient care.

Steady progress toward rehabilitation goals and functional independence is another important criterion of continued inpatient rehabilitation. Referring back to Figure 5, one can see that the patient made consistent progress. Further examination of therapists' progress notes is unnecessary for this global evaluation, because the functional assessment profile conforms to our expectations of consistent functional progress.

Program Evaluation

Thus far, this section has presented methods of using functional assessment data to track the progress of individual patients toward rehabilitation goals. These data can also be useful in evaluating the effectiveness of entire programs in an effort to refine program practices and improve treatment outcomes.

The United States Commission on Accreditation of Rehabilitation Facilities (CARF) identifies two components of any system for evaluating program effectiveness: "(1) Explicit criteria or expectancies must be applied to each result measured so that program performance can be properly judged . . . [and] (2) Results presented must provide for a comparison against a standard such as base rate performance, last quarter's performance, cumulative performance, actual vs. expected performance, etc."[8] A program evaluation system, therefore, must perform three functions:

1) *Measure* the performance of programs.

2) *Establish* explicit standards for performance of programs.

3) *Compare* the actual performance with the expected performance to detect deviations from expectations.

A comprehensive discussion of using functional assessment data to evaluate rehabilitation medicine programs is beyond the scope of this chapter (see Keith, 1984, and Silverstein et al., 1990, for a more complete presentation).[17,32] However, briefly described below are two program evaluation methods of varying usefulness. The first addresses the magnitude of progress

Figure 7. Status and goal profile of a possible discharge candidate.

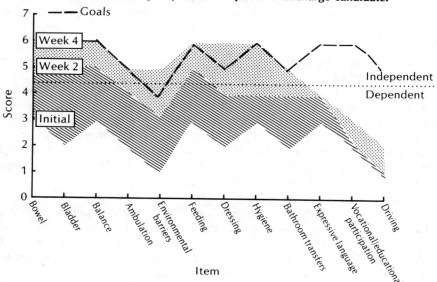

patients have made. The second examines the extent to which explicit goals set by the rehabilitation team have been achieved.

Progress measurement requires evaluators to measure patients' performance at least twice: at admission and discharge. The mean programwide difference is used as a measure of effectiveness. Using the Barthel Index of FIM, for example, this method requires adding the category numbers assigned to the respective items and interpreting the difference between the totals at admission and at discharge as the magnititude of gain achieved during rehabilitation.

This approach presents problems in satisfying each of the three CARF program evaluation criteria. The measurement problems associated with lack of unidimensionality and additivity have already been discussed. Because the totals are not derived from intervally related phenomena, a hypothetical mean difference of, say, 24 "Barthel Index units" or "FIM points" is difficult to interpret. As the previous section demonstrated, one cannot be confident that a group with a mean difference of 24 units has improved twice as much as a group with a difference of 12 units. Similarly, one cannot be certain about the magnitude of functional improvement represented by a group's increase from a mean of 40 to a mean of 50. Have they improved by 25%? It is impossible to say. Other factors in the measurement of change, such as the reliability of measures, standard errors of measurement, and regression effects, can affect the interpretation of each difference score.[4,9]

The second program evaluation requirement, explicit standards, is difficult to establish with difference scores. How much gain is enough? What functional assessment totals should be expected at discharge of patients who vary in initial functional level, age, diagnosis, disabilities, medical complications, levels of family support, socioeconomic status, and other variables that affect rehabilitation outcome? Addressing such questions requires sophisticated statistical modeling using a large data base that contains information on thousands of representative patients, and that was built with carefully standardized and closely monitored data collection procedures.

Only after, first, constructing reliable and valid measures and, next, building extensive data bases yielding valid outcome expectations can program evaluation analyses determine the extent to which the observed outcomes deviate from statistically derived expectations. Data analyses addressing the issue typically employ multivariate models to project expected outcomes from optimal combinations of variables that affect discharge level of functioning. Silverstein et al.[32] have delineated practicable methods of modeling expected outcome using intervally scaled functional assessment data. As can be seen by the preceding discussion, however, these methods require a large data base, powerful computing capability, and sophisticated statistical software.

Goal-based program evaluation offers a more universally accessible and readily interpretable approach. It follows directly from the interdisciplinary patient care conference at which functional independence goals are set for each patient's hospital stay. Using rehabilitation goals and patient progress data in the context of program evaluation requires aggregated data on the percentage of patient goals that are achieved and the percentage of patients who attain independent functioning by the time of discharge. These statistics must be compared against a standard level of success deemed acceptable and against the program's past performance. Data can then be aggregated and sorted by any topic of interest: specific medical programs, therapeutic disciplines, disability groups, etc.

The goal-based method has strong intuitive appeal, in that the program is evaluated based on what it plans to do. Use of inpatient rehabilitation is most often justified by the expectation that the patient will achieve functional milestones in such key areas as ambulation, bowel and bladder management, feeding, dressing, and hygiene. This method considerably simplifies the evaluation question, which becomes: "Did the patients accomplish what the rehabilitation teams decided was required and feasible?"

Figure 8 presents an example of how such goal attainment data can be used for program evaluation. Upon admission, the rehabilitation team in this example establishes goals for each patient in all of the functional areas displayed in the histogram. Patients are assessed biweekly throughout their stay and a final time at discharge. The top graph in Figure 8 shows the percentage of patients who attained set goals in each of the functional areas during the quarter under evaluation. The expected level of goal attainment is shown by the transverse line. The bottom graph shows the percentage of

Figure 8. Goal-based evaluation of a rehabilitation program.

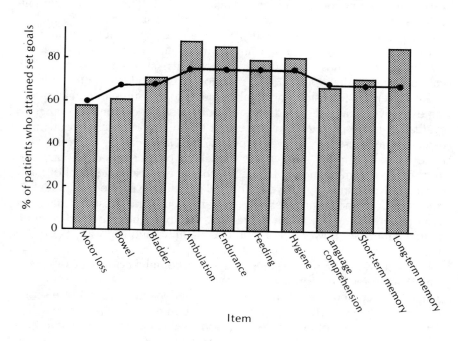

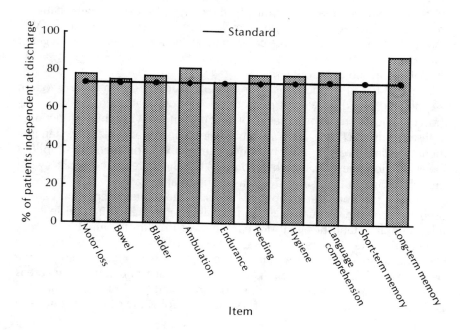

these same patients who had achieved the independent level of functioning at discharge. The top graph shows that the brain injury program achieved its standard in all areas except bowel control, motor loss, and language comprehension. The finding that an unacceptably low percentage of patients are achieving functional independence in these areas suggests that initial goals are being set too high—perhaps giving patients and families unrealistic expectations.

Goal attainment does not tell the whole story. For each functional item for which the goal attainment standard is met, evaluators also should examine the "% independent at discharge" data (see Figure 8, bottom). If programs are meeting goal attainment criteria but are showing substandard "% independent at discharge," the team may be setting goals too low.

CONCLUSION

This chapter has presented several uses of functional assessment in rehabilitation and has discussed some of the problems that can arise from ambitious but inappropriate applications of ordinal-level functional assessment data. Used correctly, these data can provide an empirical basis for professional communication about patient progress in rehabilitation. They can also help identify interventions for individual patients and medical programs that require further review or improvement.

REFERENCES

1. Agre JC, Magnus JL, et al. Strength testing with a portable dynamometer: reliability for upper and lower extremities. *Arch Phys Med Rehabil.* 1987;68:454–458.
2. Ashworth B. Preliminary trial of carisoprodol in multiple sclerosis. *Practitioner.* 1964;192:540–542.
3. Buskirk ER. Exercise, fitness and aging. In: Bourchard C, et al, eds. *Exercise, fitness and health: a consensus of current knowledge.* Champaign, IL: Human Kinetics Books; 1990.
4. Bereiter C. Some persisting dilemmas in the measurement of change. In: Harris CW, ed. *Problems in measuring change.* Madison: University of Wisconsin Press; 1967.
5. Brunnstrom S, Dennen M. *Round table on muscle testing; annual conference of the American Physiotherapy Association.* New York: Federation of Crippled and Disabled; 1931:1–12.
6. Chaffin DB, Herrin GED, Keyserling WM. Pre-employment strength testing: an update position. *J Occup Med.* 1978;20:403–408.
7. Cole T. Goniometry. In: Kottke FJ, Lehmann JF, eds. *Krusen's handbook of physical medicine and rehabilitation.* 4th ed. Philadelphia: WB Saunders; 1990:20–32.
8. Commission on Accreditation of Rehabilitation Facilities. *Program evaluation: utilization and assessment principles.* Tucson; 1981.
9. Cronbach L, Furby L. How we should measure "change"—or should we? *Psychol Bull.* 1970;74:68–80.
10. Engelberg A, ed. *AMA guide to the evaluation of permanent impairment.* 3rd ed. Chicago: American Medical Association; 1988.
11. Feldman R, et al. *Spasticity: disordered motor control.* Chicago: Year Book Medical; 1980.
12. Fischer A. Diagnosis and management of chronic pain in physical medicine and rehabilitation. In: Ruskin AP, ed. *Current therapy in physiatry.* Philadelphia: WB Saunders; 1984:123–145.

13. Fregly AR, Graybiel A. An ataxia test battery not requiring rails. *Aerosp Med.* 1982;39:277.
14. Hamilton B, Granger C, Sherwin F, Zielezny M, Tashman J. A uniform national data system for medical rehabilitation. In: Fuhrer M, ed. *Rehabilitation outcomes analysis and measurement.* Baltimore: Paul H. Brookes; 1987:137–150.
15. Harvey R, Jellinek H. Functional performance assessment: a program approach. *Arch Phys Med Rehabil.* 1981;62:456–461.
16. Kamon E, Goldfuss AJ. In-plant evaluation of the muscle strength of workers. *Am Indus Hyg Assoc J.* 1978;39:801–807.
17. Keith R. Functional assessment of program evaluation for rehabilitation medicine. In: Granger C, Gresham G, eds. *Functional assessment in rehabilitation medicine.* Baltimore: Williams & Wilkins; 1984.
18. Livneh H. Person-environment congruence: a rehabilitation perspective. *Int J Rehabil Res.* 1987;10:3–19.
19. Loebl WY. Measurement of spinal posture and range of spinal movement. *Ann Phys Med.* 1967;9:103–110.
20. Marianjoy Rehabilitation Center. Protocol for the Center of Occupational Rehabilitation. Wheaton, IL; 1989. [Unpublished document].
21. Mayer TG, et al. Progressive isoinertial lifting evaluation I and II. *Spine.* 1988;13:993–1001.
22. Mayer TG, et al. Objective assessment of spine function following industrial injury: a prospective sudy with comparison group and one year follow up. *Spine.* 1985;10:482–493.
23. Mayer TG, et al. A prospective two-year study of functional restoration in industrial low back injury: an objective assessment procedure. *JAMA.* 1987;258:1763–1767.
24. Mayerson NH, Milano RA. Goniometric measurement reliability in physical medicine. *Arch Phys Med Rehabil.* 1984;65:92–94.
25. Mayo Clinic. *Clinical examination in neurology.* 4th ed. Philadelphia: WB Saunders; 1976.
26. Merbitz C, Morris J, Grip JC. Ordinal scales and foundations of misinference. *Arch Phys Med Rehabil.* 1989;70:308–312.
27. Merritt JL, et al. Measurement of trunk flexibility in normal subjects: reproducibility of three clinical methods. *Mayo Clinical Proc.* 1986;61:192–197.
28. Montaye HJ. Assessment of physical activity during leisure and work. In: Bouchard C, et al, eds. *Exercise, fitness and health: a consensus of current knowledge.* Champaign, IL: Human Kinetics Books; 1990.
29. Nashner LM. *Data interpretation manual for the Equitest dynamic posturography system 1–47.* Clackamas, OR: NeuroCom International; 1989.
30. National Institute for Occupational Safety and Health. *A work practices guide for manual lifting.* Cincinnati, OH: US Department of Health and Human Services; 1981. (Tech rep 81–122).
31. Parkside Associates. *LORS American Data System (LADS) data manual.* Park Ridge, IL; 1986.
32. Silverstein B, Kilgore K, Fisher W. *Implementing patient tracking systems and using functional assessment scales.* Wheaton, IL: Center for Rehabilitation Outcome Analysis; 1990.
33. Snook SH. The design of manual handling tasks. *Ergonomics.* 1978;39:963–985.
34. Tunks E, Crook J, Norman G, Kalaher S. Tender points in fibromyalgia. *Pain.* 1988;34:11–19.
35. Walker JM, Sue D, Miler-Elkousy N, Ford GF, Trevelyan H. Active mobility of the extremities in older subjects. *Phys Ther.* 1984;64:919–923.

Chapter 12

ADVANCES IN REHABILITATION FOR VISUALLY IMPAIRED AND BLIND PERSONS

Stanley F. Wainapel and Donald C. Fletcher

Visual loss is one of the most dreaded of all disabling conditions. It is also one of the more common. The 1977 National Health Survey included information on 10 chronic conditions in the United States, of which visual impairment was the second most prevalent and also the fastest growing.[18] More recently, the U.S. Bureau of the Census reported that in 1986 there were 13,000,000 citizens aged 15 or older who had difficulty reading print due to vision problems, and that 1,700,000 of them were so impaired that they could not read words at all.[10] Among older persons, the prevalence of severe visual impairment is even more notable. An analysis of data collected in 1984 by the U.S. National Center for Health Statistics (NCHS) showed that more than 2,000,000 people over age 65 had difficulty reading (or were unable to read) newsprint. This represents 7.8% of the elderly, and the prevalence of such severe visual impairment rises to 25.0% among people aged 85 or older.[16]

Visual impairments result in significant functional limitations. Ambulation is compromised, the risk of potentially harmful falls increases, and activities of daily living (ADL) cannot be performed without special training and/or equipment. Those who develop visual problems often experience significant depression and social isolation as a result of loss of independence and of previously pleasurable avocational activities (e.g., reading, sewing, running). This is a classic description of a person for whom the multidisciplinary rehabilitation model of comprehensive care is appropriate, yet such a person is unlikely to be seen by a physiatrist.

It seems rather ironic that this common and devastating physical disability is one of the few not served by a medical specialty created expressly to help manage disabling illness—physical medicine and rehabilitation (PMR). The second edition of the *Handbook of Physical Medicine and Rehabilitation* included a chapter on vision problems by Goodpasture,[9] but the third edition[15] covered no similar subject matter, and recent major rehabilitation texts have similarly neglected the topic except insofar as it relates to other types of disability (for example, the homonymous hemianopsia associated with stroke and the diplopia produced by multiple sclerosis). Likewise, the journal *Archives of Physical Medicine and Rehabilitation* has published very few articles relating to visual impairment.

Why has this exclusion occurred, and should it continue? The main reason for its occurrence probably relates to the history of care of the blind, which developed separately from care for other disabling conditions, perhaps because blindness does not directly affect a person's physical health (the same is true of deafness). Care of the blind was seen as more of a social and/or educational service than a medical one, and until recent times the medical establishment had little to offer in the way of restorative interventions. Interestingly, the impetus for modern vision rehabilitation was identical to that which spurred the development of PMR—the war-injured veterans of the 1940s. Over the next half-century a distinct vision rehabilitation system evolved, with agencies at local, state, and national levels. At least two journals have become the main professional forum for research in this area: the *Journal of Visual Impairment and Blindness* and the more recent *Journal of Vision Rehabilitation*.

Recent developments and trends suggest that the historic insularity of blindness rehabilitation from the medical and PMR community is ripe for change. Dramatic breakthroughs in the treatment of eye disorders with medication (eyedrops for glaucoma) or surgery (cataract extraction, laser photocoagulation) have altered the proportion of blind versus low-vision patients to markedly favor the latter; concurrently, the technology for low-vision care has greatly advanced. Moreover, the aging of the population has meant that a growing proportion of the visually impaired are in the older age range: according to NCHS statistics, the average age of patients visiting an ophthalmologist's office is 64.[10] Under these circumstances, visual impairment is likely to become but one of a constellation of functional limitations found in an increasingly aged patient population. It can be expected that physiatrists will encounter such multisystem disability with increasing frequency. Therefore, it is necessary for the physiatrist to gain greater familiarity with the causes, consequences, and rehabilitation of irreversible vision loss. This chapter is written to provide a foundation for that knowledge.

VISION IMPAIRMENT: ITS CAUSES, CLASSIFICATION, AND FUNCTIONAL IMPLICATIONS

From a physiatrist's perspective, the etiology of visual loss is of lesser significance than its degree of severity, its prognosis, and its resulting functional disabilities or handicaps. Nevertheless, a brief mention of the major causes of blindness or severe visual impairment is warranted. Among patients under age 21, these include hereditary or congenital conditions such as congenital toxoplasmosis, congenital cataract, albinism, and retinopathy of prematurity (formerly called retrolental fibroplasia); four additional etiologies are tumors, trauma, infection, and juvenile-onset diabetes mellitus.[10] Diabetic retinopathy is also the major cause of blindness among adults aged 21 to 60, along with progressive hereditary conditions such as retinitis pigmentosa (RP). Among those aged 70 or older, four diagnoses account for 98% of all cases of loss of visual function: age-related macular degeneration (AMD), cataracts, glaucoma, and diabetic retinopathy.[11] Of these disorders, AMD is the only one for which no successful ophthalmologic intervention exists, and it has become the number one cause of blindness in the geriatric population.

The two major forms of visual loss are central (loss of visual acuity) and peripheral (loss of visual fields). Central losses can be diffuse or discreet; the latter situation is called a scotoma and can occur as a result of disciform scars, drusen formation, or optic nerve involvement in multiple sclerosis. Peripheral loss can be concentric, as in RP, with resulting "tunnel vision," in which the patient can see straight ahead but cannot detect objects in the periphery. Such patients also have the associated symptom of night blindness due to impaired dark adaptation mechanisms. The opposite of a concentric field loss is loss of the central visual field with preservation of peripheral vision, which is characteristic of AMD.

Degree of visual impairment is classified on the basis of level of acuity and/or field restriction. Since 1935 the United States has defined "legal blindness" (a term which entitles those so labeled to special services and to tax advantages) as 1) visual acuity of 20/200 or less in the better eye despite maximal corrective lenses, or 2) visual field of 20 degrees or less in the better eye. Such a definition excludes a large proportion of the visually impaired population, particularly those with corrected visual acuities between 20/70 and 20/200 or with significant field restriction that has not reached 20 degrees. This degree of visual impairment has been termed *low vision,* and persons with low vision have been recognized as a particularly underserved group in terms of medical and social services. The World Health Organization (WHO) has further classified low vision as follows:[10]

- Moderate low vision: Corrected acuity of 20/70 to 20/160 in the better eye.
- Severe low vision: Corrected acuity of 20/200 to 20/400 or visual field of 20 degrees or less in the better eye.

Acuity and field values represent only the impairment (abnormal function of an organ, in this case the eye); they do not indicate the resulting disability (problems with task performance) or handicap (problems in fulfilling a social role), and it is these levels of difficulty that most engage the physiatrist's attention and efforts. Each individual will respond differently to a visual loss based on lifestyle, vocation, and the environment in which he/she lives. However, some general observations can be made about the functional effects of certain types of visual impairment. Central visual field loss (as in AMD) severely affects the ability to read, to drive an automobile, and to identify faces, but mobility on foot is less impaired because of the preservation of peripheral vision. Conversely, the person with a peripheral visual field deficit (as in RP or glaucoma) may be able to read using preserved central vision, but will find independent travel more difficult and hazardous because of the combination of lost peripheral vision and impaired visual ability in dark surroundings. Loss of central acuity results in difficulty with discrimination of detail—reading, recognition of street signs, and needlework, for example. A corrected central acuity of 20/70 or less implies that the person will have difficulty in reading standard newspaper print.

The emotional consequences of vision loss can be profound, but their type and severity are very much determined by the lifestyle, goals, support systems, and premorbid coping patterns of the affected individual. Especially when its onset is sudden or rapidly progressive, vision loss can produce such fear and despair that the visually impaired person is virtually as paralyzed as if he/she had had a stroke and as immobilized as if he/she had had a leg amputated. Awareness and utilization of residual vision or of the other senses is at this point relatively minimal. Firm, supportive counseling is needed to help direct the visually impaired person into the rehabilitation system and, ultimately, back into a meaningful life. Fortunately, the surgical and technological advances of the past decade have made such a goal far more realistic than it was before.

VISION REHABILITATION: TECHNIQUES AND TECHNOLOGIES

Recent advances in ophthalmologic surgery have been dramatically successful in salvaging or restoring functional vision in individuals who formerly could anticipate progressive deterioration leading to total or near-total blindness. These procedures can be considered forms of surgical rehabilitation. Cataract extraction with intraocular lens implantation has revolutionized the management of this extremely common accompaniment of the aging process. The benefits of such surgery on physical and mental (as well as visual) functions are highlighted in a paper by Applegate et al.,[2] who prospectively studied 293 elderly (aged 70 or older) patients before and after intraocular lens implantation. They found that subjective ADL improved slightly; mental status measurements had improved four months postoperatively and reached statistical significance one year after surgery; and timed manual task performance was also significantly improved. Patients with diabetic retinopathy and, to a lesser extent, age-related macular degeneration have benefited from the use of laser technology. Particularly for diabetic retinopathy, the visual prognosis has been markedly improved through the use of laser treatments, and many years of useful vision have been gained.

Notwithstanding these surgical successes, many visual impairments are not amenable to such rapid and lasting interventions. For individuals with nonremediable impairments the techniques of low-vision rehabilitation and (in the case of near-total vision loss) blindness rehabilitation are essential. A full discussion of these measures is beyond the scope of this chapter, but can be found in texts by Faye[5] and Fonda.[7] Interventions can be classified as either vision enhancement (for low vision) or vision substitution (for near total blindness), and are outlined in Table 1.

Vision Enhancement

Apart from standard glasses for near and distant vision, the most available, affordable, and widely used vision enhancement devices are magnifiers, which can magnify the object up to 15 times its normal size.[14] High-power spectacles are the most commonly prescribed low vision magnifier; they focus reading material at a closer than normal distance. Hand-held magnifiers come in numerous designs (Figure 1) and may include a built-in source of incandescent or (more recently) halogen light for optimal illumination. They can be placed at varying distances from the object or reading material being viewed. Stand magnifiers are used from a fixed distance and are less portable than hand-held magnifiers, but have advantages when the patient has hand tremors or deformities such as those caused by arthritis.[4]

Table 1. Outline of vision rehabilitation techniques.

I) Vision enhancement
  A) Acuity enhancers
    1) Magnifiers
    2) Telescopes
    3) Closed-circuit television (CCTV)
  B) Field expanders
    1) Prisms
    2) Reverse telescopes
  C) Illumination devices
  D) Antiglare devices
  E) Contrast enhancing devices
  F) Enlarged print
II) Vision substitution
  A) Mobility devices
    1) White cane
    2) Laser cane
    3) Ultrasonic mobility aids
  B) Reading and writing aids
    1) Recorded books and periodicals
    2) "Talking" devices
    3) Computers with synthetic speech
    4) Kurzweil Reading Machine
    5) Optical-tactile converter (Optacon)

Figure 1. Hand-held magnifiers.
(Photograph courtesy of Resources for Rehabilitation, Lexington, Mass.)

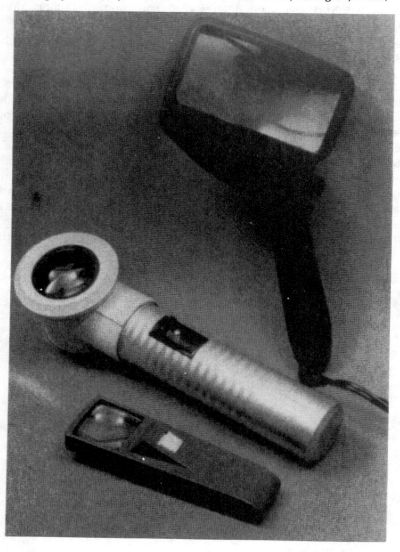

They are particularly useful as reading aids since they can be placed on a desk or table. In general, one can recommend magnifiers for patients with central visual acuity as low as 20/800; the treatment goal varies based on the severity of vision loss and individual patient needs, for example, reading newspaper, labels, etc.

Telescopes also provide selective magnification. Small hand-held monocular telescopes for distance vision are useful for reading street signs when walking. Spectacle-mounted models can be monocular or binocular; they are useful for stationary viewing, but one of their disadvantages is that they cover a narrow field of vision. Telescopes for near vision have the same disadvantage and most people do not accept them for this reason.[4]

The closed-circuit television (CCTV) videomagnifier consists of a variable sized television screen (small portable models are now available) with a reading table and small video camera with zoom lens. Although it is considerably more expensive than magnifiers or telescopes, with prices varying from US$1,000 to $3,000 depending on the features included, the CCTV has become one of the most effective magnification devices for individuals with severe low vision (acuity as low as 20/2000). It can magnify print up to 60 times normal size[14] and can produce a white-on-black (reversal) picture that provides enhanced contrast for easier reading (Figure 2). It also allows people with low vision to read for prolonged periods with little of the fatigue associated with using other magnifiers, and is therefore of particular value to students and professionals whose daily activities entail significant amounts of reading.

All the above devices are applicable to the patient with impaired central visual acuity. Fewer options are available for those with visual field defects such as homonymous hemianopsia following cerebrovascular accident, extensive loss of central vision with preserved peripheral vision due to AMD, or peripheral field loss (tunnel vision) due to glaucoma or RP. Some special prisms have been developed that, when mounted on glasses, allow the patient to look one way and see in another direction; prisms for hemianopsia are a case in point. Reverse telescopes (the equivalent of looking in the wrong end of a pair of binoculars or opera glasses) and special fish-eye lenses mounted on glasses can expand the remaining central field of patients with RP or glaucoma,[7] but in doing so they make objects appear much farther away, a situation that can prove difficult for most users. Adequate lighting is also of particular importance in these latter two conditions, which also produce impaired dark adaptation.

Appropriate illumination is, in fact, one of the most basic requirements for successful function in the face of low vision. A well-directed incandescent or halogen lamp is as important a piece of technology as a magnifier, telescope, prism, or CCTV. However, the illumination needs of each patient are quite different; for example, patients with AMD usually benefit from maximally bright lighting, while those with cataracts often note excessive

Figure 2. Closed-circuit television (CCTV) used for reading newspaper; note white-on-black image.

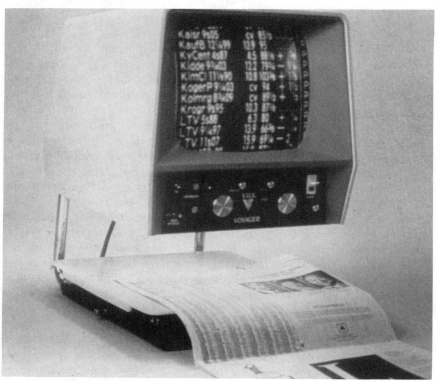

glare when illumination is too strong. The home and work environments of anyone with low vision need to be analyzed from the point of view of consistent and even lighting to maximize residual abilities. To reduce glare, devices such as simple sunglasses, sun visors, clip-on sun shades, and yellow- or orange-tinted filters can be used; the latter block the blue end of the light spectrum, which contributes to glare. Another factor important for optimal visibility is adequate color contrast. Contrast can be enhanced by simple aids such as bold print pens, paper with extra-dark lines, and typoscopes—black plastic templates with apertures that facilitate the writer's ability to fill out checks, address envelopes, or write entire pages of script (Figure 3). Heightened contrast of colors at home or at work can also facilitate daily activities and mobility.

A final form of vision enhancement involves not magnification of pre-existing material but rather presentation in enlarged form. A number of periodicals—the *New York Times* and *Readers Digest,* for example—have

**Figure 3. Typoscopes (writing guides) for writing letters
and addressing envelopes.**

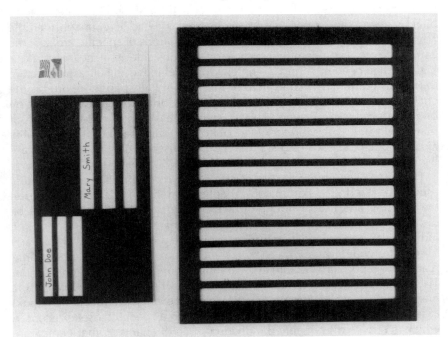

large-print editions. Many organizations that serve the visually impaired and/or elderly population now publish materials in large-print format. Computer output can also be modified to produce larger-sized print on hard copy in addition to enlargement of the print seen on the computer screen.

Vision Substitution

At least 80% of the legally blind population has some usable vision;[12] the remaining 20% must turn to vision substitution rather than vision enhancement techniques. However, the delineation between groups and techniques is not a strict one. Many individuals with severe low vision will use and benefit from the mobility and reading aids designed for those lacking any eyesight.

Mobility is a prerequisite for independent living by the blind individual, and he/she can choose between two major mobility options: the guide dog or the long white cane. Both have been in use for many years and are well-described in the vision rehabilitation literature.[21] Both require the user to receive extensive training for optimal success. In recent years several new mobility technologies have been developed, but they are much more costly than the standard white cane. The laser cane sends three laser beams ahead of the user; one detects drop-offs in his/her path, a second indicates objects directly ahead, and a third warns of obstacles at head level (a considerable advantage over the standard white cane). Vibrations of specific areas of the cane indicate an upcoming obstacle; if the obstacle is at head height, a high-pitched beeping sound is emitted. Three devices using ultrasound rather than laser output are also available: the Russell Pathsounder (worn on the chest, leaving hands free), the Sonicguide (mounted on glasses, object on one side produces a sound in the ipsilateral ear), and the Mowat Sensor (hand held unit with vibratory feedback).[4] Although each of these mobility aids has potential advantages, none has been used widely enough to establish it as preferable to the more affordable white cane.

The loss of the ability to read is one of the most upsetting and isolating aspects of blindness. Fortunately, reading options have extended beyond the learning and use of Braille (a tactile language). Braille should not be dismissed as outdated, however, since it has many important uses for blind individuals, particularly those whose blindness is congenital or of early onset. The wide availability of books and magazines in recorded form has made tape a popular medium even among the normally sighted population. The National Library Service for the Blind and Physically Handicapped, a branch of the Library of Congress, maintains an extensive collection of books in four-track tape format that can be played on a special cassette recorder, which is provided to qualified individuals free of charge. Other companies offer rental or purchase of standard cassette recordings of contemporary or classic literature, often read by professional actors. Because of this availability, and the overall importance of recorded formats in the workplace (e.g., dictation of memos), a compact cassette recorder is basic equipment that is recommended for almost all blind individuals.

The advent of "talking" technology has been an enormous asset to blind persons and has spawned many devices with synthetic speech output: watches, clocks, calculators, scales, blood pressure machines, thermometers, and blood glucose meters (for diabetics with retinopathy), to name but a few. Computers can also be equipped with speech synthesizers to allow greater access for blind or severely visually impaired users. Braille output is also an option for those who prefer it. The ultimate in current technology is the Kurzweil Reading Machine, which reads print and then renders it into synthetic speech.[4] Although the newer desk-top Kurzweil model is less bulky and less than half the cost of the original Reader, it remains out of the financial reach of most individuals. However, it could be made available to multiple individual users through libraries or other large institutions.

A final example of modern technology harnessed for the service of blind people is the optacon, an optical-tactile convertor which translates letters or diagrams into vibratory signals that can be perceived by the fingers of one hand. This small device is portable and is useful for "reading" columns of data or diagrams. A blind physician can use it to "read" electrocardiograms. The optacon's cost is similar to that of the more widely applicable CCTV devices described above.

Physiatrists desiring more detailed descriptions, specifications, and commentary on vision enhancement and/or vision substitution can refer to the resource list found in the Annex at the end of this chapter. This Annex is not intended as a comprehensive list but rather as a selection of information sources with which the authors are familiar.

COMBINATIONS OF NEUROMUSCULAR AND VISUAL IMPAIRMENT

The rehabilitation literature on combined visual and neuromuscular disease is remarkable mainly for its paucity, but a few articles have been published in the past decade concerning blind amputees,[1,6] blind stroke patients,[19] and visually impaired head injury patients.[8] A survey of the prevalence of severe visual problems in rehabilitation inpatients has also been published.[20] It seems likely that double disability is an underreported phenomenon in medical rehabilitation settings and that it may well be encountered with increasing frequency, particularly among older patients. And based on evidence from the aforementioned literature, these doubly disabled patients do surprisingly well in terms of the functional outcome of their rehabilitation. This fact is most apparent among elderly patients.

Altner and associates[1] reported on the results of their experience with 12 blind lower-extremity amputees. Seventy-five percent of these patients became successful users of prosthetic devices. Fisher[6] reported similarly successful results with two blind diabetic below-knee amputees, both of whom returned to their homes after hospitalization able to use a prosthesis functionally.

Blind stroke patients have also done remarkably well in their rehabilitation. A two-year survey of 220 consecutive stroke admissions included nine admissions (4.1%) involving seven previously blind individuals.[19] These patients were all elderly, ranging from 71 to 84 years of age (mean age 76.1 years), and had been blind for considerable periods prior to their stroke. Six of the seven became ambulatory with supervision or minimal assistance by the time of their discharge from the rehabilitation unit, and four were able to be discharged to their homes. Mean length of stay (LOS) was 54 days as compared to 30.5 days for all rehabilitation inpatients during the period of study.

Other examples of successful rehabilitation of doubly disabled elderly patients were found in a prospective survey of 191 consecutive admissions to a general rehabilitation inpatient unit, 11 of which involved patients with severe visual impairment combined with neuromuscular disabilities.[20] Eight of these 11 elderly (mean age 79.7 years) patients could ambulate with a cane or walkerette by the time they were discharged, after a mean LOS that was actually shorter than that for all admissions (33.1 versus 35.9 days). Two patients had to be sent to medical-surgical units for complications (one subsequently died), and a third had to be placed in a skilled nursing facility.

The common thread that links these articles, and the patients they depict, is the age of the patients (almost exclusively elderly, mostly 75 or older) and the time sequence of the disabilities, that is, vision loss preceded neuromuscular disability. It is possible that the latter fact is the key to these patients overcoming their impairments so successfully. Visual loss, a purely sensory disability, preceded the development of neuromuscular impairment (usually purely motor but at times, as with stroke, a mixed sensorimotor disability) in almost every case in each of the studies alluded to above. Also significant is the fact that visual loss was sometimes gradual rather than sudden in its onset; thus, patients had the experience—often at a comparatively younger age—of a progressive functional loss for which they were able to compensate and develop new strategies for independent function. This rehabilitative experience may have been helpful at a later time when the now-elderly individual found himself or herself with a second disabling problem. It was striking how often mention was made of already-blind patients who, after a stroke or amputation, reached a level of mobility comparable to their status as blind ambulators.

Could visual loss actually be helpful to some of these patients? This may be true in the case of stroke patients whose brain injury produces significant visual dysperception, as in right parietal cerebral infarction. Such patients often become confused and do poorly in physical or occupational therapy tasks. These problems were strikingly absent in three of the four left hemiparetic patients studied by Wainapel.[19] Upper extremity dressing difficulties were not present, and patients were extremely alert; the one exception was the patient who had the greatest amount of residual visual function. It was hypothesized that the prolonged and profound visual loss present in these patients prior to their stroke protected them from the potentially devastating visual-motor sequelae commonly associated with right brain damage.

Lest the above discussion suggest that visual impairment occurs only in older patients in rehabilitation settings, the experience of Gianutsos et al. should be cited.[8] They prospectively reviewed 55 consecutive brain-injured residents of a head injury recovery center; the patients were mostly (73%) male, with a median age of 26.7 years. Careful (and often prolonged) optometric screening tests were performed, and more than half of those tested were felt to have visual problems that would be amenable to treatment. A total of 26 individuals received rehabilitative optometric services for problems that included inadequately corrected visual acuity, visual field deficits, and binocular vision problems (e.g., diplopia). Optometric treatment had a beneficial effect on the subsequent rehabilitation of affected patients.

The implications of the cited rehabilitation literature are that vision problems occur in many rehabilitation patients. Physiatrists routinely do tests of strength, joint range of motion, peripheral sensation, and cranial nerve function (which does include visual function), but the systematic and careful assessment of visual function has not been a standard part of physiatric evaluation. Clearly it should be, and more frequent use of ophthalmologic or optometric consultants is recommended. Moreover, when a visual impairment is discovered, it is incumbent upon the physiatrist to have at least sufficient familiarity with the principles of vision enhancement and/or substitution (as outlined above) to be able to appropriately advise and encourage such patients. This would represent a first step in the closer integration of medical rehabilitation and vision rehabilitation services.

TOWARD A MORE INTEGRATED APPROACH TO VISION REHABILITATION

Modern vision rehabilitation had its genesis in the experience gained from working with blinded veterans during World Wars I and II—young, male, and usually totally blind. The vision rehabilitation service system that evolved from this experience tended to focus on vocational issues, and favored the young, totally blind client while relegating older individuals to a much lower priority. This situation was vividly examined by Scott in his 1969 book *The Making of Blind Men*,[17] which criticized vision services for fostering dependency among their clients. Meanwhile, it was becoming increasingly evident that the majority of visually impaired persons were older, and that most were not totally blind. Has the system changed in the two decades since Scott's critique? Recent survey data by Kirchner and Aiello[13] suggest that there is more awareness of and attention to the partially sighted (low vision) client. However, Biegel et al.,[3] who surveyed agencies that serve the elderly and those for the visually impaired in Pennsylvania, have suggested that the older person with vision impairment may still be receiving disproportionately fewer services from either of these types of agencies.

As for the vision and PMR service systems, their interaction and cross-fertilization has been negligible. This is particularly ironic since there are so many similarities between them. The orientation and mobility instructor teaches the blind or visually impaired client how to walk using a cane or guide dog, much as the physical therapist trains a stroke patient to ambulate with a walker or cane. The rehabilitation teacher in the vision rehabilitation system resembles the occupational therapist; both focus on ADL tasks. Low-vision aids for vision enhancement can be considered orthotic devices which, like a brace or splint, support the affected body part (in this case the impaired eye). And vision substitution aids are analogous to prosthetic devices; the speech synthesizer "replaces" the absent vision as surely as a lower extremity prosthesis replaces the amputated limb. The importance of psychosocial and vocational interventions in either system is obvious. Lastly, the multidisciplinary rehabilitative team approach is equally applicable to the blind and to those with other physical disabilities.

The physical medicine and rehabilitation specialty is sensitive to the needs of people with physical disabilities, and its multidisciplinary perspective is ideally suited to include the care of visually impaired or blind individuals. Heretofore the vision rehabilitation and medical rehabilitation systems have developed to resemble two parallel lines: they go in the same basic direction but never intersect. However, the growing awareness that vision impairment is often only one of several limiting conditions in many patients, particularly the elderly, is beginning to change this pattern of mutual exclusivity. A closer relationship between the two care systems is a highly desirable goal for the final decade of this century. Given current trends in aging and disability statistics, it can be anticipated that physiatrists of the 21st century will become more frequent providers of rehabilitation care for the visually impaired.

REFERENCES

1. Altner PE, Rusin JJ, DeBoer A. Rehabilitation of blind patients with lower extremity amputations. *Arch Phys Med Rehabil.* 1980;61:82–85.
2. Applegate WB, Miller ST, Elam JT, et al. Impact of cataract surgery with lens implantation on vision and physical function in elderly patients. *JAMA.* 1987;257:1064–1066.
3. Biegel DE, Petchers MK, Snyder A, Beisgen B. Unmet needs and barriers to service delivery for the blind and visually impaired elderly. *Gerontologist.* 1989;29:86–91.
4. DiStefana AF, Aston SJ. Rehabilitation for the blind and visually impaired elderly. In: Brody SL, Ruff GE, eds. *Aging and rehabilitation: advances in the state of the art.* New York: Springer; 1986:203–217.
5. Faye EE. *Clinical low vision.* Boston: Little, Brown; 1984.
6. Fisher R. Rehabilitation of the blind amputee: a rewarding experience. *Arch Phys Med Rehabil.* 1987;68:382–383.
7. Fonda GE. *Management of low vision.* New York: Thieme-Stratton; 1981.
8. Gianutsos R, Ramsey G, Perlin RR. Rehabilitative optometric services for survivors of acquired brain injury. *Arch Phys Med Rehabil.* 1988;69:573–578.
9. Goodpasture RC. Rehabilitation of the blind. In: Krusen FH, Kottke FJ, Ellwood PM, eds. *Handbook of physical medicine and rehabilitation.* 2nd ed. Philadelphia: WB Saunders; 1971.
10. Greenblatt SL, ed. *Providing services for people with visual loss.* Lexington, Massachusetts: Resources for Rehabilitation; 1989.
11. Kahn HA, Leibowitz HM, Ganley JP, et al. The Framingham Eye Study 1: outline and major findings. *Am J Epidemiol.* 1977;106:17–32.
12. Kahn HA, Moorehead HS. *Statistics on blindness in model reporting area, 1969-70.* Washington, DC: US Government Printing Office; 1973; Department of Health, Education, and Welfare publication no 73-427.
13. Kirchner C, Aiello R. Services available to blind and visually handicapped persons in the US: a survey of agencies. *J Vis Impairment Blindness.* 1980;74:241–244.
14. Kornzweig AL. Rehabilitation ophthalmology for the aged. In: Williams TF, ed. *Rehabilitation in the aging.* New York: Raven Press; 1984:229–234.
15. Kottke FJ, Stillwell GK, Lehmann JF, eds. *Krusen's handbook of physical medicine and rehabilitation.* 3rd ed. Philadelphia: WB Saunders; 1982.

16. Nelson KA. Visual impairment among elderly Americans: statistics in transition. *J Vis Impairment Blindness.* 1987;81:331–334.
17. Scott R. *The making of blind men.* New York: Russell Sage; 1969.
18. United States Department of Health and Human Services (DHHS). *Prevalence of selected impairments: United States—1977; data from the National Health Survey.* Hyattsville, Maryland: National Center for Health Statistics; 1981; DHHS publication no (PHS) 81-1562. (Vital and health statistics; series 10; no 134).
19. Wainapel SF. Rehabilitation of the blind stroke patient. *Arch Phys Med Rehabil.* 1984; 65:487–489.
20. Wainapel SF, Kwon YS, Fazzari PJ. Severe visual impairment on a rehabilitation unit: incidence and implications. *Arch Phys Med Rehabil.* 1989;70:439–441.
21. Walsh R, Blasch BB. *Foundations of orientation and mobility.* New York: American Foundation for the Blind; 1983.

APPENDIX: RESOURCES AND SOURCES OF INFORMATION RELATED TO VISUAL IMPAIRMENT

General Information

1. American Foundation for the Blind, 15 W 16th St, New York, NY 10011
2. National Library Service for the Blind and Physically Handicapped (including Talking Books Program), Library of Congress, Washington, DC 20542
3. Vision Foundation Inc, 2 Mt Auburn St, Watertown, MA 02171
4. Resources for Rehabilitation, 33 Bedford St, Suite 19A, Lexington, MA 02173

"Talking" and Other Electronic Devices

1. American Foundation for the Blind, 15 W 16th St, New York, NY 10011
2. Boston Information and Technology, MIT Branch, PO Box 7, Cambridge, MA 02139
3. Innovative Rehabilitation Technology Inc (IRTI), 1605 W El Camino Real, Mountain View, CA 94040.
4. Science Products, Box A, Southeastern Facility, Chester, PA 19399
5. Vox-Com, 100 Clovergreen, Peachtree City, GA 30269 (also available from other distributors)

Low-vision Optical Aids

1. LS and S Group, PO Box 673, Northbrook, IL 60065
2. Center for the Partially Sighted, 1250 16th St, Santa Monica, CA 90404
3. Low Vision Service, New York Association for the Blind, 111 E 59th St, New York, NY 10022
4. Ocu-aid Enterprises, Box 5772, Columbus, GA 31906

Electronic Vision Aids

1. Pelco Sales Inc, 351 E Alondra Blvd, Gardena, CA 90248
2. Telesensory Systems Inc, 455 N Bernardo, Mountain View, CA 94043

Optical-tactile Converter and Other High-technology Sensory Aids

1. Kurzweil Computer Products, 185 Albany St, Cambridge, MA 02139
2. Telesensory Systems Inc, 455 N Bernardo, Mountain View, CA 94043

Sources of Brailled and Cassette-recorded Materials

1. National Braille Association Reader Transcriber Registry, 5300 Hamilton Ave, Cincinnati, OH 45231
2. National Library Service for the Blind and Physically Handicapped, Library of Congress, Washington, DC 20542
3. Recordings for the Blind, 20 Rozel, Princeton, NJ 08540

Information Concerning Computers Adapted for Vision Impairment

1. *Technical Innovations Bulletin,* Innovative Rehabilitation Technology Inc (IRTI), 1605 W El Camino Real, Mountain View, CA 94040
2. *Second Beginner's Guide to Personal Computers for the Blind and Visually Impaired, 1984,* National Braille Press Inc, 88 St Stephen's Street, Boston, MA 02115

Chapter 13

GERIATRIC REHABILITATION

Stephen F. Noll

THE GERIATRIC IMAGE

The image of aging is often linked to negative perceptions: that age 65 is old; that older people are all about the same, and usually somewhat unattractive or sexless; that with old age come poor health and senility. In fact, these perceptions are far from the truth. In one poll, when asked about their health, the majority of elderly persons responded that they felt well. Only slightly more than 20% indicated that they were debilitated by health problems. Yet, in the same poll, young people estimated that 50% of the elderly suffered from serious illness.[16]

Names or adjectives used to describe older persons—even those of the same age—can connote entirely disparate images: patriarch/matriarch, golden-ager, senior citizen, elder, or dean versus old duffer, dotage, aged, senescent, palsied, or wizened. The difference lies in the quality of life maintained by the persons to which the words refer, and that quality of life depends primarily upon whether or not they have maintained their independence in activities of daily living (ADL), mobility, and communication through appropriate programs of rehabilitation and maintenance.

Unfortunately, negative stereotypes may persuade physicians and the laity that aging is a progressively disabling state, that quality of life for the elderly with chronic illnesses is dismal, and that care of the elderly is palliative and unrewarding. Such perceptions are false. Many of the changes attributed to the "disease" of aging are in fact due to modifiable influences such as inactivity, diet, and personal and psychosocial factors.[47]

Health care professionals may presume that health is the sole determinant of quality of life in the older population. Yet Pearlman and Uhlmann[41] found that older persons rated their quality of life as good enough to be free of major complaints despite the presence of chronic illness. This viewpoint was in contrast to the perception of their physicians.

Perceptions are changing. The interaction of true age-related changes with true disease states sets the stage for geriatric clinical practice,[7] a domain that offers as much if not more intrigue as other fields in medicine. When the elements of functional impairment and the need to restore function are added to the formula for health care, geriatric rehabilitation emerges with a dominant role in maintaining the quality of life of the elderly. Principles of rehabilitation are applicable to many of the problems encountered in the treatment of older persons.

THE GERIATRIC APPROACH

While the diagnostic evaluation of disorders remains essential to optimal care, the identification of associated functional impairment has recently been recognized as equally important in comprehensive management of the elderly. To that end, several tools have been developed in an attempt to evaluate functional impairment.[4] Many of these tools are derived from rehabilitation literature, especially those which address physical function such as the Katz ADL scale, the Barthel index, and the Kenny Self-Care scale. Some tools have evolved from other specialties and address specific areas such as cognitive function (e.g., Folstein Mini-Mental State Examination,[20] Kokmen Mini-Mental Status Examination[31]) or emotional status (e.g., Hamilton Depression Inventory[26]).

Assessment tools offer several features important in clinical practice. First, they provide a data base by which changes in an individual patient can be monitored over time—for example, to see whether there has been functional improvement or regression and whether established functional goals have been met. Second, they provide a data base by which the outcome from an individual program can be monitored over time—for example, to see whether the patients under treatment have shown functional improvement or regression in a particular area, such as transfers, dressing, etc. Third, if used uniformly, they may provide a data base to compare and contrast programs in different facilities.

Figure 1 shows a composite diagram of tools exemplifying these three functions. The institution-specific tool (A) represents segments from a patient evaluation profile designed to monitor those items which the facility's staff (Mayo Clinic Department of Physical Medicine and Rehabilitation) has determined are important. The program evaluation graph (B) represents data taken from one item in the tool to demonstrate functional performance of an entire cohort of patients for that item, i.e., the percentage of a population whose score increased by one, increased by two or more, or remained the same in performance of transfers. Finally, the Functional Independence Measure (C) represents a standardized tool taken from the Uniform Data Set for Medical Rehabilitation[25] which can stand alone or as a component of an institution-specific tool. This measure, when utilized uniformly and in conjunction with a uniform data base, allows comparison of outcomes between various institutions.

One tool seldom meets all assessment needs. Shortcomings vary: some are too narrow in scope, failing to address all the necessary issues; some are too insensitive to change, failing to reflect small yet significant functional

Figure 1. Samples of functional assessment tools.

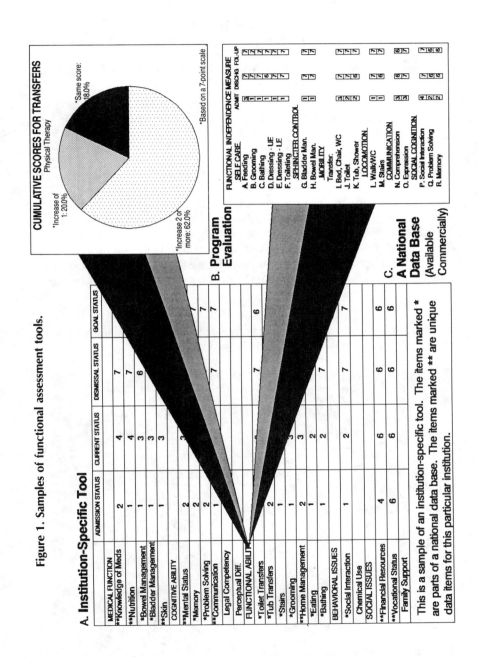

A. Institution-Specific Tool

	ADMISSION STATUS	CURRENT STATUS	DISMISSAL STATUS	GOAL STATUS
MEDICAL FUNCTION				
**Knowledge of Meds	2	4	7	
*Nutrition	1	4	7	
*Bowel Management	1	3	6	
*Bladder Management	1	3		
**Skin	1	3		
COGNITIVE ABILITY				
**Mental Status	2	3		7
*Memory	2			7
*Problem Solving	2		7	7
**Communication	1			
Legal Competency				
Perceptual Diff.				
FUNCTIONAL ABILITY				
*Toilet Transfers			7	6
*Tub Transfers	2			
*Stairs				
*Grooming	1	3		
**Home Management	2	3		
*Eating	1	2	7	7
*Bathing	1	2		
BEHAVIORAL ISSUES				
*Social Interaction	1	2	7	
Chemical Use				
SOCIAL ISSUES				
**Financial Resources	4	6	6	6
*Vocational Status	6	6	6	6
Family Support				

B. Program Evaluation

CUMULATIVE SCORES FOR TRANSFERS
Physical Therapy

*Increase of 1: 200%

*Same score: 18.0%

*Increase 2 or more: 62.0%

*Based on a 7-point scale

C. A National Data Base
(Available Commercially)

FUNCTIONAL INDEPENDENCE MEASURE

	ADMIT	DISCHG	FOL-UP
SELF CARE			
A. Feeding	6	6	7
B. Grooming	1	6	7
C. Bathing	1	6	7
D. Dressing - UE	1	6	7
E. Dressing - LE	6	6	7
F. Toileting	1	6	7
SPHINCTER CONTROL			
G. Bladder Man.	1	7	7
H. Bowel Man.	1	7	7
MOBILITY			
Transfer:			
I. Bed, Chair, WC	3	7	7
J. Toilet	2	6	7
K. Tub, Shower	2	6	7
LOCOMOTION			
L. Walk/WC	1	6	7
M. Stairs	1	6	7
COMMUNICATION			
N. Comprehension	3	6	6
O. Expression	3	6	7
SOCIAL COGNITION			
P. Social Interaction	4	6	6
Q. Problem Solving	2	6	6
R. Memory	2	6	6

This is a sample of an institution-specific tool. The items marked * are parts of a national data base. The items marked ** are unique data items for this particular institution.

progress; and some may be too complex or time-consuming to administer in clinical practice.

More importantly, comprehensive geriatric assessment implies more than evaluation using a standardized scale. It also implies the coordinated input of a team of professionals representing several disciplines to carry out a comprehensive program of rehabilitation. The interaction of the interdisciplinary team makes the rehabilitation approach unique.

AGE-RELATED ISSUES IN GERIATRIC REHABILITATION

Decubiti

Physiological changes in the skin that accompany aging include a decrease in elasticity, a decrease in vascularity, and often a decrease in subcutaneous adipose tissue. These expected changes, in conjunction with other risk factors, predispose an older person to pressure sores. Pressure sores characteristically occur over boney prominences, which, in an elderly person at bed rest or seated in a chair, are commonly the sacrum, trochanters, ischial tuberosities, and heels (see Figure 2). Pressure sores develop owing to a host of factors that impair the metabolism of the tissues, including

Figure 2. Typical appearance and location of decubitus ulcers on the heels (left) and sacrum of a debilitated elderly patient.

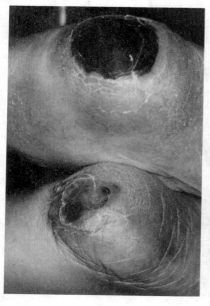
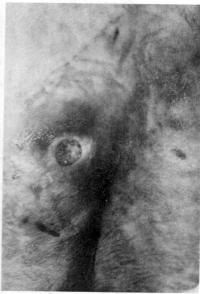

mechanical, medical, and biochemical factors, but pressure and shear forces are most frequently noted.[3,32] Breakdown of the skin also can occur in the elderly from abrasion due to friction or from maceration due to moisture.

Prevention is the most desirable management, and to this end a tool to assess risks has been developed.[55] Rating an elderly patient on a scale of potential risks provides a useful profile to identify the necessary skin management practices (see Figure 3). Once the components of risk have been identified, then the level of intervention with equipment, nursing care, and protocols can be prescribed.

There are a host of prescribed treatments for decubiti, but general principles apply to all. Classification of the sore by depth (Grades I–IV) and measurement of its diameter are essential for monitoring the effect of treatment. Treatment may include systemic antibiotics if there is evidence of sepsis, cellulitis, or osteomyelitis; local care with hydrotherapy and various dressings to keep the wound debrided, clean, and protected; and possible surgical repair for ulcers that extend into fascia and muscle.[3]

The cornerstone of prevention and treatment is relief of pressure. Protection in bed ranges from frequent changes of position and use of a foam pad for the low-risk patient to use of an air-fluidized or low-air-loss bed for the high-risk patient. Appropriate foam, gel, or air-celled wheelchair cushions[19] are necessary for the debilitated elderly, rather than the usual vinyl sling seat. It has been shown that with repeated loading, there is impaired recovery of oxygen tension in the tissue of debilitated patients as compared to healthy persons and thus a significantly greater risk of skin breakdown.[5] Limiting

Figure 3. Factors contributing to risk of skin breakdown.

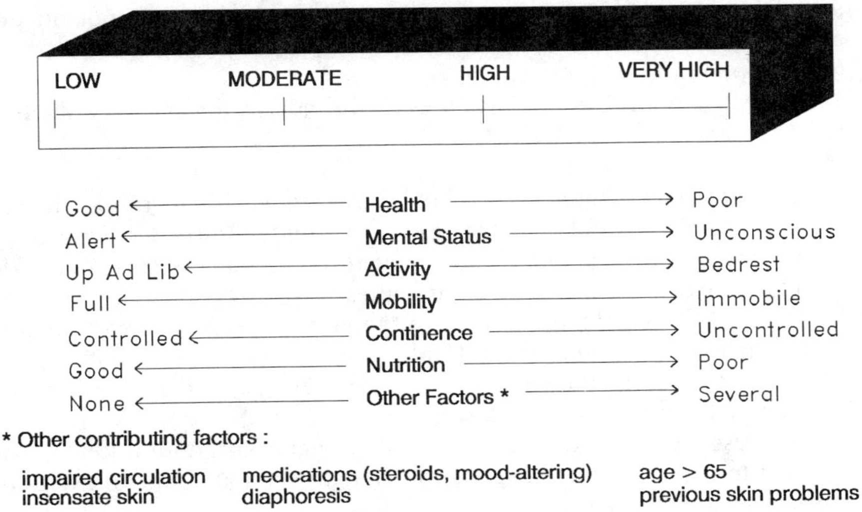

Good ←	Health	→	Poor
Alert ←	Mental Status	→	Unconscious
Up Ad Lib ←	Activity	→	Bedrest
Full ←	Mobility	→	Immobile
Controlled ←	Continence	→	Uncontrolled
Good ←	Nutrition	→	Poor
None ←	Other Factors *	→	Several

* Other contributing factors :

impaired circulation	medications (steroids, mood-altering)	age > 65
insensate skin	diaphoresis	previous skin problems

the amount of sitting time allowed and ensuring optimal wheelchair positioning to diminish shear forces are as important as providing the proper cushion.

Deconditioning

Aged persons have decreased strength, endurance, and joint mobility, although with a wide range of variation.[27,44] A 70-year-old man has approximately the same strength as a 15-year-old boy, but without the endurance or flexibility. Deconditioning becomes significant when it results in the older person being unable to perform self-care, carry out activities of daily living, or move about safely.

The decrease in physical activity and exercise that frequently accompanies aging may be a major influence in the loss of strength and endurance. Unfortunately, exercising provokes images of the young, of equipment, and of strenuous workouts. In fact, exercise does not need to be vigorous to be effective. For example, a light stretching program, exercises against gravity (but without weights), and regular aerobic walking have been documented to increase strength and flexibility in older women.[2,42] Furthermore, it has been shown that maximal oxygen consumption responds to low-intensity aerobic training; thus, it is unnecessary for an older person to risk injury with higher intensity training.[21]

Benefits of a regular exercise program can be both physical and psychological. Elderly persons participating in group exercises perceive themselves more favorably than those who do not exercise.[10] In addition, they may experience less pain following exercise, not more, as one might expect. Benefits are not limited to the healthiest of the elderly.[42] Frail elderly residing in nursing homes show similar benefits, including increased spontaneous activity and decreased dependence, especially if programs are initiated before profound loss of function has occurred.[39]

When prescribing exercise regimens for the elderly, the general principles to be considered are as follows:

- Strengthening programs should focus on key functional groups, such as the "crutch" muscles in the upper extremities (shoulder depressors, triceps, and wrist muscles) and the quadriceps, hip extensors, and ankle plantar extensors in the low extremities.
- Because of its potential to elevate blood pressure, sustained isometric strengthening should be used only with caution in those with hypertension. An isometric contraction need not be longer than 3–5 seconds to be effective in increasing strength.
- Because isotonic exercises may further aggravate arthritic joints, it is best to use isometric exercises for strengthening and kinetic exercises to develop endurance.

- Aerobic programs in an older person require modification. They should begin at approximately 40% or less of maximum oxygen consumption or heart rate for age, rather than 60%. A program should initially be divided into 2–5 minute intervals rather than carried out over a sustained period. Exercise that makes a person breathless represents 60–70% of maximum oxygen consumption. Usual chosen walking speed is 35–40% of maximum oxygen consumption.[49]
- The risk of falling during exercise can be minimized through the use of gait aids for safety as necessary and avoidance of uneven, wet, or slippery surfaces.

With these considerations in mind, exercise can be recommended with the goal of improving overall functional performance safely.

Falls

Falling is a feared but often preventable incident for elderly persons. Even those falls that are not associated with injury often take a toll in decreasing an older person's level of activity by leading to fear of further falls.[60] Therapeutic intervention requires identification of the risks and reasons for falling for each individual. Risk factors can be intrinsic, activity-related, or environmental.[56] Development of a risk profile for each elderly person is helpful in prevention (Figure 4).

Intrinsic factors are medical conditions that impair a person and predispose him or her to fall. Gait characteristics in themselves do not identify the high-risk patient,[22] but decreased balance, decreased strength, and decreased flexibility are all factors related to risk of falling.[23] Older persons impaired because of a stroke or a lower-limb amputation are also in high-risk categories.[57] Acute illness, postural hypotension, and decreased alertness because of medication are three transient intrinsic factors that are always important to take into account.[56]

Activity-related falls usually occur during routine daily activities, not during unusual or "risky" tasks. In the rehabilitation setting, falls frequently occur when an older person leans or reaches from a wheelchair, or during a transfer.[56] Falls are especially frequent when elderly persons get out of bed at night.

Finally, environmental factors increase the risk of a fall. Of the risk factors mentioned, these are the most amenable to corrective intervention. Factors such as inadequate lighting, a slippery, uneven, or rough floor surface, stairs, an inaccessible tub, and icy walkways are just a few of the items to be considered in a comprehensive risk assessment.[56]

Prevention is always the best intervention. A home assessment by the therapist will allow appropriate placement of grab bars, bathroom accessories such as a bath bench, and other home modifications to enhance

Figure 4. Sample checklist of risk factors for falling.

Mental Status	**Elimination**
Confused/disoriented _____	Incontinence _____
Emotional disability _____	Urgency/frequency _____
Impulsive behavior _____	
High need for	
independence _____	**Orthostatic**
	Hypotension _____
Mobility (circle Right or Left)	
R/L UE paresis/paralysis _____	**Sleep Pattern**
R/L LE paresis/paralysis _____	**Disturbance** _____
Generalized weakness _____	
Ataxia _____	
R/L below-knee amputation _____	**Sensory Deficits**
R/L above-knee amputation _____	Visual _____
	Speech _____
	Auditory _____
Seizure Disorder _____	Perceptual alteration _____
Other _____	

safety.[56] If on assessment a problem with balance is identified, or strength and flexibility are significantly decreased, then gait training with a gait aid is advisable. Gait aids vary in design, but all enhance stability by increasing the size of the base of support.[30] A rolling walker, which provides a constant base since it never leaves the ground, is often the aid of choice for the frail elderly. If orthostatic hypotension is a problem, elastic compression garments are useful to help to maintain effective blood pressure. Insertion of zippers in these garments will make them easier to put on (Figure 5).

Urinary Incontinence

Urinary incontinence is a problem frequently encountered by older persons. It may be due to significant medical disease, but to the person affected it is often symbolic of personal and social regression. It also affects an older person's acceptance in the family and the community.

Before treatment begins, the functional performance and health of the urinary system should be assessed. A routine laboratory screen (urinalysis,

Figure 5. Leotard pressure garment used in the management of orthostasis, adapted with zippers for ease of donning.

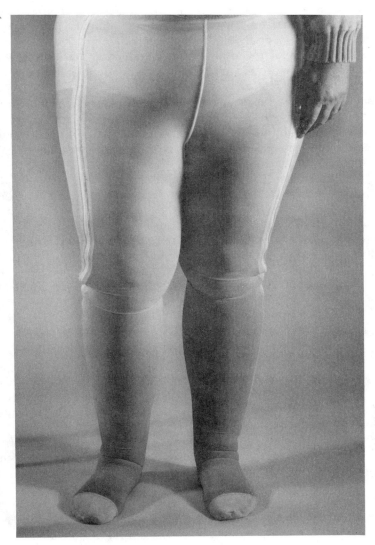

serum creatinine, blood urea nitrogen, and urine culture/sensitivity) can indicate the health status of the urinary system.[43] A measurement of post-voiding residual urine by catheterization or by ultrasound provides information about mechanical function. If the postvoiding residual is greater than approximately 100 cc, some mechanical dysfunction of the system is suspected.[40]

Abramson[1] summarized bladder mechanics in a formula that helps explain the dynamics of bladder function: $(P - R)T \sim V$, where P = pressure within the bladder, R = outflow resistance, T = time of voiding, and V = percent bladder volume voided. In the context of this formula, the postvoiding residual volume is inversely related to the percentage of the volume voided (V). When the postvoiding residual is abnormally high, the percent volume voided is low due to causes well explained by the formula. First, the bladder pressure (P) may be too low, as is the case in lower motor neuron bladder dysfunction or in an "overstretched" bladder. Second, the resistance (R) may be too high, such as in prostatic hypertrophy or detrusor-sphincter dyssynergia. In both of these circumstances, further urological evaluation to define a specific problem is warranted, since the incontinence is likely an overflow phenomenon.

On the other hand, if the postvoiding residual is approximately 100 cc or less, incontinence is often caused by stress or uninhibited detrusor contractions that push the vesicular pressure (P) intermittently above the outflow resistance (R). In these situations, and if the screening data are normal, initiation of a behavioral bladder retraining program without further evaluation is reasonable.[18] Bladder retraining programs vary, but they usually consist of structured components including a fluid schedule (which directs the timing and amounts of oral fluids, a voiding schedule (which directs the time intervals for voiding), and feedback for the patient.[40] Voiding intervals may begin at 30 to 60 minutes and be lengthened to two to three hours provided continence is maintained.

A behavioral program alone is effective in at least 50% of older persons with incontinence.[17,18] The addition of Kegel exercises and biofeedback muscle reeducation may enhance effectiveness.[12,59] If adequate improvement is not realized with a behavioral program, or if there is suspected underlying neurogenic bladder dysfunction, further urologic evaluation including urodynamics is indicated to direct treatment. Pharmacologic intervention is typically next on the treatment pyramid and consists of drugs which: (a) decrease detrusor contractility, such as anticholinergics, smooth muscle depressants, and calcium antagonists; (b) increase outflow resistance, commonly alpha-adrenergic agonists; (c) alter more than one function, such as tricyclics and estrogen.[58] Because pharmacokinetics is significantly different in the older population, when drugs are used for the treatment of urinary incontinence the optimal procedure is to begin with a low dose and titrate upward until the desired effect or side effect is reached.

Constipation

Older patients' attention to their bowel habits often seems exaggerated, but, in fact, the focus is not unwarranted. Constipation may become increasingly problematic with age and may lead to fecal impaction, a condition causing significant morbidity.[61] The cause for this problem is not necessarily age itself but rather other precipitating factors, which include poor diet, inadequate fluid intake, too little physical exercise, and medications such as narcotics or anticholinergics. If neurological disease impairs sensation, mentation, or motor function, the problem is compounded.

Constipation can be defined in a variety of ways, but a stool frequency of less than three per week is an operational definition that provides a guideline indicating when to intervene. Rehabilitation principles of neurogenic bowel care can apply to prevention and/or treatment of constipation in the elderly; strategies include timed evacuation, preferably after a meal to incorporate the influence of the gastrocolic reflex, and a diet high in fiber, supplemented with a bulk agent and a stool softener. Fluid intake and physical activity are two major considerations in the older person. If a bowel movement does not occur spontaneously every other day, the use of a rectal suppository and/or anal stretch to stimulate peristaltic reflexes is helpful and does not result in bowel dependency on oral laxatives. If fecal impaction occurs, more aggressive measures are necessary, such as Hypaque enemas, sigmoidoscopic disimpaction, or rarely surgery.[61] In the older person the possibility of neoplasm as a cause of constipation also exists.[48]

Osteoporosis

Fractures secondary to osteoporosis are disabling because of the chronic severe pain caused by vertebral compression fractures and the loss of ability to walk following fracture of the hip. With age, both cortical and trabecular bone mass decrease. Trabecular losses begin earlier (about age 30) and in postmenopausal women exceed cortical losses. Typically, bone loss occurs in a pattern that predisposes an older person to hip, wrist, and vertebral fractures.[45]

Based on clinical characteristics, osteoporosis is classified as either postmenopausal (Type I) or senile (Type II). The former syndrome primarily affects women age 45 to 75 who show especially rapid trabecular bone loss. Senile osteoporosis constitutes a serious threat of fractures in women and men over the age of 75, at a 2:1 female to male ratio.[45] Often, estrogen and calcium supplements are employed to treat Type I osteoporosis, and calcium alone for Type II, as well as appropriate exercise for both. However, optimal treatment is prevention. To that end, a risk inventory that classifies factors as modifiable or nonmodifiable will assess areas in which the possibility of intervention exists (see Table 1).

The rehabilitation considerations for osteoporosis are fivefold: diet, exercise, physical therapy, orthotics, and endocrines. Figure 6 presents the measures to be considered. In the case of vertebral fractures, the acuteness or chronicity of the problem dictates which interventions are most appropriate.[50] Exercise plays more than one role: it may stimulate new bone

Table 1. Risk factors for osteoporosis.

Modifiable	Nonmodifiable
Estrogen deficiency	Race
Inactivity	Age
Endocrine disease	Sex
Alcoholism	Body habitus
Immobility[a]	Steroids (exogenous)[a]
Low calcium intake	Family history
	Nulliparity
	Anticonvulsants[a]

[a]May be in either category.

Figure 6. Rehabilitation options for osteoporosis.

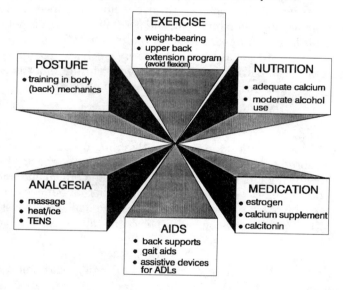

formation to increase bone density and also improves posture. Since vertebrae wedge anteriorly when they fracture, a back extension strengthening program should be used.[51]

Dementia

Forgetfulness is a characteristic of aging, and fear of senile dementia commonly accompanies growing old. In fact, intellectual functions are relatively well maintained in normal aging. Consequently, if an older person shows mental impairment on psychological testing, the finding cannot be considered "normal for age."[46]

Clinically, it is important to differentiate dementia from delirium and depression. These latter two conditions may masquerade as dementia or, perhaps more commonly, accompany and aggravate dementia. Typically, delirium is an abrupt phenomenon that shows variability, while dementia is more stable in its course. Consciousness is not usually clouded in dementia as it is in delirium.[14] Delirium may result from improper or excessive medication. Because of multiple medical problems, the older person is more likely to have multiple medications prescribed; because of altered pharmacokinetics and pharmacodynamics, the older person is also more prone to have adverse drug reactions. When prescibing medication for an older person, it is important to first review drugs already prescribed, to start with small dosages, to simplify the dosage schedule, to provide devices to assist with accurate administration, and to educate the patient and family about the medications.[38]

A decreased ability to think or concentrate is as characteristic of a major depression as it is of dementia. However, pseudodementia, or depression mimicking dementia, is less common in the elderly than dementia presenting with an associated depression. Older persons with depression typically show physical signs such as loss of appetite, weight loss, apathy, and inability to initiate activity. Of great concern is the fact that they are at high risk for suicide.[9]

Cognitive impairment also may be due to other treatable causes such as thyroid disease, vitamin B_{12} deficiency, anemia, renal failure, and normal-pressure hydrocephalus. The more common dementias, however, are due to Alzheimer's disease, a progressive disorder of unclear etiology, or to cerebrovascular disease resulting in multiple infarcts.

Experience in the rehabilitation of traumatic brain injury has aided understanding of ways to mitigate the problems associated with dementia. Such measures as compensatory memory aids, a structured environment that includes a calendar and a clock, and rehearsal techniques may help a person with dementia to carry out necessary daily activities. Studies have shown that cognitive training may diminish or reverse losses in an older person's cognitive function.[47]

AGE IN RELATION TO IMPAIRMENT GROUPS

Stroke

Several variables have been correlated negatively with rehabilitative outcome after stroke.[15] Age is identified as one of those variables in some studies but not in others. Jongbloed[29] points out that confusion regarding age and functional outcome may be related to how outcome is measured. If outcome is measured as function at discharge, the correlation with age is likely negative. If outcome is measured as positive change in function resulting from rehabilitation, the correlation with age is likely positive. As an independent variable, age has not been shown to correlate well enough to predict individual outcome, and therefore cannot be the sole factor weighed in determining whether rehabilitation is indicated or not. By virtue of age, however, a person may be more likely to have other characteristics which correlate negatively with rehabilitation potential, such as previous strokes, cardiovascular disease, and lack of family or social support.

The atypical presentation of disease states in the older patient adds to the challenge of patient care during rehabilitation. Frequently, the onset of illnesses in the elderly may present with nonspecific symptoms such as confusion, fatigue, or merely a failure to thrive, rather than specific symptoms such as fever in an infection or chest pain in a myocardial infarction.[8]

Traumatic Brain Injury

Age is a factor in predicting outcome following traumatic brain injury. Increased morbidity and a poorer overall functional outcome are reported for injuries occurring after the age of 60. The influence of age is theorized to be due to reduced plasticity of the older nervous system, but it is likely also due to the higher incidence of medical complications related to traumatic brain injury in the older age group.[37] Outcome from anoxic coma appears to be poorer in older individuals than in younger ones,[24] a finding that has implications for consideration of cardiopulmonary resuscitation.

Spinal Cord Injury

Spinal cord injuries (SCI) in the older population more often result from falls than from motor vehicle accidents, the major cause in younger persons. Moreover, the ratio of quadriparesis to paraparesis is greater in the older population.[54] When compared to the younger cohort, older spinal cord-injured persons are more likely to have medical complications such as pneumonia, gastrointestinal hemorrhage, and pulmonary emboli, and they also have a poorer two-year survival rate.[13] However, when matched for impairment, only in certain areas of daily living skills does advancing age correlate negatively with functional independence.[62] In and of itself, then, age is not an indication to limit rehabilitation services for spinal cord injury. For the elderly SCI patient, chronic use of a wheelchair over several years may result in degenerative changes or nerve entrapment syndromes.[34] Furthermore, chronological age is related to an overall decline in activity (decrease in sitting tolerance and weekly outings).[33]

Amputation

Success in the rehabilitation of an elderly amputee may not be so much related to age as to a number of associated factors. One such factor is level of amputation. The energy requirements for walking with an above-knee prosthesis are significantly higher than for a below-knee prosthesis. Steinberg[53] has shown success, as measured by full-time prosthetic wear, in approximately 75% of a group of geriatric below-knee amputees. The success rate falls to 50% in above-knee amputees and to 33% in bilateral amputees. In the evaluation of the geriatric patient for prosthetic fitting, important considerations include visual acuity, upper extremity strength, lower extremity flexion contractures, the health of the other limb, cardio-pulmonary disease, and cognitive status.[11]

Musculoskeletal Limitations

Chronic musculoskeletal problems are common in the elderly. Evidence of osteoarthritis is said to be universal in persons over the age of 65.[36] In persons with loss of strength and range of motion, Jette et al.[28] have found an interesting relationship between specific sites of impairment and type of physical disability. Basic ADLs are most affected by impaired hand function and instrumental ADLs by lower extremity function. Limited range of motion alone is not unusual in the elderly, but it may have little effect on performance of ADLs. One study documented that 80% of 79-year-old persons were able to perform their basic ADLs and 50% their own housework, despite restricted ranges of motion of joints.[6]

QUALITY OF LIFE FOR THE AGED

In *The Angle of Repose*,[52] the character Lyman Ward is an elderly amputee in a wheelchair, with limited neck motion due to arthritis, who is living independently. Early in the book, he reflects on the attitude of his family:

> "They keep thinking of my good, in their terms. . . . So I may anticipate regular visits of inspection and solicitude while they wait for me to get a belly full of independence. . . . I would have them understand that I am not just killing time during my slow petrifaction. I am neither dead nor inert."

Just as it is for the rest of us, the quality of his or her life is of utmost importance to the elderly person. The right to make one's own decisions is a key determinant of quality of life. Where to live, how to live, what to do—all are decisions of primary importance to the elderly just as they are to the rest of us. The most significant contribution of rehabilitation is the restoration of capacity for a greater degree of independent living, which gives the individual greater freedom of choice and prolongs the period of independence.

On the other hand rehabilitation professionals, in their enthusiasm to help the elderly, have the potential to strip them of control, decision making, and dignity. The impact of having control versus not having control over one's life is striking. Studies in nursing homes suggest that residents given a part in decision making and in performance of tasks are more satisfied, more active, and in better general health. Furthermore, studies suggest that unnecessary direct assistance to older persons encourages helplessness.[47] Therefore, just as the goal of rehabilitation is functional independence in mobility and in activities of daily living, so too the goal for older persons should be functional independence in setting their own objectives and in controlling or arranging their own schedules whenever possible.

Frederic Verzar, a Swiss dean of gerontologists, once said: "Old age is not an illness, it is a continuation of life with decreasing capacities for adaption."[35] It may be said then that the focus of geriatric rehabilitation is to augment these capacities for adaption so that each elderly person may have more freedom to set and achieve his or her own goals.

REFERENCES

1. Abramson AS. Neurogenic bladder: a guide to evaluation and management. *Arch Phys Med Rehabil.* 1983;64:6–10.
2. Agre JC, Pierce LE, Raab DM, McAdams M, Smith EL. Light resistance and stretching exercise in elderly women: effect upon strength. *Arch Phys Med Rehabil.* 1968;69:273–276.
3. Allman RM. Pressure ulcers among the elderly. *N Engl J Med.* 1989;320:850–853.
4. Applegate WB, Blass JP, Williams TF. Instruments for the functional assessment of older patients. *N Engl J Med.* 1990;322:1207–1214.
5. Bader DL. The recovery characteristics of soft tissues following repeated loading. *J Rehabil Res Dev.* 1990;27:141–150.
6. Bergstrom G, Aniansson A, Bjelle A, et al. Functional consequences of joint impairment at age 79. *Scand J Rehabil Med.* 1985;17:183–190.
7. Besdine RW. The maturing of geriatrics. *N Engl J Med.* 1989;320:181–182.
8. Besdine RW. Rehabilitation of the elderly stroke victim: a primer for geriatric medicine. In: Erickson RV, ed. *Medical management of the elderly stroke patient.* Philadelphia: Hanley and Belfus and Company;1989:453–456. (Physical Medicine and Rehabilitation: State of the Art Reviews).
9. Blazer D. Current concepts: depression in the elderly. *N Engl J Med.* 1989;320:164–166.
10. Blumenthal JA, Emery CF, Madden DF, et al. Cardiovascular and behavioral effects of aerobic exercise training in healthy older men and women. *J Gerontol.* 1989;44(5):147–157.
11. Brown PS. The geriatric amputee. In: Maloney FP, Means KM, eds. *Rehabilitation of the aging population.* (Physical Medicine and Rehabilitation: State of the Art Reviews. 1990;4:67–76).
12. Burns PA, Pranikoff K, Nochajski T, et al. Treatment of stress incontinence with pelvic floor exercises and biofeedback. *J Am Geriatr Soc.* 1990;38:341–344.
13. DeVivo MJ, Kartus PL, Rutt RD. The influence of age at time of spinal cord injury on rehabilitation outcome. *Arch Neurol.* 1990;47:687–691.

14. *Diagnostic and statistical manual of mental disorders* (DSM-III-R). 3rd ed. revised. Washington, DC: American Psychiatric Association; 1987.
15. Dombovy ML, Sandok BA, Basford JR. Rehabilitation for stroke: a review. *Stroke.* 1986;17:363–369.
16. Dychtwald K, Flower J. *Age wave: the challenges and opportunities of an aging America.* Los Angeles: Jeremy P. Tracher, Inc; 1989:30–34.
17. Fantl JA, Wyman JF, Harkins SW, Hadley EC. Bladder training in the management of lower urinary tract dysfunction in women; a review. *J Am Geriatr Soc.* 1990;38:329–332.
18. Fantl JA, Wyman JF, McClish DK, et al. Efficiency of bladder training in older women with urinary incontinence. *JAMA.* 1991;265:609–613.
19. Ferguson-Pell MW. Seat cushion selection. *J Rehabil Res Dev.* 1990;(Clin Suppl 2):49–73.
20. Folstein MF, Folstein SE, McHugh PR. Mini-mental state: a practical method for grading the cognitive state of patients for the clinician. *J Psychiatr Res.* 1975;12:189–198.
21. Foster VL, Hume GJ, Byrnes WC, Dickinson AL, Chatfield SJ. Endurance training for elderly women: moderate vs low intensity. *J Gerontol.* 1989;44(6):M184–M188.
22. Gehlsen GM, Whaley MH. Falls in the elderly: part I, gait. *Arch Phys Med Rehabil.* 1990;71:735–738.
23. Gehlsen GM, Whaley MH. Falls in the elderly: part II, balance, strength, and flexibility. *Arch Phys Med Rehabil.* 1990;71:739–741.
24. Grosswasser Z, Cohen M, Costeff H. Rehabilitation outcome after anoxic brain damage. *Arch Phys Med Rehabil.* 1989;70:186–188.
25. *Guide for the use of the uniform data set for medical rehabilitation,* Research Foundation, Buffalo, New York, State University of New York, 1990.
26. Hamilton M. Development of a rating scale for primary depressive illness. *Br J Soc Clin Psychol.* 1967;6:278–296.
27. James B, Parker AW. Active and passive mobility of lower limb joints in elderly men and women. *Am J Phys Med Rehabil.* 1989;68:162–167.
28. Jette AM, Branch LG, Berlin J. Musculoskeletal impairments and physical disablement among the aged. *J Gerontol.* 1990;45:M203–M208.
29. Jongbloed L. Prediction of function after stroke: a critical review. *Stroke.* 1986;17:765–776.
30. Joyce BM, Kirby RE. Canes, crutches, and walkers. *Am Fam Physician.* 1991;43:535–542.
31. Kokmen E, Nassens JM, Offord KP. A short test of mental status: description and preliminary results. *Mayo Clin Proc.* 1987;62:281–288.
32. Kosiak M. Etiology and pathology of ischemic ulcers. *Arch Phys Med Rehabil.* 1959;40:62–69.
33. Krause JS, Crewe MM. Chronological age, time since injury, and time of measurement: effect of adjustment after spinal cord injury. *Arch Phys Med Rehabil.* 1991;72:91–100.
34. Lammertse DP, Yarkony GM. Rehabilitation in spinal cord disorders; 4, Outcomes and issues of aging after spinal cord injury. *Arch Phys Med Rehabil.* 1991;72:S309–S311.
35. Leaf A. Getting old. *Sci Am.* 1973;229:44–53.
36. Lewis RB, Applin JW. Degenerative joint disease. In: Maloney FP, Means KM, eds. *Rehabilitation of the aging population.* (Physical Medicine and Rehabilitation: State of the Art Reviews. 1990;4(1):49–55).
37. Mack A, Horn LF. Functional prognosis in traumatic brain injury. In: Horn LJ, Cope DN, eds. *Traumatic brain injury.* (Physical Medicine and Rehabilitation: State of the Art Reviews. 1989;3(1):13–26).
38. Montamat SC, Cusack BJ, Vestal RE. Management of drug therapy in the elderly. *N Engl J Med.* 1989;321:303–309.
39. Naso F, Carner E, Blankfort-Doyl W, Coughey K. Endurance training in the elderly nursing home patient. *Arch Phys Med Rehabil.* 1990;71:241–243.
40. Opitz JL. Bladder retraining: an organized program. *Mayo Clin Proc.* 1976;51:367–372.
41. Pearlman RA, Uhlmann RF. Quality of life in chronic diseases: perceptions of elderly patients. *J Gerontol.* 1988;43:M25–M30.
42. Raab DM, Agre JC, McAdam M, Smith EL. Light resistance and stretching exercise in elderly women: effect upon flexibility. *Arch Phys Med Rehabil.* 1988;69:268–272.

43. Resnic NM. Initial evaluation of the incontinent patient. *J Am Geriatr Soc.* 1990;38:311–316.
44. Rice CL, Cunningham DA, Patterson DH, Rechnitzer PA. Strength in an elderly population. *Arch Phys Med Rehabil.* 1989;70:391–397.
45. Riggs BL, Melton LJ. Involutional osteoporosis. *N Engl J Med.* 1986;314:1676–1686.
46. Rowe JW. Health care of the elderly. *N Engl J Med.* 1985;312:827–835.
47. Rowe JW, Kahn RL. Human aging: usual and successful. *Science.* 1987;237:143–149.
48. Shamburek RD, Farrar JT. Disorders of the digestive system in the elderly. *N Engl J Med.* 1990;322:438–443.
49. Shepard RJ. Prescribing exercise. In: Ham RJ, ed. *Geriatric medicine annual, 1987.* Oradell, NJ: Medical Economics Company; 1987:117–134.
50. Sinaki M. Exercise and osteoporosis. *Arch Phys Med Rehabil.* 1989;70:220–229.
51. Sinaki M. Postmenopausal spinal osteoporosis: physical therapy and rehabilitation principles. *Mayo Clin Proc.* 1982;57:699–703.
52. Stegner W. *Angle of repose.* New York: Valentine Books; 1971.
53. Steinberg FU, Sunwoo IS, Roettger RF. Prosthetic rehabilitation of geriatric amputee patients: a follow-up study. *Arch Phys Med Rehabil.* 1985;66:742–745.
54. Stover S, ed. *Spinal cord injury: the facts and figures.* Birmingham, AL: University of Alabama at Birmingham; 1986.
55. Taylor KJ. Assessment tools for the identification of patients at risk for the development of pressure sores: a review. *J Enterostomal Ther.* 1988;15:201–205.
56. Tinetti ME. Prevention of falls among the elderly. *N Engl J Med.* 1989;320:1055–1059.
57. Vlahov D, Myers AH, Al-Ibrahim MS. Epidemiology of falls among patients in a rehabilitation hospital. *Arch Phys Med Rehabil.* 1990;71:8–12.
58. Wein AJ. Pharmacological treatment of incontinence. *J Am Geriatr Soc.* 1990;38:317–325.
59. Wells TJ. Pelvic (floor) muscle exercise. *J Am Geriatr Soc.* 1990;38:333–337.
60. Wolf-Klein GP, Silverstone FA, Basavaraju N, Foley CJ, et al. Prevention of falls in the elderly population. *Arch Phys Med Rehabil.* 1988;69:689–691.
61. Wrenn K. Fecal impaction. *N Engl J Med.* 1989;321:658–662.
62. Yarkony GM, Roth EJ, Heinemann AW, Lovell LL. Spinal cord injury rehabilitation outcome: the impact of age. *J Clin Epidemiol.* 1988;41:173–177.

Chapter 14

ADVANCES IN PHYSIATRIC MANAGEMENT OF PATIENTS TO PREVENT AND HEAL DECUBITI

John F. Ditunno, Jr., and William E. Staas, Jr.

Decubitus ulcers or pressure sores are a major problem for those who have neurological impairments of weakness and sensory loss, as well as other chronically ill and debilitated patients. The illness for which pressure sores have been most studied in regard to their incidence, epidemiology, and severity is spinal cord injury. A review of the literature reveals that the incidence is from 25% to 85% and that this complication accounts for 7% of deaths. Even in today's best programmed systems of care, pressure sores still occur; data from close to 10,000 cases reported in the National Spinal Cord Injury (NSCI) data base will be cited. The cost of nursing care increases 50% with the development of these lesions. The cost of treatment ranges from $15,000 to $19,000 (in 1980 U.S. dollars) for severe ulcers. The insurance industry, based on 1969 figures, designates 25% of anticipated expenses for patients with spinal cord injury specifically for management of decubitus ulcers. These include the direct cost of medical care, but do not include indirect costs of loss of employment and other expenses incurred by prolonged illness. When one examines the experiences in Canada, Australia, and the United States, the costs of treating decubiti based on these assumptions can be estimated to be in excess of two billion dollars per year. This monetary cost is in addition to the emotional costs and frustration of the individuals and families who must interrupt their normal lifestyle for six weeks or frequently longer for treatment of a severe ulcer.

Prevention of pressure sores should be of high priority. It requires knowledge, strategy, skilled personnel, attention to detail, and resources. A thorough understanding of the pathophysiology and factors that contribute to development of pressure sores is critical for effective prevention and subsequent treatment. Although pressure is the predominant causal factor in most cases, shear, friction, moisture, spasticity, poor nutrition, and various psychosocial problems contribute to the sores' development. In order to have a reasonable approach toward prevention and treatment, a classification of pressure sores is desirable.

The classification currently used by the National Spinal Cord Data Collection System utilizes four grades:

Grade I—limited to superficial epidermis and dermal layers.

Grade II—involving the epidermal and dermal layers and extending into the adipose tissue.

Grade III—extending through superficial structures and adipose tissue down to and including muscle.

Grade IV—destruction of all soft tissue structures down to bone. There is communication with bone or joint structures or both.

Another common classification lists five grades; however, Grades 1 and 2 of this system are included under Grade I of the system outlined above, and Grades 3, 4, and 5 correspond essentially to Grades II, III, and IV above. Figure 1 shows the depth of involvement of each grade. This latter system

Figure 1. The depth of tissue involvement for each grade of pressure sores.

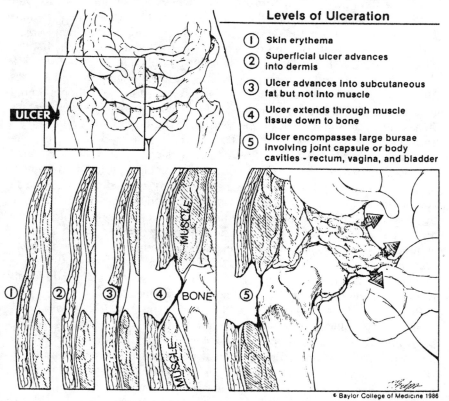

Levels of Ulceration

1. Skin erythema
2. Superficial ulcer advances into dermis
3. Ulcer advances into subcutaneous fat but not into muscle
4. Ulcer extends through muscle tissue down to bone
5. Ulcer encompasses large bursae involving joint capsule or body cavities - rectum, vagina, and bladder

© Baylor College of Medicine 1986

Reproduced from Donovan, W.H. et al., "Pressure Sores," in DeLisa, J.L., ed., *Rehabilitation Medicine*: *Principles and Practice* (Philadelphia: J.B. Lippincott, 1989), p. 482 (Figure 25-4), with the permission of the publisher.

will probably supplant the former, but the data shown in Figures 2 and 3 are based on the 4-grade classification.

FACTORS CONTRIBUTING TO PRESSURE SORES[4]

Pressure

Several authors have shown the importance of pressure as a major factor contributing to decubitus ulcers. Lindan[6] demonstrated that pressure causes tissue damage by closure of blood vessels resulting in ischemic necrosis, while Koziak[5] described the time/pressure relationships as well as the clinical and histologic changes that occur throughout tissue. In work on animals, 70 mm of pressure applied continuously for two hours resulted in pathological changes. An inverse relationship was defined between amount of pressure and duration of pressure in the development of decubiti. Intense pressure for a brief duration could be as damaging to tissue as less pressure for a more prolonged period of time. Tissue ischemia and anoxia developed when pressure exceeded capillary pressure. Capillary pressures under normal circumstances are 32 mm on the arterial side and 13 to 15 mm on the venous segment.

Ischemic necrosis was marked by venous sludging and thrombosis, edema with cellular infiltration and extravasation, increased membrane permeability, and damage to muscle fibers as part of the histologic picture. Muscle fiber damage included loss or decrease of cross striations and myofibrils, white cell infiltration, and phagocytosis by macrophages and neutrophils.

Initially, reactive hyperemia or redness of the skin occurs when the pressure is relieved. The response occurs over the compressed skin and subcutaneous tissue and lasts for close to half the length of time during which the pressure was applied. Usually within 24 hours the skin will return to normal. More prolonged pressure is followed by the formation of edema and a vascular inflammatory response that precedes the ulceration by two to four days. Unlike the initial hyperemia, this redness will not blanch when pressure is applied. While the initial ulceration may appear to be localized to skin, most often it is much deeper, and over the subsequent days and weeks liquefaction occurs and reveals the full thickness of the injury. These lesions have been characterized as the tip of the iceberg; the skin ulceration has a small diameter, but there is significant undermining of deeper tissues, with fissures and sinus tract invasion of bone and joints typical of Grades 4 and 5 ulcers.

Sensory Impairment

With sensation to pinprick, pressure, and other modalities absent or diminished due to damage to afferent tracts, the individual is unaware of discomfort resulting from prolonged pressure. Because the patient has difficulty shifting weight due to weakness and is unaware of the need to relieve pressure due to lack of sensation, continued pressure may lead to ischemic necrosis of the tissue.

Motor Impairment

As noted above, weakness of muscles in the upper extremities may result in difficulty in shifting weight off of skin that is subject to prolonged pressure. In patients with intact upper extremities but paralysis of the lower extremities, edema may also contribute to skin breakdown. Prolonged dependency of the legs may result in interstitial edema, which can compromise circulation in the presence of pressure.

Shear Pressure

When the upper layers of tissue area slide against the lower layers with an angular force, this shear pressure may lead to decubiti. Continuous friction of skin surfaces may result in abrasion and compromise circulation when pressure is applied. The extent of the friction or shearing is significant in determining the size and grade of the ulcer.

The role of pressure and friction in the development of decubitus ulcers was studied by Dinsdale in paraplegic swine.[3] He showed that friction in combination with pressure as low as 45 mm caused ulceration. He was able to demonstrate that friction did not produce ulcers by an ischemic mechanism by use of isotope clearance studies.

With pressure in excess of 500 mm, friction did not increase the likelihood of ulcers. However, friction was shown to predispose to ulcers when pressure was less than 500 mm. In most clinical situations, pressure of less than 500 mm is typical; therefore, friction must be considered an important contributing factor.

Spasticity, Moisture, Infection

The increased muscle tone subsequent to recovery from spinal shock will result in spasticity. This may cause problems with hygiene, may increase shear pressure, and may be intensified by infection or other noxious stimuli including a preexisting pressure sore. Adductor spasms draw knees and ankles together, creating shear and pressure. Flexor spasms will draw heels across sheets in bed or pull heels against heel loops in a wheelchair, which may lead to decubiti.

Poor techniques for transfer or bed movement stemming from increased spasms may result in shearing of skin over hips or buttocks. Halo-vests and body jackets may increase shear if there is poor fit or increased patient mobility.

Hip adductor spasticity plus soiling can lead to poor cleansing of skin with resultant maceration. Any break in the skin that becomes infected can further compromise impaired circulation and, with pressure and shearing, contribute to decubiti.

Chronic infectious states of the urinary or respiratory systems associated with poor nutrition will compromise general health and the ability to repair tissue damage.

Psychosocial Factors

Cull[2] was unable to demonstrate a relationship between numerous psychosocial variables and the incidence of decubiti, but did find that the incidence was lower in females than in males. Another study by Anderson and Andberg,[1] however, was most informative. They examined various psychosocial factors related to pressure sores. Initially, the patient's history of decubiti was documented and then the occurrence of skin breakdown was recorded, as reflected in number of days hospitalized. Each patient was questioned regarding his or her feelings about measures taken to care for the skin. In addition, other variables, such as satisfaction with education classes, avocational activities, organization or group activities, living arrangements, and sexual activities, were studied. Self-esteem was examined utilizing the Tennessee Self-Concept Scale. Interestingly, quadriplegics showed fewer days lost than paraplegics. Those quadriplegics who were independent in caring for their skin had the fewest days lost. Paraplegics who needed help to care for their skin had the highest number of days interrupted. Those who lost no time scored higher on their feelings and attitudes about skin care and on satisfaction with the activities listed above than individuals who did experience time lost. No significant difference was demonstrated on the Tennessee Self-Concept Scale in the comparison patient groups. Satisfaction with life activity was most closely correlated with the presence or absence of disabling skin problems and attitude toward the importance of skin care.

Anemia and Hypoalbuminemia

Anemia contributes to tissue breakdown and plays a role in delaying wound healing. Anemia may be due to multiple factors, among them blood loss as a result of the pressure sore or a peptic ulcer. Iron deficiency and anemia of chronic disease are frequently identified. A hemoglobin in the range of 13 to 15 g/dl is more compatible with the maintenance and repair of healthy skin than hemoglobin less than 10 g/dl.

Decreases in serum albumin below 3.0–3.5 g/cm³ are quite common in patients with pressure sores, even when body weight is normal. Therefore, hypoalbuminemia and body weight are not directly related. The constant drainage of serum from a pressure sore can deplete the body stores of protein, especially albumin. The relationship between decreased albumin and tissue necrosis has been well documented, but the specific mechanisms responsible for the development of pressure sores remain unclear.

* * *

The factors enumerated above must be understood and discussed by the health care team, particularly the nurse, physician, and dietitian, so that appropriate measures may be instituted to prevent the development of this complication. Prevention is the cornerstone of good skin care.

USUAL SITES OF PRESSURE SORES

The sites most commonly at risk for pressure sores have been reported in the literature for spinal cord injured subjects included in the NSCI data base (1971–1985). Figure 2 shows the distribution of pressure sores of all grades, the three most common sites being the sacrum, heels, and ischium, in that order. Figure 3 illustrates the most common locations of severe sores (Grades III and IV). Over 50% of all Grade III and IV pressure sores occur in the sacral area. Below are listed the vulnerable sites, with a brief description of forces and activities that contribute to pressure sores there.

Sacrum

Direct pressure: In supine position, pressure unrelieved by turning, or insufficient time off back; poor wheelchair posture when sitting.
Shearing force: Sliding down in bed when head of bed is raised; poor turning technique in bed.
Maceration: Prolonged contact with urine, sweat, feces, or all of these.

Trochanters

Direct pressure: Prolonged lying on one side; trauma during wheelchair transfer when trochanter is hit against wheel of chair; scoliosis, causing weight to be shifted to opposite hip; heterotopic ossification; poor wheelchair fit.
Shearing: Lower extremity spasticity causing hips to be drawn across bedsheets.

Ankles

Direct pressure: Lateral malleolus—secondary to lying on side with in-

Figure 2. Distribution of pressure sores (all types).

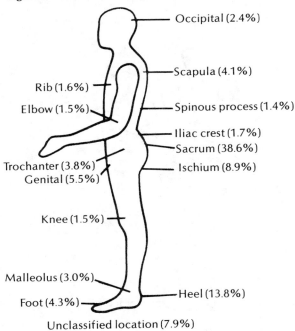

Occipital (2.4%)

Scapula (4.1%)

Rib (1.6%)

Elbow (1.5%)

Spinous process (1.4%)

Iliac crest (1.7%)

Sacrum (38.6%)

Trochanter (3.8%)

Ischium (8.9%)

Genital (5.5%)

Knee (1.5%)

Malleolus (3.0%)

Heel (13.8%)

Foot (4.3%)

Unclassified location (7.9%)

Based on Figure 20 in Stover, S.L., and P.R. Fine, eds., *Spinal Cord Injury: The Facts and Figures* (Birmingham, AL: University of Alabama at Birmingham, The National Spinal Cord Injury Statistical Center, 1986), p. 43. Used with the permission of Samuel L. Stover, M.D.

sufficient turning or to trauma during transfer activity; poor footrest position, such as medial ankle resting on pins of heel loops.

Shearing: Medial malleolus—adductor spasms drawing ankles together and across one another.

Heels

Direct pressure: Insufficient pressure relief.

Shearing: Posterior aspect of the heels drawing across bedsheets during movement in bed or due to lower extremity spasticity.

Ischial Tuberosities

Direct posture: Prolonged pressure without relief in sitting position; poor position of wheelchair footrests (if too high, weight is shifted onto ischium).

Shearing: Poor sliding board transfers, dragging skin and tissue over board.

Figure 3. Most common locations of severe pressure sores (Grades III and IV).

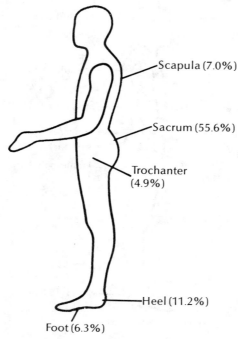

Scapula (7.0%)

Sacrum (55.6%)

Trochanter (4.9%)

Heel (11.2%)

Foot (6.3%)

Based on Figure 21 in Stover, S.L., and P.R. Fine, eds., *Spinal Cord Injury: The Facts and Figures* (Birmingham, AL: University of Alabama at Birmingham, The National Spinal Cord Injury Statistical Center, 1986), p. 43. Used with the permission of Samuel L. Stover, M.D.

Knees

Direct pressure: Anterior knee—secondary to prone position; insufficient pressure relief. Lateral knee—lying on side with insufficient turning.

Elbows

Direct pressure: Leaning, especially in prone position; trauma when elbows are used for leverage and to change position.

Feet

Direct pressure: Against end of bed due to poor bed positioning.

Toes

Direct pressure: Trauma from bumping toes when in wheelchair; poor prone position; poorly fitting shoes or tight elastic hose.

Scapulae

Direct pressure: Prolonged supine positioning.
Shearing: Sliding down in bed.

* * *

No commercially available cushion or device in use at this time will adequately prevent pressure sores by itself when the patient is in the sitting position. Regardless of the type of cushion used, there is no substitution for regular weight shifts to relieve pressure. The most effective method to regularly shift weight when in the sitting position is to perform a wheelchair push up. For those patients who are unable to do a push up because of weak arms or other problems, a lateral weight shift is suggested. Other patients simply lean forward and then backward. High quadriplegics who are unable to perform the above maneuvers can use a motorized reclining wheelchair which allows them to shift position from sitting to supine and semisitting at regular intervals. Relief of pressure every 30 minutes or more often is mandatory when the patient is in the sitting position.

PREVENTION

Prevention strategies will depend on the phase of illness and the capacity and knowledge that the patient and/or those who have been assigned to help him possess regarding proper care.

During the prehospital, acute hospital, and early rehabilitation phases of traumatic spinal cord injury, the patient is solely dependent on paramedical and hospital personnel. However, patients with cognitive impairment due to traumatic brain injury or dementia may be unable to participate in the prevention program at later phases of rehabilitation. Patients who are cognitively intact and can communicate should be able to direct their own prevention program following training, even if they are physically incapable of participation. Although pressure sores are easy to develop and difficult to heal, they should be preventable. Prevention requires continuous monitoring and an education program involving the physicians, nurses, therapists, attendants, patient, and family. The patient, however, must be the center of the prevention program in the rehabilitation phase and must be well informed and able to direct his own care. Prior to rehabilitation, the system of care must provide an adequate number of well-qualified and knowledgeable staff in the prehospital and acute hospital setting to prevent decubiti. The patient and family must be educated, with emphasis on the following steps:

1. Frequent inspection of skin for possible pressure problems and proper cleansing technique.

2. Use of appropriate pressure relief.
3. Awareness of potential hazards to the skin.

Inspection and Cleansing

Skin care includes careful inspection, which must be done as frequently as every two hours while the patient is in bed and more often if a new activity such as sitting or transfers with a sliding board is initiated. As a minimum, inspection should be done in the morning and evening on a daily basis by the patient alone or with some assistance. If the patient cannot inspect his own skin because he is unable to manipulate a mirror due to weakness in the upper extremities, he should be trained to have another person hold the mirror so they both can inspect the skin. The skin must also be cleansed promptly of urine and feces with a mild soap and water. Perspiration may be excessive and require frequent attention, but the patient should be kept dry with cleansing to prevent maceration of tissue.

Pressure Relief

As mentioned in the section on common sites of sores, bony prominences are the areas most prone to breakdown, and proper bed positioning is essential to relieve pressure to these sites. Relief of pressure and avoidance of friction or shear depend on anticipation and use of appropriate methods of turning and shifting and on proper equipment. When a patient is turned or assisted in transfer, he must be lifted and not dragged across sheets or other surfaces. Heels should be protected with foam blocks. Sheepskin pads have no value in pressure relief. Use of mattresses filled with air or foam is not a substitute for turning, and patients should be cautioned that although they may feel comfortable, they should not become lulled into a false sense of security. Water mattresses, on the other hand, if properly inflated so that the body is supported by buoyance rather than the tension of the top membrane, will allow mean capillary pressure of 11 mm of Hg per cm^2 of body surface in the supine position. Not all water mattresses will achieve flotation resulting in these low pressures, so care must be taken in their use and prescription. In addition, the patient on the mattress may require additional attention in relief of perspiration or in turning if the patient is very dependent. Therefore, its use should be relegated to the patient with special needs in the hospital, such as those with existing pressure sores, individuals who resist the prone position, or those with orthoses and halo-vest jackets who are difficult to turn. Similar indication for use in the home is reasonable when there is chronic skin breakdown and inability to turn or to tolerate the prone position.

When the patient is sitting upright, the sites bearing the greatest weight are over the ischial tuberosities and thighs. Pressure is greater when sitting than when recumbent since the same body weight is being supported by a decreased surface area. This surface area has been calculated to be approximately 150 square inches. Pressure would exceed 26 mm/cm^2 if one assumed only a 75% load and the weight evenly distributed. A number of studies with pressure measurement devices have shown that the area over the ischial tuberosity is subjected to the highest pressure, and no cushion has been found which will reduce this pressure below capillary pressure.

A number of cushioning products are on the market, varying from cushions filled with air, water, or plastic material that simulates body fat to polyurethane foam. Each has advantages and disadvantages. Polyurethane foam is the least expensive, is lightweight, and can be cut to any size or thickness. Unfortunately, it cannot be washed or cleansed and wears out in six months.

Hazards

Excessive exposure to heat or cold may cause damage to insensate skin. Safety precautions are the mainstay of a prevention program. Prolonged exposure to cold can result in frostbite of distal extremities, whereas prolonged exposure to sun may result in severe burns. Use of hot water when bathing can be a hazard, and water temperature should be monitored and regulated. Inadvertent contact with hot objects, such as water pipes or radiators, may result in severe burns to the hands, feet, elbows, or thighs.

MANAGEMENT OF PRESSURE SORES[7]

The same measures utilized in prevention form the bases for management of pressure sores. Pressure relief must be accomplished; if not, the decubitus will worsen or fail to heal. Good nutrition and adequate hemoglobin and albumin levels are also essential for healing, regardless of the need for surgery. Many different methods have been advocated for treatment over the years, but few have been subjected to controlled studies. Virtually every method reported is of value in healing ulcers, probably because attention is given to the ulcer and other fundamental measures are taken. The debridement of necrotic tissue and local cleansing are essential.

The approach to treatment will vary based on the severity of the pressure sore. The grading of severity is important for recording incidence, establishing guidelines for treatment, and determining the effects of treatment. We will use the four-grade system adopted by the Spinal Cord Injury Model Centers, which was defined in the first section of this chapter.

The majority of decubiti will heal with conservative methods and do not require surgery, given the proper circumstances. Patient compliance with staff and physician recommendations is essential. Grade IV sores, however, will usually require surgery, particularly if located over the ischial tuberosities. Grade IV pressure sores in other areas may heal without surgery.

The management of the pressure sore involves both local wound treatment and surgical intervention. The principal goal of management is to keep the wound clean and uninfected with complete relief of pressure. The pressure sore should be debrided and cleansed of all necrotic tissue as soon as possible to allow for adequate drainage and reduce the number of bacteria in the wound.

The management of pressure sores based on severity is as follows:

Grade I: Cleanse the wound, relieve pressure, monitor change by weekly measurement of size and depth.

Grade II: Cleanse the wound, pack with gauze for drainage, perform sharp and/or enzymatic debridement of necrotic tissue, relieve pressure, measure and grade weekly.

Grades III and IV: Cleanse the wound, pack with gauze, debride necrotic tissue, relieve pressure, measure and grade weekly. However, patient should also be referred to a spinal cord injury center or plastic surgeon skilled in decubiti, or both.

A review of topical agents to suppress infection, various types of debridement, wound cleansing, and dressing techniques is presented below.

Topical Agents

Most topical agents applied to wounds are for the purpose of reducing the number of bacteria or stimulating granulation tissue. Numerous preparations exist, many of which make claims of "curing" pressure sores. These agents range from some very expensive products to home remedies such as honey and sugar. Some of the more common preparations discussed in the literature are dextranomer, gel foam, benzoyl peroxide, and various sugar preparations. They are most often used with topical antibiotic agents.

In addition to the overall principles of pressure relief and maintenance of good health, cleansing of the wound is a major objective. A variety of agents may be used. These include normal saline, hydrogen peroxide 3%, povidone iodine, collagenase ointment, Neosporin powder, and hydrophilic sugar polymers.

Povidone Iodine

Povidone iodine has an antibacterial action, but also stimulates granulation tissue due to irritation to the tissues in the wound. These properties make it a good agent for treating Grade I and II sores. It facilitates the sloughing of fibrous tissue when present in Grade I and II pressure sores and the development of granulation tissue. In addition to its antibacterial action, it further decreases immediate contamination through the drying effect.

Certain precautions are important to observe in the use of povidone iodine:

1. Signs of irritation and local sensitization of the wound to iodine must be monitored. The appearance of bleeding into the wound and resultant thrombosis of newly formed capillary buds is an indication of wound sensitization. The development of a blue-black color to the wound, particularly if deep, indicates that the povidone iodine should be cut to a 1:2 solution with normal saline or its use discontinued.

2. In superficial Grade I ulcers, povidone iodine may keep the wound open and prevent epithelialization. In such cases peroxide and saline should be used for cleaning instead.

3. Povidone iodine is drying and irritating to normal skin and therefore should be applied only to the open wound edges and not the surrounding normal tissues. This drying effect may also cause fissuring of wound edges and possible extension of the wound.

Collagenase Ointment and Neosporin Powder

These agents are commonly used together in wound management. The collagenase enzyme produces liquefaction of necrotic tissue which serves as a medium for bacterial growth. This could result in a delay of healing, although the wound is sloughing necrotic material and in spite of frequent cleansing and change of dressings. The application of Neosporin powder immediately prior to the collagenase ointment should control bacterial counts. These agents are particularly indicated in Grade III pressure sores with a large amount of necrotic tissue.

Debridement

The debridement of wounds can be achieved by one of three methods or combinations thereof: 1) mechanical debridement with cleansing and dressings; 2) enzymatic debridement; 3) sharp debridement.

Various topical agents are used in local cleansing, and dressing technique will depend on the agents used for cleansing and debridement. If necrotic tissue fills the wound, it must be debrided to allow a clean wound base. This will speed the healing process, since allowing the tissue to slough prior to granulation takes longer without mechanical assistance. When eschar covers the wound it should be removed to allow free drainage of infected material. Otherwise, the wound may worsen, with more extensive tissue involvement.

Mechanical Debridement

Mechanical debridement is accomplished while cleansing and dressing the ulcer. Flushing the wound with solution, wiping it with gauze, and removing gauze packing that has dried and adhered to the wound surface mechanically removes dead tissue and bacteria. This type of debridement should be done several times a day together with wound dressing.

Gauze sponges with cotton lining should be avoided since cotton will adhere to the wound surface. Saline should be poured directly into the wound to rinse the peroxide or onto the gauze. The gauze should then be applied in a circular motion with friction, which cleanses the wound from the center to the periphery. The mechanical action of wiping with the gauze is more important in the removal of necrotic tissue and bacteria than the topical agent being used. Although soap and water are perhaps more economical than some agents, they may be more difficult to remove from deeper wounds. Saline and hydrogen peroxide are both economical and easily rinsed from the wound.

Enzymatic Debridement

When sharp debridement is difficult due to secondary sinus formation in deep wounds, enzymatic preparations should be utilized. There are two types of enzymatic debridement agents: fibrinolytic and collagenolytic. Fibrinolytic preparations tend to produce more local wound irritation; therefore, we prefer the use of collagenolytic agents. However, these agents do not penetrate eschar. The eschar must be removed or scored to allow application of enzymatic agents. It is important to recognize that these agents may be used in conjunction with, but not as a substitute for, sharp debridement. The liquefaction of necrotic material by enzymatic preparations permits easier mechanical and sharp debridement. The enzyme preparations are particularly useful to assist daily debridement in patients who are not hospitalized and may be seen only once or twice a week.

Sharp Debridement

Eschar and underlying necrotic tissue should be removed by sharp debridement. Sharp debridement with scissors, forceps, and scalpel can be performed daily at the bedside until a clean wound base is achieved. Excessive bleeding that cannot be controlled by pressure or is related to anticoagulant therapy should be avoided in deep wounds. If excessive bleeding occurs or the patient is undergoing anticoagulant therapy, the wound should be packed with gel foam, pressure applied, and consideration given to reversal of anticoagulation. Hemoglobin and hematocrit levels should be followed for several days following such an episode.

Wound Cleansing

Again, many different agents are used to clean wounds. We have already mentioned soap and water, hydrogen peroxide, and povidone iodine; Dakin's and Burow's solutions are also used. Three percent hydrogen peroxide to cleanse the wound followed by normal saline to rinse the wound is our preference. If the oxidizing action of the peroxide results in a large amount of "foam," we prefer to dilute the peroxide to a 1:3 ratio with normal saline. The hydrogen peroxide is more easily removed from the wound if diluted with saline.

Hydrophilic agents such as sugar polymers have a good cleansing and drying action. However, they can cause wound irritation and may be considerably more expensive than saline and peroxide.

Dressing Techniques

Grade I and II pressure sores

These ulcers most often only require cleansing with peroxide and normal saline. While the area of nonepithelial tissue can be "painted" with povidone iodine, the areas of pink, healthy epithelial tissue should not be painted, to avoid irritation. The edges of Grade II pressure sores may become thickened with fibrous tissue. To control this condition, the edges of the wound should be irritated daily with the end of a sterile cotton swab or forceps. The wound should be covered with two layers of all-gauze type sponge, and those with cotton lining should be avoided, since the cotton adheres to the wound. The dressing should be changed a minimum of twice a day and more frequently if drainage is excessive. When the drainage penetrates the gauze dressing, the entire dressing should be removed and the wound cleansed and redressed. Covering an already-saturated dressing with added dressing should be avoided, since it adds bulk and pressure to the wound site and the dressing saturated with exudate provides a medium for bacterial growth.

Grade III and IV pressure sores

When necrotic tissue is present, the wound should be dressed utilizing a wet to dry technique. In this technique, the dressing is wet with normal saline and then the excess is squeezed out. When the dressing dries, the gauze will adhere to the necrotic tissue, which will then be removed as the gauze is removed from the wound, thus achieving debridement when the dressing is changed, twice a day. This technique may be used with or without collagenolytic agents.

Packing the Wound

Caution in packing deep wounds is important. The coarse weave of rolled gauze is preferred over gauze in sponges because it will adhere better to necrotic tissue. The use of gauze sponges may result in too tight a packing in a sinus, drainage obstruction, or, at times, the "loss" of the sponge. In order to insure no loss of dressings, the edges of the rolled gauze should be tied together when more than one length is required to pack a wound. In smaller wounds, one may use "fluffs," which are made from gauze sponges and permit more contact with the wound surface for the purpose of debridement. The wound should be adequately covered with two layers of dry gauze sponges.

Dressing Changes

The preferred time to remove dressings is after they have been in place a sufficient period to allow drying in order to achieve debridement, but prior to their saturation with exudate. For this reason dressing changes may be required more often than the minimum of twice a day. If drainage is allowed to soak through and saturate the gauze packing, the dressing should be changed and the wound thoroughly cleansed. As stated above, adding or reinforcing the dressing with additional gauze promotes further bacterial growth and the extension of the pressure sore to deeper tissues.

The local treatment of pressure sores should involve simple techniques of cleansing with frequent debridement and dressing changes. If treatment of the sores is not complicated, it will be performed more often and will constitute a program that the patient and family can learn and apply at home if necessary. More complicated regimes of mixing pastes and covering with plastic wrap can take many hours and have not been proven to be more successful than simpler techniques.

Surgical Management

The indications for surgical intervention involve failure of pressure sores to heal spontaneously, poor quality of the skin following healing, and the need to mobilize the patient. Not all pressure sores heal and, depending on their depth, those that do may heal without hair follicles or sweat glands, with thin epithelial tissue, and without normal dermal papillae. Scar tissue may adhere to underlying bone, making it more susceptible to friction and pressure.

On some occasions a Grade II pressure sore will not epithelialize and will require surgery. Grade III and IV pressure sores over the ischial tuberosities, sacrum, and trochanters will usually require skin grafting. The formation of fibrous tissue, which occurs secondary to healing, will become more extensive the longer the sore takes to heal, and will tend to produce a wound with an avascular base rather than healthy granulation tissue. Therefore, patients with Grade III and IV pressure sores that are resistant to closure should be referred to spinal cord injury centers and/or a skilled plastic surgeon.

Prior to surgical intervention, patients should receive a diagnostic workup, presurgical management of contractures and spasticity, and conditioning to determine if they can tolerate the postsurgical positioning. This evaluation and preoperative management is best accomplished at an established spinal cord injury center, in which staff are available for and knowledgeable in this routine. Lack of attention to these pre- and postoperative details may result in failure of skin flaps or grafts.

The preoperative diagnostic workup should include a detailed medical evaluation; monitoring of hemoglobin, hematocrit, and serum protein levels; and serial x-rays of the pressure sore to define wound depth and fistulae and to rule out the presence of heterotopic ossification. Blood transfusion and hyperalimentation may be necessary if hemoglobin, hematocrit, and serum protein levels are not within normal limits.

The management of contractures, spasticity, and heterotopic ossification will not be discussed in this chapter. It is essential, however, to recognize the importance of these associated conditions in pre- and postoperative management. Spasticity may create shear pressure which will cause the flaps to displace, while contractures may interfere with the positioning of the patient. Ideally, heterotopic bone should be mature prior to surgery. Attempts to repair a pressure sore over active heterotopic ossification may fail. Continued formation of new bone beneath the repaired decubitus may lead to stress and pressure on the operative site.

Since the prone position is the most common one postoperatively, it is important to condition patients to this position prior to surgery. Problems of discomfort and patient compliance are more effectively dealt with before surgery because the staff can work with the patient and build up his tolerance. Failure to condition the patient to the prone position prior to surgery may jeopardize the skin graft or flap if patient discomfort leads to excessive turning and repositioning.

CONCLUSION

Prevention of pressure sores is by far the most effective management, but prevention requires an intimate knowledge by patients, family, and staff of predisposing factors and strategies for coping with hazards and unpredictable circumstances. As previously cited, many factors—ranging from the physiological to the psychological and sociological—contribute to pressure sore formation. The primary physician must be capable of reviewing these factors and translating them into an education and treatment program. This program must be based not only on sound physiological principles, but in addition must take into consideration the specific emotional and psychosocial needs of the patient and family.

Patient compliance remains one of the most important factors in both operative and nonoperative management. Patient compliance, appropriate evaluation and workup, and skilled preoperative, operative, and postoperative care can invariably achieve a healed wound and a restored patient. Unfortunately, if any of these important elements is lacking, complications of chronic infection, abscess, osteomyelitis, sepsis, and death may be the result.

REFERENCES

1. Anderson TP, Andberg MM. Psychosocial factors associated with pressure sores. *Arch Phys Med Rehabil*. 1979;60:341–346.
2. Cull JF, Smith OH. Preliminary note on demographic and personality correlates of decubitus ulcer incidents. *J Psychiatr*. 1973;88:225–227.
3. Dinsdale SM. Decubitus ulcers in swine: light and microscopic study of pathogenesis. *Arch Phys Med Rehabil*. 1973;54:51–56.
4. Donovan WH, Garber SL, Hamilton SM, Kroreskop A, Rodrigues GP, Stal S. Pressure ulcers. In: DeLisa J, ed. *Rehabilitation medicine: principles and practice*. Philadelphia: JB Lippincott; 1989:476–491.
5. Koziak M., Etiology of decubitus ulcers. *Arch Phys Med Rehabil*. 1961;42:19–26.
6. Lindan O. Etiology of decubitus ulcers: an experimental study. *Arch Phys Med Rehabil*. 1961;42:774–783.
7. Staas WE, LaMantia J. Decubitus ulcers. In: Ruskin A, ed. *Spinal cord injury: current therapy in physiatry*. Philadelphia: WB Saunders; 1984:410–419.

Chapter 15

ADVANCES IN SPORTS MEDICINE

Karen Snowden Rucker and Ralph Buschbacher

INTRODUCTION

The purpose of this chapter is to provide an update for the physiatrist of advances made in the past 10 years in sports medicine. While musculoskeletal medicine is a cornerstone of physiatry, the physiatric literature has, in the past, provided little information geared specifically toward treating the competitive athlete. This chapter will discuss some common injuries, syndromes, and medical problems encountered in an office practice of sports medicine, placing emphasis on those entities in which advances have been made in the last decade. A good discussion of sideline management of injuries may be found in *Sports Medicine: Prevention, Evaluation, Management and Treatment.*[32] In-depth illustrations of the pathophysiology of injury and recovery are available in the 4th edition of *Krusen's Handbook of Physical Medicine and Rehabilitation.*[21]

Controlling Inflammation

A large portion of the morbidity from athletic injuries is due not to the injury itself, but rather to the body's response to injury, mainly inflammation. Inflammation is a necessary prelude to healing, but it can delay healing following an injury if not controlled. Inflammation decreases the tensile strength of tendons and ligaments.[26,29] Loose connective tissue, when not maintained mobile, is transformed into dense connective tissue, a process accelerated and exacerbated by edema, bleeding, and additional trauma to the area. The RICE protocol (*Rest, Ice, Compression,* and *Elevation*) decreases soft tissue swelling, bleeding, and muscle spasm and provides analgesia.[26] Thus, controlling inflammation minimizes both subsequent tissue weakness and stiffness. Ice, in particular, is important in the first 24–48 hours after injury. It is applied for 20–30 minutes three or more times a day. Ice is also helpful before and after exercise in the early period of resumption of activity to prevent further exacerbation of the inflammation.

Nonsteroidal anti-inflammatory drugs (NSAIDs) are used in the acute phase of injury to improve healing of ligamentous injuries. Table 1 reviews the beneficial effects and the adverse side effects of NSAIDs.

Table 1. Effects of nonsteroidal anti-inflammatory agents.

Beneficial	Adverse
Analgesic	Gastrointestinal irritation
Anti-inflammatory	Renal disease (cause or exacerbate)
Anti-pyretic	Allergic reactions
	Bronchospasm
	Tinnitus (aspirin only)
	Prolonged bleeding time

Early Mobilization

Early mobilization has significantly changed the management of ankle sprains and ligamentous knee injuries in the past few years. Ligaments that have been immobilized show a loss of parallelism of collagen fibers, distorted cellular alignment, and increased randomness of matrix organization. These changes lead to decreased strength, reduced lineal stiffness, and lessened energy-absorbing capacity of the ligament.[26,36] Early mobilization is thought to increase the parallelism and elasticity of the healing collagen fibers. Specific active range of motion exercises are instituted in the first 48 hours in certain ankle and knee ligamentous injuries.

Various mechanical devices have been designed to promote mobilization. These continuous passive motion machines are most often used after knee surgery to passively move the joint repeatedly through a range of motion (ROM). Also, ankle braces and knee supports that allow movement but restrict mediolateral displacement permit earlier weight-bearing and mobilization.

Overuse Injuries

Overuse injuries are among the most common athletic problems. They involve repetitive microtrauma to the soft tissue and bones, which can lead to chronic inflammation, stress reactions, more extensive tears, or stress fractures. The more chronic the injury, the more difficult it is to treat because of randomly arrayed collagen in the scar tissue. The mainstays of treatment include rest, NSAIDs, gentle ROM exercises, ice in the early stages, and ice alternated with heat in the later stages. Factors that predispose to such injury are briefly outlined in Table 2.[14]

SPECIFIC CONDITIONS

The following sections describe recent advances in the diagnosis and treatment of specific conditions and affected body parts.

Table 2. Risk factors for overuse injuries and areas likely to be involved.

Extrinsic risk factors
- Any endurance training with repetitive motion
- Too rapid an increase in training activity (repetitions, intensity, distance, time)
- Poor training conditions and equipment (hard running surface, uncushioned shoes, ill-fitting equipment)
- Improper training technique (excessive uphill or downhill running, poor follow-through after throwing)
- Application of force in a new direction (shear, twisting, direct pressure)

Intrinsic risk factors
- Abnormal joint alignment (pronation, supination, leg length discrepancy)
- Muscle strength imbalances or weakness
- Poor flexibility
- Underlying degenerative change from aging or past injury
- Increase in muscular size (supinator syndrome)

Areas likely to be involved
- Weight-bearing structures
- Musculotendinous junction
- Areas of friction, especially in an enclosed space (coracoacromial arch, carpal tunnel, tarsal tunnel)
- Abnormal cartilagenous compression (radiocapitellar joint in valgus stress at elbow)

Source: Herring, S.A., and K.L. Nilson, "Introduction to overuse injuries," *Clin Sports Med* 6(2), 1987.

Shoulder

The glenoid labrum was once believed to be a discrete fibrocartilaginous rim around the glenoid fossa, but it is now regarded as a redundant fold of the joint capsule.[25] This has implications in the treatment of subluxations and dislocations. When the rim was thought to be a discrete entity, dislocation could be viewed as a simple slipping of the humeral head over the rim, causing little lasting damage. The muscles around the joint could be strengthened to prevent recurrence; however, this conservative approach often had disappointing results. Regarding the labrum as a redundant fold of the capsule readily illustrates why this has been the case. During dislocation, the head of the humerus, instead of merely slipping over an obstacle, usually tears the insertion of the joint capsule at the glenoid fossa. In fact, in anterior instability caused by acute trauma or repetitive stretching, up to 85% of the cases have a resultant labral tear.[28] Controversy exists regarding the need for immobilization following a labral tear.

In diagnosing labral injuries, plain radiographies (Westpoint axillary view) may show an area of ectopic calcification where the capsule was torn. Computerized axial tomography and arthroscopy are also helpful.

The last decade has witnessed development of a better understanding of impingement and rotator cuff injuries. The supraspinatus tendon contains an area of anastomosis of the blood vessels supplying it from above and below. This watershed area, located 1–2 cm proximal to the humeral insertion of the tendon, is particularly prone to ischemia and is the area most likely to undergo degenerative changes, tendonitis, calcification, and rupture.[5] The tendon in this area becomes inflamed and swollen as it is damaged by repetitive overuse or acute trauma. This condition contributes to impingement of the tendon under the coracoacromial arch and starts a vicious degenerative cycle that can lead to rotator cuff tears. Individuals with subacromial spurs, a prominent distal clavicle, a flattened slope of the acromion, and a nonunion of the acromial epiphysis are believed to be at risk for impingement.[6]

Jobe and Jobe in 1983[18] described an examination to isolate the supraspinatus for manual testing, as demonstrated in Figure 1. The arm is abducted 90° and flexed 30° to lie in the plane of the scapula, and is then rotated internally to point the thumb down. Pain or weakness to downward pressure in this position suggests supraspinatus pathology. When the arm is abducted between 60° and 120°, the rotator cuff passes below the coracoacromial arch. Pain during abduction through this interval is suggestive of cuff pathology or subacromial bursitis.

Figure 1. Supraspinatus test: pain or weakness on downward pressure on the arm abducted 90°, flexed 30°, and rotated internally.

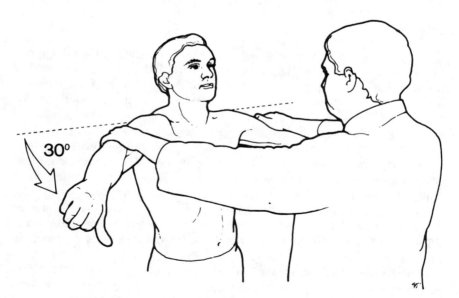

Reprinted from Jobe, F.W., *Clinics in Sports Medicine*, 8(3):424 (Figure 1), 1989, with the permission of W.B. Saunders Co.

Recognition of acromioclavicular osteophytes, a narrowing of the supraspinatus outlet, or an unfused acromial epiphysis on plain x-ray can support the diagnosis of impingement. Cuff tears are suggested by the drop-arm test and can be confirmed by arthrogram or arthroscopy. The initial treatment of impingement is to minimize inflammation and avoid exacerbating activities (usually overhead and throwing activities). Anti-inflammatory drugs and isometric rotator cuff (RTC) exercises are useful early in treatment. Conservative care is the treatment of choice, but if this fails to provide benefits after six to nine months, surgical decompression of the underside of the coracoacromial arch can be done, either by open surgery or by arthroscopy. Operative treatment, however, is not always successful in allowing the athlete to return to his or her former level of competition. The decision of whether to refer an older individual to a surgeon for treatment of an RTC tear that has not responded to conservative treatment may be determined by the individual's level of activity. A golfer, for example, or a very active person may be significantly limited by pain and dysfunction and may benefit greatly from surgery.

A large proportion of shoulder injuries among throwing athletes occur during the deceleration or follow-through phase of the throw. Throwing athletes tend to be flexible in external rotation and somewhat less flexible though stronger in internal rotation. This imbalance predisposes them to posterior muscle and capsule injury. The posterior glenoid labrum can become calcified from this repeated traction stress, and the unequal strength and loading may lead to posterior subluxation.[2,28] Rehabilitative and preventive efforts must be directed toward strengthening the external shoulder rotators as well as developing proper throwing motion of the torso to minimize the deceleration stress on the posterior shoulder.

Elbow

A major cause of elbow joint pathology in athletes is valgus stress, especially that associated with baseball pitching. The medial elbow structures tend to be stretched and the lateral ones compressed. Also, in the throwing motion or in racket sports, the anterior elbow can be stretched by hyperextension and the posterior elbow can be forcibly compressed. Loose bodies can form within the elbow joint; they are usually accompanied by a catch, a click, or joint crepitus, which may help to differentiate this condition from tendonitis. These fragments must be removed by arthroscopy or surgery.[28]

Lateral epicondylitis is common in athletes performing racket sports. It is due to repetitive damage to the common extensor tendon, usually secondary to poor stroke mechanics and overuse. Current treatment emphasizes initial rest from the exacerbating activity, with icing of the lateral epicondyle and anti-inflammatory medications. If the occupation or recreational activity forces continued wrist extension, immobilization of the wrist in a volar cock-up splint or short-arm cast for three to five days is an effective means of enforcing rest. This treatment should be followed by gentle stretching of the wrist extensors, followed by progressive strengthening. The persistently painful lateral epicondyle can be injected with steroids to allow tolerance to gentle stretching. Prior to return to previous activities or sport, the upper extremity and torso should be evaluated for weakness. Weakness, especially in the rotator cuff, can contribute to overuse of the wrist extensors and should be corrected. If conservative management is unsuccessful, a common extensor tendon release may be performed.[28]

Posterior elbow pain is often caused by olecranon bursitis, which can be the result of acute trauma or repetitive trauma and pressure. It is treated with ice, rest, protection, and nonsteroidal anti-inflammatory agents. Consistent padding and protection of the posterior elbow is very important. If the bursa is severely swollen, the fluid may be aspirated. Steroid injections may be used once infection is ruled out. If conservative management fails, or if the bursal fluid is infected, the bursa is surgically drained or removed.[28]

Hand

Fractures of the hand and fingers are common sports injuries; however, most are beyond the scope of this chapter. The physiatrist should have a high index of suspicion for two commonly missed fractures: those of the hook of the hamate and of the scaphoid. Hook of the hamate fracture usually occurs when an object held in the hand meets unexpected resistance, such as during a golf swing if the golfer strikes the ground instead of the ball. It is accompanied by pain and decreased grip strength. Conservative treatment with 10–12 weeks of immobilization may allow healing to take place, but often the fragment must be removed surgically.[28]

Navicular (scaphoid) fractures are frequently missed because they are not easily seen on initial x-rays. They require prolonged immobilization for healing and have a high rate of complications, such as nonunion and avascular necrosis. Scaphoid fractures are usually due to a fall on an extended wrist and present with tenderness in the "snuff box."[32]

"Game keeper's thumb" or "skier's thumb," a sprain of the ulnar collateral ligament of the thumb, is very common. This ligament is necessary for stabilization of the thumb-to-index finger pinch. Inadequate treatment of this injury will result in a loss of pinch ability and chronic pain. The ligament should be tested for laxity in positions of both extension and flexion and should be compared to the nonsymptomatic thumb. A first degree sprain can be taped. Second degree sprains should be immobilized in a splint for four to six weeks, and third degree sprains should be treated surgically.[28]

"Mallet finger"—rupture of the extensor tendon of the distal phalanx— occurs by a force to the fingertip, usually as a ball is caught. The ball strikes the extended finger, forcing it into flexion and avulsing the tendon. Active extension at the distal interphalangeal (DIP) joint is lost. If the avulsion fracture is small, and specifically if it does not involve the joint surface, the DIP joint can be splinted in extension for six to eight weeks.[32]

"Jersey finger"—rupture of the flexor tendon of the distal phalanx—occurs by grabbing an opponent's jersey, forcing the flexed finger into extension. Active flexion of the DIP joint is lost, especially when the proximal interphalangeal joint is held in extension. This injury requires surgery.[32]

Foot and Ankle

Running, jumping, and kicking frequently cause injuries to the feet and ankles of athletes. It has been known for some time that proprioceptive ability is impaired after an ankle injury.[12] A number of devices have been used to retrain the proprioceptive sense as well as to improve range of motion and muscular strength.

The biomechanical ankle platform system, or BAPS board (see Figure 2) consists of a round piece of plywood with half a sphere attached to the bottom center. By balancing while progressively shifting weight back and forth on the device the athlete regains proprioception. Similarly, a teeter board, essentially a rocking platform, can be used for the same training. Drills such as running backward and up and down stairs on the toes will also improve proprioception.

As always, after the initial treatment of rest, ice, elevation, and compression, mobilization is instituted. A brace providing mediolateral support may be used in the beginning to allow early weight-bearing and mobilization.

Figure 2. The biomechanical ankle platform system.

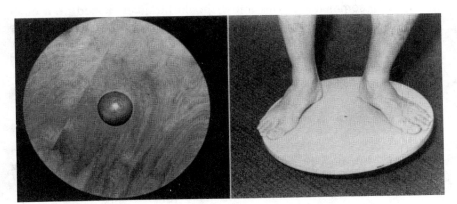

Reproduced from Nicholas, J.A., and E.B. Hershman, *The Lower Extremity and Spine in Sports Medicine*, vol. 1 (St. Louis: The C.V. Mosby Co., 1986), by permission of the publisher.

New devices, such as plastizole molds that can be heated and molded to the individual in the office and air splints that are inflated around the heel and ankle, allow early resumption of athletic activity. Adequate flexibility, specifically in the gastroc-soleus complex, is important for maximizing return to activity and decreasing the risk of ankle reinjury.

Plantar fasciitis is a common overuse injury of the foot in running athletes, which typically presents as morning pain at the insertion of the plantar fascia into the calcaneus. It should initially be treated with heel cups, rest, ice, and NSAIDs. Malalignment or biomechanical running abnormalities such as excessive pronation should be minimized. Moldable in-shoe orthotic devices can be fitted to the patient's shoe in the office to correct excessive foot pronation. A tight triceps surae increases pronation, and calf stretching should be started early. If the above measures are unsuccessful, steroid injections may be administered. Surgical release may be the last resort if there is no improvement in six to nine months.[26]

Stress fractures are common in the bones of the foot, especially the second and third metatarsals and the calcaneus. Often, the initial x-rays are negative, but repeat films show areas of new bone formation. Bone scan imaging can help in diagnosis if plain films are inconclusive. Treatment consists of rest from the causative activity and correction of contributing biomechanical abnormalities. An alternative aerobic conditioning program should be substituted until healing is complete.

Fifth metatarsal fractures are said to be the most common fractures in dancers and are frequent fractures in other athletes as well. A fracture of the proximal diaphysis (base) of the fifth metatarsal (Jones' fracture) heals slowly with unpredictable union. Controversy exists as to whether non-weight-bearing, cast immobilization, or early internal fixation is the treatment of choice. In highly competitive athletes, consideration of early internal fixation is recommended. This injury should be differentiated from other fifth metatarsal fractures such as tuberosity and avulsion fractures. More common is fracture through the tuberosity produced by an inversion injury of the plantar flexed foot. These fractures heal well and can be treated symptomatically with a walking cast for two or three weeks. Care must be taken to differentiate the tuberosity fracture from a normal apophysis.[27]

Orthotics

In-shoe orthotics are used to control excessive or prolonged pronation and other mechanical problems of the lower extremity. Taping and padding can be done in the office to ascertain how well an individual will respond to orthotics. Particularly useful is "low dye strapping" to provide arch support in plantar fasciitis, medial arch strain, and excessive pronation (Figure 3).

Heel cups that cushion the heel are useful in plantar fasciitis and heel

Figure 3. Low dye taping technique: (a) Tape is applied from the lateral foot just proximal to the fifth metatarsal head, around the heel to just proximal to the first metatarsal head. The foot is held neutral and relaxed. (b) Metatarsal heads two through five are supported by the thumb of the person doing the taping, and the first metatarsal head is depressed with the fingers while the tape is secured. (c) This process is repeated three to four times. (d) Straps are tied down with strips running from the dorsolateral to the dorsomedial foot to support the arch.

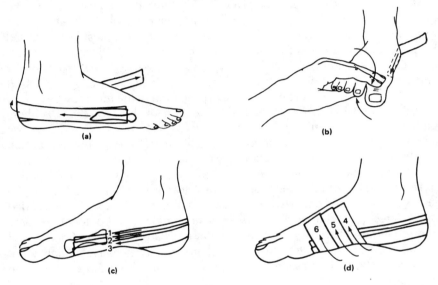

From Roy, S., and R. Irvin, *Sports Medicine: Prevention, Evaluation, Management and Rehabilitation*, p. 58, © 1983. Reprinted by permission of Prentice-Hall, Inc., Englewood Cliffs, N.J.

pain. Heel lifts decrease the stretch on the achilles tendon and gastroc-soleus to allow less painful walking in cases of achilles tendonitis or strain of the gastroc-soleus.

Leg

"Shin splints" is a term that has been used to describe any pain in the lower extremity associated with overuse. The American Medical Association suggests that this term be limited to inflammatory conditions of any of the musculotendinous units in the anterior or posterior compartments of the lower leg. Shin splints often occur during initiation of training or when the athlete's activity level increases, before the muscles and tendons have had time to strengthen in response to the greater activity. They are most likely to occur when the running surface is hard, or when shoes are uncushioned or improperly fitted. Pain usually appears soon after exercise is begun. Early treatment consists of rest, ice massage, and nonsteroidal anti-inflammatory drugs. When pain is reduced, stretching and strengthening exercises are started. For anterior shin splints, the anterior muscles are strengthened and posterior muscles are stretched. Posterior shin splints are treated with anterior muscle and heel cord stretching and posterior muscle strengthening.[26]

Medial tibial stress syndrome is a condition of pain and tenderness in the posteromedial distal tibia, usually occurring after activity and relieved by rest. Pain may persist for hours or days after activity. It is most likely caused by periostitis or a stress fracture created by overuse.[19] Diagnosis can occasionally be made by plain films, which may show cortical hypertrophy and periosteal reaction, or by bone scan, which may show an increased uptake in the area in question. Excessive pronation of the foot may be found. Treatment consists of rest, ice, and correction of the pronation. Athletic participation can resume when the symptoms have resolved and after the athlete has completed an appropriate stretching and strengthening program emphasizing the tibialis posterior, flexor hallucis longus, and flexor digitorum longus muscles. Heel cord and tibialis posterior stretching is helpful.[26]

The above conditions must be differentiated from stress fractures in the leg. Stress fractures occur when the bone's ability to remodel is exceeded by the stress placed on it. They present with gradual onset of localized pain and tenderness. Percussion of the bone at a distance from the fracture still causes pain at the fracture site. X-rays are usually negative initially, but eventually show signs of new bone formation. A bone scan confirms the diagnosis.[26]

Treatment of stress fractures is by rest from the causative activity until the pain resolves, usually three to eight weeks. Return to activity must be slowly progressive, with an increase of not more than 25% per week.

Compartment syndromes in the leg can occur acutely after trauma or chronically secondary to exertion. In chronic exertional compartment syndrome, pain typically occurs during exercise and subsides with rest. The changes are reversible and the muscle may be normal between episodes. Involvement is often bilateral. Measurement of anterior compartment pressure is diagnostic. Treatment is by fasciotomy of the involved compartment.[26]

Knee

The recent evolution in treatment of knee injuries has concentrated on several major areas, including change in treatment of meniscal tears and cruciate and collateral ligaments, better understanding and treatment of patellofemoral disorders, focus on the intercondylar femoral notch, new diagnostic and surgical techniques, and a better understanding of the usefulness of knee braces.

In the past, the accepted treatment for meniscal injuries was total meniscectomy.[26] The meniscus is not necessary for stability, and it was felt that without it, there was essentially no increase in knee morbidity. Since it is avascular, the meniscus was not thought to be capable of healing. It is now recognized that meniscectomy does increase future morbidity,[26,35] and some meniscal injuries do heal. This realization has drastically changed the treatment of meniscal injury.

If the knee is stable ligamentously and there is an undisplaced tear of the meniscus, treatment can be nonoperative (ice, crutches, and NSAIDs). As pain and swelling resolve a strengthening program is instituted, and when strength is regained, the athlete can return to his or her sport. The peripheral circumferential fibers are most crucial to meniscus function. It they are torn and cannot be repaired they must be removed, and indeed partial meniscectomy is now the most common meniscal surgery—often done arthroscopically. Following partial meniscectomy, the patient may ambulate in one to three days, train in one to two weeks, and return to athletics in three to four weeks. Prognosis is usually good. Displaced peripheral tears can be surgically repaired and immobilized for one month, followed by a slow remobilization and strengthening program. Return to athletic activity may be slow.[26]

Ligamentous Injury

It is helpful to view the ligaments of the knee as primary and secondary stabilizers. The primary stabilizer to valgus stress is the medial collateral ligament (MCL). The secondary stabilizers are the middle one-third of the medial joint capsule, the posterior oblique ligament, the anterior cruciate ligament (ACL), and the posterior cruciate ligament (PCL). The primary stabilizer to varus stress is the lateral collateral ligament (LCL) aided secondarily by the iliotibial band, middle one-third of the lateral joint capsule, popliteus and biceps femoris muscles, and the ACL and PCL. Anterior displacement is prevented primarily by the ACL and secondarily by the iliotibial band, the middle one-third of the medial and lateral capsules, and by both the MCL and LCL. Posteriorly, the primary stabilizer is the PCL, secondarily the posterolateral capsule, LCL and MCL, and the popliteus.[26,30] Isolated injury to one of the primary stabilizers can usually be treated conservatively, but multiple injury needs a surgical evaluation.[15,26]

The MCL is usually injured through valgus trauma. Its stability can usually be evaluated by physical exam with valgus stress testing at extension and 30° flexion of the knee. If the knee is unstable at 30 degrees but stable at extension there is usually an isolated MCL tear. Laxity at extension indicates that other structures are most likely damaged also.

A Grade I sprain (pain but no ligamentous laxity with valgus stress) can be treated with ice, anti-inflammatory agents, and avoidance of running and cutting activities until the swelling and pain resolve. A quadriceps and hamstring strengthening program is instituted early. Progressive return to athletic activity is begun when full range of motion and strength are regained and the athlete is free of pain.[26]

For a partial disruption of the ligament (Grade II sprain) the initial phase of rest and partial weight-bearing usually lasts a few weeks and rehabilitation lasts longer. A double upright brace providing mediolateral support may be used when activities are resumed. Complete MCL tears (Grade III) without other knee injury can be treated with two weeks of immobilization followed by four weeks of stabilization by brace and then gradual range of motion and strength training.[17] Some centers use protected range of motion instead of immobilization. Since the medial meniscus is attached to the MCL, a high index of suspicion for associated meniscal injury is warranted.[26]

Injury to the ACL alone is usually due to a noncontact twisting injury. Pain is immediate and swelling progresses in one to two hours secondary to hemarthrosis. Diagnosis is by pivot shift test, which causes anterior displacement of the tibia, or by the newer Lachman test, which is an anterior drawer test at 25–30° of knee flexion[26,37] (see Figures 4 and 5). This technique

Figure 4. The Lachman test for disruption of the anterior cruciate ligament.

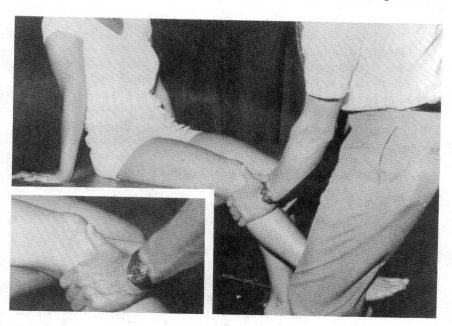

Reproduced from Nicholas, J.A., and E.B. Hershman, *The Lower Extremity and Spine in Sports Medicine*, vol. 1 (St. Louis: The C.V. Mosby Co., 1986), by permission of the publisher.

Figure 5. The direction of forces applied in the Lachman test.

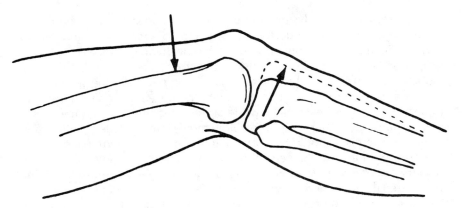

From Roy, S., and R. Irvin, *Sports Medicine: Prevention, Evaluation, Management and Rehabilitation*, p. 313, © 1983. Reprinted by permission of Prentice-Hall, Inc., Englewood Cliffs, N.J.

of examination is more useful acutely than the anterior drawer test, because it eliminates the contribution of other supporting structures to stability and tests solely the ACL.

Nonoperative treatment of ACL injury is initiated with range of motion exercises, staying within the pain-free range. When full range of motion is reached, a strengthening program is begun, emphasizing the hamstrings and avoiding terminal knee extension quadriceps exercises. A derotation brace should be used when returning to cutting activities. Up to 60–70% of acute ACL injuries have associated meniscal tears, so this possibility should be assessed carefully.[26]

The ACL is thought to be injured sometimes as athletes kick, presumably from compression of the ligament within the posterior intercondylar femoral notch. This somewhat V-shaped notch can trap the anterior cruciate ligament. Chronic damage can weaken the ligament and an acute strain from a kick may tear it. This injury may occur more often in people with a narrower or sharper intercondylar notch. Athletes who have sustained such an injury may be at risk for the same injury on the other leg.

LCL injury is caused by a hyperextension varus stress. Management is similar to that of an MCL injury. PCL injury usually occurs along with other injuries. It happens when a posterior force is directed at the tibia while the knee is flexed. On physical examination there is a positive posterior drawer sign. Treatment stresses quadriceps strengthening exercises. Surgery may be required.[26]

Patellofemoral Dysfunction

Patellofemoral joint dysfunction is usually due to chronic faulty motion of patellar tracking. To understand patellofemoral dysfunction and rehabilitation it is important to understand the biomechanics of this joint. During weight-bearing the patellofemoral joint reactive force increases the further the knee is flexed, but this increase is compensated by the greater joint surface area that is in contact. With weight-training, stress on the joint tends to be greater toward extension, while at the same time the surface contact area diminishes.[16] Therefore, in patellofemoral joint disorders, full flexion/extension exercises should be avoided and isometrics or terminal extension exercises used instead. Since subluxation and lateral tracking tend to occur with the knee in relative extension—a position in which the patella has not yet entered the intercondylar groove of the femur—it is evident that muscular forces are crucial to provide stability. The knee is normally in a position of some valgus (except in full flexion), which tends to pull the patella laterally on knee extension. The vastus medialis is of great importance in counteracting this and therefore must be strengthened. Ninety percent of patellofemoral dysfunctions can be treated conservatively with quadriceps strengthening (emphasizing the vastus medialis oblique—VMO), muscle education to ensure synchrony of the VMO and the quadriceps, and hamstring and iliotibial band stretching. Braces to hold the patella medially can also be helpful. Excessive pronation at the subtalar joint frequently exacerbates patellofemoral dysfunction and should be corrected. If a conservative program fails, surgery, with either a lateral retinacular release, debridement, or tendon repositioning, may be considered.[26]

A number of other soft tissue disorders of the knee may cause pain and impair function in the athlete. Osgood-Schlatter's disease is osteochondritis at the tibial tubercle and is a common cause of pain in adolescents. Treatment is conservative, with ice, nonsteroidal anti-inflammatory agents, and rest. Cast immobilization is sometimes required to enforce rest. Popliteal tendonitis may cause lateral knee pain during running. Pain is exacerbated by running downhill and sitting cross-legged. Treatment is again with ice, rest, ultrasound, and NSAIDs. Iliotibial band (ITB) friction syndrome causes lateral knee pain as the band crosses over the lateral femoral condyle during repeated knee flexion. Ober's test for tensor fascia lata (TFL) tightness is positive, and compression of the ITB between the palpating fingers and femoral condyle reproduces pain. Treatment emphasizing ITB and TFL stretching, before and after exercise, and ice massage should be effective. Gait evaluation and orthotics may be necessary.[26]

Pes anserinus bursitis causes medial knee pain and must be differentiated from injury to the meniscus and MCL as a source of pain. Treatment is conservative as above, with emphasis on decreasing inflammation and stretching the hamstrings. Again, lower extremity mechanical problems, such as excessive pronation, can contribute.[26]

Knee Braces

There are three categories of knee braces: prophylactic, rehabilitative, and functional. Prophylactic braces have not been shown to be of any benefit and may actually worsen injuries. Rehabilitative braces allow protected mobility. They include a hinge, hinge brace arms, and thigh and calf enclosures. The hinges may have settings to limit the range of motion allowed. Such braces offer little or no reduction of anterior laxity in anterior cruciate ligament-deficient knees. Nevertheless, this type of brace is useful since it will give some support, especially mediolaterally, and it will allow earlier mobilization and weight-bearing than would be possible without it. Functional braces, such as the double upright (Don Joy) and derotation (Lennox Hill) braces, increase stability at low loads, and thus are beneficial for returning the athletes to activity. One must be aware that these functional braces do not correct the laxity of the joint and do not significantly resist joint displacement under high loads. A knee sleeve with a lateral horseshoe and patellar tracking straps is often useful for decreasing symptoms of patellofemoral dysfunction.[24]

Hip

A "hip pointer" is the result of a blow to the iliac crest. It must be differentiated from an avulsion fracture by x-ray. Treatment is with ice, rest, compression, and padding to prevent reinjury. Only when normal motion (lateral bending and trunk rotation) returns and pain subsides should an athlete return to play. In adolescents and children hip pathology can also present as pain in the knee, especially in conditions such as avascular necrosis of the femoral head or in transient synovitis.

Back Pain

Back pain in athletes commonly results from soft tissue injuries, spondylolysis, facet inflammation, and disk herniation. Musculoskeletal and mechanical dysfunction must be differentiated from irritation of the nerve root. Athletes with pain exacerbated by lumbar extension must be evaluated for a stress fracture of the pars interarticularis (spondylolysis). Plain films may be negative early, but a bone scan will detect a recent stress fracture. If a lesion is present on x-ray and doubt exists as to acuteness of the injury, a bone scan should be performed. In such a case a negative scan indicates that the fracture is old. An acute injury will require rest from activity and possibly immobilization. An old injury may or may not be the cause of current pain.

Lumbar disk herniation with nerve root irritation is common in athletes. A patient without neurologic deficit can usually be treated conservatively with two to three days of bed rest, lumbar traction, nonsteroidal anti-inflammatory agents, and muscle relaxants.[27] If evidence of nerve root irritation is present (positive straight leg raising, Lasegue, bowstring), oral steroids can be considered to decrease nerve root inflammation. Nerve root inflammation that fails to resolve under this regimen may benefit from an epidural steroid injection.[11] If incapacitating pain persists, or if a progressive neurologic deficit develops, surgical evaluation is appropriate. Back pain in athletes should be evaluated thoroughly, with a high index of suspicion for disk herniation or spondylolysis. Back pain in children can have serious implications and should never be ignored.

Facet irritation and inflammation from lumbar hyperextension is a common cause of back pain in athletes. Pain is exacerbated by running and jumping (jarring activities) and activities requiring increased lumbar lordosis or extension, i.e., poor-technique weight lifting, gymnastics, swimming, tennis serve. Flexion strengthening exercises and correction of poor athletic techniques are effective treatments. Facet injection with steroids under fluoroscopy may also relieve pain. Acute back muscle and ligamentous injuries may be treated with short-term bed rest, nonsteroidal anti-inflammatory agents, muscle relaxants, and physiatrics modalities. In 1985 Deyo et al. published data indicating that prescribing two days of bed rest may give the same long-term outcome as longer bed rest, with less time lost from work and activity.[7]

Muscle Injury

Contusion of the quadriceps is often undertreated and can be a disabling injury in an athlete. Along with directly crushing the muscle fibers, a forceful blow to the thigh causes bleeding and swelling. This results in pain, muscle stiffness, and inability to flex the knee or contract the quadriceps. Treatment includes a cold wet elastic wrap to the thigh at the level of the injury along with ice. The athlete should lie prone with the knee being passively flexed to the point where only minimal discomfort is felt. No excessive force should be applied to flex the knee. The purpose of this is to maintain flexibility, not to increase it. Crutches should be used for ambulation. Icing should be continued intermittently for 12–48 hours. After that, icing in a prone position with the knee held flexed for 30–60 minutes should be continued until full flexibility is achieved. Quadriceps strengthening should be started when the athlete is pain free. Myositis ossificans at the site of injury is a potential complication and may permanently limit the amount of knee flexion.[32]

Head and Neck Injuries

"Stingers" or "burners" is the complaint of the athlete who has radiating pain with paresthesias in the extremity following a blow to the head, neck, or shoulder. This can be due to an injury of pain endings in ligaments, periosteum, or perineurium of the brachial plexus, nerve root, or peripheral nerve. The mechanism of injury and distribution of neurological deficits and local and referred pain help to determine the location of suspected injury.[10] The brachial plexus stretch injury is the most common and occurs when the head and shoulder are forced apart. Less commonly, entrapment at the nerve root is caused by hyperextension or hyperflexion of the neck. Protrusion of a ruptured disk is an uncommon cause of neck pain in the athlete. Prior to return to play after a neck injury the athlete must have full painless active range of motion and strength of the neck, a normal neurological examination, including strength and sensory testing, and resolution of symptoms.[32]

Recurrent minor head injury in collision sports, with all its sequelae, is underrecognized. Education of coaches, trainers, and family is important.[3] See Table 3 for a brief overview of treatment for head injuries.

Eye

The eye can be injured in contact sports and in racket sports. In one study of Canadian racket sport injuries, the most common were hyphema, lid hemorrhage and laceration, corneal abrasion, and iritis. Vitreous hemorrhage and retinal detachment were also found.[9]

Retinal detachment deserves special mention because it can present without an obvious eye deformity or specific injury. This is the condition made famous by boxer Sugar Ray Leonard, who developed such a detachment. Retinal detachment is a separation of the neural retina from the underlying pigment layer. It is painless and is heralded by vitreous floaters, flashes of light, blurred vision, and a sensation of a veil being drawn over part of the visual field. If it involves the macula, visual acuity is decreased. Impaired

Table 3. Head injury triage.

Return to immediate activity
   No loss of consciousness or amnesia
   Normal neurological examination
   No headache, nausea, or other symptoms

No return to immediate activity
   Post-traumatic or retrograde amnesia
   Loss of consciousness
   Abnormal neurological examination

Out for the season
   Three or more "dings"
   Focal neurological signs
   Persistent amnesia

Source: Besgo, J.J., and R. Lehman, "Field evaluation and management of head and neck injuries," *Clin Sports Med* 6(1), 1987.

acuity, impaired visual field to confrontation, and retinal irregularity on ophthalmoscopy are diagnostic. It can be obscured by concomitant hemorrhage. If retinal detachment is suspected, the patient should be referred to an ophthalmologist immediately and undergo hospitalization, bed rest with the head elevated, sedation, binocular eye patching, and pupillary dilatation. The condition can usually be treated with cryotherapy or photocoagulation with good results.[4]

Prevention of any eye injury is desirable. Racket sports have a high incidence of ocular trauma, since the ball may be traveling at 85–140 miles (130–225 km) per hour. It has been shown that ordinary glasses, even with hardened lenses, do not protect the player from an eye injury since they can shatter. Also, open eye guards are now known to be of little use. A ball can penetrate the open area and hit the eye. New closed-lens eye guards that meet strict standards have been shown to prevent eye injury and should be recommended for use during all potentially high-risk sports[9] (Figure 6).

DIAGNOSTIC TECHNIQUES

Magnetic resonance imaging is useful in visualizing the articular surfaces of joints, as well as soft tissues. It can detect early aseptic necrosis of the humeral head and provides noninvasive assessment of knee ligament and meniscal injuries.[28]

Computerized axial tomography is particularly useful in detecting disk herniation and in discerning a distorted patellofemoral relationship with a lateral shift and tilting of the patella. It also is used to assess glenoid labrum integrity in the shoulder.

Arthrography—the use of injected dye to facilitate x-ray viewing of tissues—allows visualization of the menisci, the articular cartilage, and the cruciate ligament in the knee. It is a less invasive and cheaper, but less accurate, alternative to arthroscopy. It also can detect complete rotator cuff tears in the shoulder.

The technicium-99m bone scan is used to detect increased bone perfusion. It is useful in detecting early stress fractures, myositis ossificans, and other conditions before they become apparent on plain x-rays.

MEDICAL CONSIDERATIONS

Nutrition

Athletes, like nonathletes, need a well-balanced diet. The athlete, however, has a much higher energy requirement—3,000 kilocalories or more a day, depending on the training level. The athlete needs little extra protein or fat, but he does need more carbohydrates to fuel his increased energy expenditure. Extra protein intake is a metabolic load on the body and will

Figure 6. Closed eyeguard to prevent injury to the eyes during racket sports.

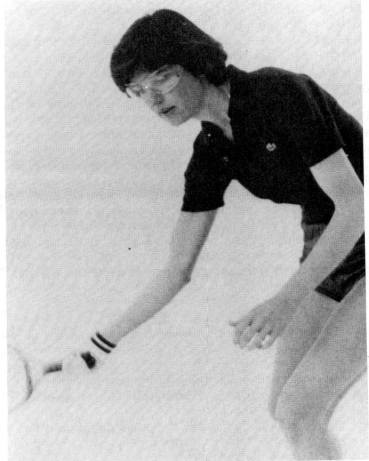

From Roy, S., and R. Irvin, *Sports Medicine: Prevention, Evaluation, Management and Rehabilitation*, p. 150, © 1983. Reprinted by permission of Prentice-Hall, Inc., Englewood Cliffs, N.J.

not, in the long run, contribute to usable energy stores. Excess fat intake leads to storage of fat. Stored fat is used for long-term energy in endurance events, but even thin athletes have plenty of fat to see them through almost any event. Carbohydrates can be stored in the body in the form of glycogen, both within the muscle and in the liver. Glycogen constitutes the most available energy store for most athletic events, after the initial short energy burst when ATP and creatine phosphate stores are depleted (1–6 seconds). Glycogen is not a long-term energy source like fat, however, and must be replenished daily. Glycogen stores provide adequate energy for up to two or three hours. For longer events, dilute sugar solution taken during the activity may be beneficial. More concentrated solutions should be avoided, however, since they are more difficult to absorb. Carbohydrate loading is an attempt to use the body's ability to store glycogen to benefit the athlete during a particular event. The carbohydrate loading schedule is timed to saturate or supersaturate glycogen stores by a targeted time. Its starts eight days before the event: the first four days are marked by vigorous training and low carbohydrate intake, and the following four days by light training and a high-carbohydrate diet. In theory, this schedule provides extra glycogen for maximal available energy without altering the athlete's peak performance level. In practice, it is often difficult to adhere to and is frequently modified to eliminate the four days of low carbohydrate intake. In both a carbohydrate loading schedule and a regular training schedule simple sugars should be avoided in favor of complex carbohydrates, since simple sugars stimulate insulin release and can cause hypoglycemia several hours later. Before athletic events and training sessions meals high in protein or fat should also be avoided since they require a long passage time to clear the stomach and small intestine. Similarly, high-bulk foods should not be eaten since they cause a feeling of fullness but add little to useful energy stores.[32,34]

Fluid Requirements

A loss of 3% of body weight from sweating during exercise can easily be replaced with adequate fluid intake. A loss of 3–5% puts the athlete at increased risk of subsequent heat injury, and a greater than 5% loss places the athlete in danger of developing significant heat-related problems. It is helpful to routinely measure pre- and post-training weights to pinpoint those athletes most susceptible to dehydration.

A general guideline for fluid intake to prevent dehydration and related heat injury is outlined in Table 4. It should be amended based on an individual athlete's size and requirements.

The fluid of choice is usually cool water. Sugar solutions are to be avoided since they delay the absorption of fluid.[32]

Table 4. Recommended fluid intake before and during athletic competition.

Time	Amount of fluid
2 hours before activity	1 liter
15 minutes before activity	400–500 ml
Every 15 minutes during activity	400–500 ml
After activity	5–6 large glasses

Source: Roy, S., and R. Irvin, *Sports Medicine: Prevention, Evaluation, Management, and Rehabilitation*, Englewood Cliffs, NJ: Prentice-Hall, 1983.

Exercise-induced Asthma

Exercise-induced asthma is a fairly common condition and should be considered a possible cause of wheezing by an athlete. It is usually caused by hyperirritability of the airways, leading to bronchoconstriction on contact with cold air. It often affects runners, who may be counseled to try swimming as an alternate form of exercise since the warm air and high humidity of indoor pools decreases the incidence of asthmatic attacks. A large variety of pharmacological treatments are available that may benefit asthmatic athletes, or those prone to exercise-induced asthma.

Exertional Rhabdomyolysis

Exertional rhabdomyolysis is a condition of skeletal muscle injury that causes the cellular contents to be released into the circulation. Abnormalities of energy production, hypoxia, primary muscle injury, infection, or toxins, among other factors, can cause this condition. During exhausting exercise, a depletion of energy stores can damage the muscle, leading to a disruption of cellular integrity and subsequent release of cell components, including myoglobin, creatinine, phosphorus, potassium, and enzymes.

During endurance exercising, exertional rhabdomyolysis occurs rather frequently in a mild form with no significant symptoms. However, more severe rhabdomyolysis can be a life-threatening illness. It appears to be a more serious problem in hot climates. Clinical signs of rhabdomyolysis include weakness, pain, and muscle tenderness. More severe injury leads to muscle swelling, loss of deep tendon reflexes, tetany, acute renal failure, compartment syndrome, and disseminated intravascular coagulation. Hyperkalemia may cause life-threatening arrhythmias. Acute renal failure may occur in people who are dehydrated, those exercising in a hot climate, or those who are not usually athletically active. It appears to be caused by myoglobin breakdown products, aciduria, dehydration, hyperuricuria, and a decrease in renal blood flow. Muscle necrosis causes edema, with an increase in the volume of the muscle that can lead to a compartment syndrome in the susceptible areas and possible resultant nerve damage.[27]

Rhabdomyolysis is diagnosed through discovery of myoglobinuria and an elevation of serum creatine phosphokinase and aldolase. Myoglobin can cause a urine dip stick to be read as positive for blood even in the absence of red blood cells on urinalysis.[39] Treatment for rhabdomyolysis should be instituted early to avoid major complications. Hydration and correction of metabolic abnormalities are of primary importance to prevent renal and cardiovascular complications. Fluid repletion of up to 10 liters within 12 to 24 hours may be necessary.[20,27]

Exercise and Hypertension

Both normal and hypertensive individuals have an increase in mean arterial blood pressure during exercise. This increase is exaggerated in the hypertensive[13] and has been suggested as an early indicator of the development of hypertension.[8]

Regular aerobic exercise appears to reduce the resting blood pressure of both normal and hypertensive participants and may be beneficial in preventing hypertension from developing in those who have the predisposing risk factors. Therefore, a regular schedule of aerobic exercise is advisable as part of a hypertensive treatment plan. Young patients and borderline hypertensives respond better than older or more severe hypertensives.[23,31]

When prescribing or recommending an exercise program for the hypertensive patient or athlete, it is best to avoid isometric exercises such as weight lifting. Isometrics have been associated with elevated blood pressure and left ventricular hypertrophy.[33,38]

When an athlete requires antihypertensive medication, a number of side effects of the drug must be taken into consideration to maximize function and health. Beta-blockers reduce heart rate and cardiac output. They may be used with less detriment to performance in athletes whose sport requires intermittent exertion. In most athletes, endurance will suffer when these drugs are used, but in those with concomitant coronary artery disease, endurance may actually be improved. Beta-blockers also predispose to hypoglycemia and may increase sweating.[23]

Thiazide diuretics reduce blood pressure by lowering plasma volume and decreasing cardiac output. Over time they reduce peripheral resistance. These drugs present the complications of fluid and potassium depletion, which can be devastating in athletes at risk for dehydration.[22,23]

Central alpha-adrenergic blockers decrease resting heart rate and cardiac output but permit a near-normal response to exercise. They are likely to be beneficial during endurance exercise.[23]

Alpha$_1$-blockers reduce peripheral vascular resistance while having little effect on heart rate and cardiac output. Prazosin is the preferred agent in this group and is generally well tolerated in athletes, but the first dose often causes hypotension.[23]

Angiotensin-converting enzyme inhibitors are also usually well tolerated in athletes. They decrease peripheral vascular resistance but produce little effect on heart rate and an increase in stroke volume. They act by inhibiting an angiotensin II-mediated increase in peripheral resistance and renal sodium retention.[23] They would seem to be advantageous in the established older hypertensive who tends to have an elevated peripheral vascular resistance.

Diabetes

An in-depth discussion of diabetes and exercise is beyond the scope of this chapter, but a few points deserve brief mention. During exercise a diabetic patient requires less exogenous insulin. Exercise uses up glucose; thus, one should always watch for hypoglycemia and treat it appropriately in diabetic athletes, especially those taking insulin. The insulin-dependent diabetic, usually juvenile, will learn to judge his or her body's insulin requirements with and without exercise and can plan the insulin dosage accordingly. This patient should be encouraged to participate in athletics, but must be aware that exercise will change food and insulin requirements.

The noninsulin-dependent diabetic should also be encouraged to participate. Frequently the patient's diabetes is exacerbated by obesity. Exercise may lead to weight loss and promote general well-being. Again, hypoglycemia is a potential complication, and the dosage of oral hypoglycemics, if the patient is taking them, may need to be reduced.

Anabolic Steroids

Anabolic steroids do seem to increase muscle mass and strength in certain well-trained athletes. The strength gain is small but significant. However, anabolic steroids have been associated with adverse effects on the liver, cardiovascular system, reproductive system, and psychological status. Their use is "contrary to the rules and ethical principles of athletic competition as set forth by many of the sports governing bodies. The American College of Sports Medicine supports these ethical principles and deplores the use of anabolic-androgenic steroids by athletes."[1]

CRITERIA FOR RETURN TO ATHLETIC ACTIVITY

Before returning to his/her previous level of performance, the injured athlete should demonstrate a full range of motion and strength. Balance and coordination must be assessed and trained with sports-related activities and with proprioceptive stimulators to determine that the basic kinematic requirements of the sport can be fulfilled without risk of reinjury. The athlete must also be instructed in and understand improved body motions to minimize risk of reinjury. He must be trained in a basic exercise-maintenance program for the long term. When reentering the sport, supportive bracing or taping is often beneficial. Functional progression (see Table 5) is a stepped program to increase the complexity of activity and to assess readiness to return to the demands of the sport.

**Table 5. Progression of functional criteria to be met before
return to a sports activity.**

After shoulder injury in throwing athletes:
- Painless active and passive range of motion, including full flexibility in both internal and external rotation
- Full strength of the deltoid, pectoralis major, latissimus dorsi, serratus anterior, biceps, triceps, as well as rotator cuff
- Full strength and flexibility of trunk and lower extremities
- Successful progression through a program of:
  a) alternate day light throwing at 15 meters;
  b) throwing 2 out of 3 days;
  c) throwing half speed;
  d) unrestricted throwing.

This program should begin with 50 throws divided by a rest period every day, and advance to 100 throws slowly and only as long as the athlete experiences no pain.[28]

After lower extremity injury:
- Painless active and passive range of motion
- Full muscular strength
- Pain-free weight-bearing and walking
- Painless straight ahead half-speed running
- Painless slalom and figure-8 running pattern
- Cutting activities without pain or instability
- Gradual return to full-speed straight-line running, progressing to slalom, figure 8, and cutting without pain

REFERENCES

1. American College of Sports Medicine. Position statement on the use of anabolic-androgenic steroids in sports. Indianapolis: American College of Sports Medicine; 1984.
2. Barnes DA, Tullos HS. An analysis of 100 symptomatic baseball pitchers. *Am J Sports Med.* 1978;6:62.
3. Besgo JJ, Lehman R. Field evaluation and management of head and neck injuries. *Clin Sports Med.* 1987;6(1).
4. Berkow R, ed. *The Merck manual.* 14th ed. Rahway, NJ: Merck and Co; 1982.
5. Cailliet R. *Shoulder pain.* 2nd ed. Philadelphia: FA Davis; 1981.
6. Chapman MW, ed. *Operative orthopedics.* Philadelphia: JB Lippincott; 1988.
7. Deyo RA, Diehl AK, Rosenthal M. How many days of bed rest for acute low back pain? A randomized clinical trial. *N Engl J Med.* 1986;315:1064–1070.
8. Dlin RA, Hanne N, Silverberg DS, Bar-Or O. Follow-up of normotensive men with exaggerated blood pressure response to exercise. *Am Heart J.* 1983;106:316–320.
9. Easterbrook M. Eye protection in racquet sports. *Clin Sports Med.* 1988;7:2.
10. Feinstein B, Langton JNK, Jameson RM, Schiller F. Experiments on pain referred from deep somatic tissues. *J Bone Joint Surg [Am].* 1954;36A:981.
11. Fletcher GF, ed. *Exercise in the practice of medicine.* Mount Kisco, NY: Futura Publishing; 1982.
12. Freeman MAR, Dean MRE, Hanham LWI. The etiology and prevention of functional instability of the foot. *J Bone Joint Surg [Br].* 1965;47B:678.
13. Haskell WL. The influence of exercise on the concentrations of triglyceride and cholesterol in human plasma. *Exerc Sports Sci Rev.* 1984;12:205.
14. Herring SA, Nilson KL. Introduction to overuse injuries. *Clin Sports Med.* 1987;6(2).
15. Holden DL, Eggert AW, Butler JE. The nonoperative treatment of Grade I and II medial collateral ligament injuries to the knee. *Am J Sports Med.* 1983;11:340.

16. Hungerford DS, Lennox DW. Rehabilitation of the knee in disorders of the patellofemoral joint: relevant biomechanics. *Orthop Clin North Am.* 1983;14(2).
17. Indelicato PA. Nonoperative treatment of complete tears of the medial collateral ligament of the knee. *J Bone Joint Surg [Am].* 1983;65A:323.
18. Jobe FW, Jobe CM. Painful athletic injuries of the shoulder. *Clin Orthop.* 1983;173:117.
19. Johnell O, Rausing A, Wandeberg B, Westlin N. Morphological bone changes in shin splints. *Clin Orthop.* 1982;167:180.
20. Knochel JP. Rhabdomyolysis and myoglobinuria. *Semin Nephrol.* 1981;1(1).
21. Kottke FJ, Lehmann JF, eds. *Krusen's handbook of physical medicine and rehabilitation.* 4th ed. Philadelphia: WB Saunders; 1990.
22. Lund-Johansen P. Hemodynamic changes in long-term diuretic therapy of essential hypertension. *Acta Med Scand.* 1970;187:509.
23. Mellion MB, ed. *Office management of sports injuries and athletic problems.* Philadelphia: Hanley and Belfus; 1988.
24. Millet CW, Drez DJ. Principles of bracing for the anterior cruciate ligament-deficient knee. *Clin Sports Med.* 1988;7(4).
25. Moseley HF, Overgaard B. Anterior capsular mechanism in recurrent anterior dislocation of shoulder: morphological and clinical studies with special reference to glenoid labrum and glenohumeral ligament. *J Bone Joint Surg [Br].* 1962;44B:913–927.
26. Nicholas JA, Hershman EB, eds. *The lower extremity and spine in sports medicine.* Vol 1. St Louis: CV Mosby; 1986.
27. Nicholas JA, Hershman EB, eds. *The lower extremity and spine in sports medicine.* Vol 2. St Louis: CV Mosby; 1986.
28. Nicholas JA, Hershman EB, eds. *The upper extremity in sports medicine.* St Louis: CV Mosby; 1990.
29. Noyes FR, et al. Biomechanics of ligament failure; II, an analysis of immobilization, exercise and reconditioning effects in primates. *J Bone Joint Surg [Am].* 1974;56A:1406.
30. Noyes FR, Grood ES, Butler DL, Pavlos L. Clinical biomechanics of the knee—ligament restraints and functional stability. In: Funk FJ, ed. *Symposium on the athlete's knee: surgical repair and reconstruction.* St Louis: CV Mosby; 1980.
31. Ramus MU, Mundale MD, Awad EA, Witsoe DA, Cole TM, Olson M, Kottke FJ. Cardiovascular effects of spread of excitation during prolonged isometric exercise. *Arch Phys Med Rehabil.* 1973;54:496.
32. Roy S, Irvin R. *Sports medicine: prevention, evaluation, management, and rehabilitation.* Englewood Cliffs, NJ: Prentice-Hall; 1983.
33. Schaible TF, Scheuer J. Cardiac adaptations to chronic exercise. *Prog Cardiovasc Dis.* 1985;27:297–324.
34. Smith NJ. Nutrition and the athlete. *Orthop Clin North Am.* 1983;14(2).
35. Tapper EM, Hoover NW. Late results after meniscectomy. *J Bone Joint Surg [Am].* 1969;51A:517–526.
36. Tipton CM, et al. The influence of physical activity on ligaments and tendons. *Med Sci Sports.* 1975;7:165.
37. Torg JS, Conrad W, Kalen V. Clinical diagnosis of anterior cruciate ligament instability in the athlete. *Am J Sports Med.* 1976;4:84.
38. Viitasalo JT, Komi PV, Karvonen MJ. Muscle strength and body composition as determinants of blood pressure in young men. *Eur J Appl Physiol.* 1979;42:165–173.
39. Wyngaarden JB, Smith LH, eds. *Cecil Textbook of Medicine.* 17th ed. Philadelphia: WB Saunders; 1985.

Chapter 16

Clinical Advances in Assistive Devices, Orthotics, and Prosthetics

Yeongchi Wu

This chapter presents a brief review of the advances made in the past decade in orthotics, prosthetics, and other assistive devices. The devices discussed were selected according to their potential usefulness, clinical practicality, availability, and effectiveness in developing countries. Thus, it may be expected that many good ideas, products, or procedures are not covered in this review, but that absence is not intended to devalue their potential for clinical application. The information may also be applicable to developed societies, where cost-effectiveness is becoming an issue because of the growing population with disability and limited health care funding.

ASSISTIVE DEVICES

User-Friendly Communication Board

It is a frustrating experience for individuals with severe disabilities not to be able to write or talk. The simple and user-friendly communication board (Figure 1) can be used by patients with brain stem infarct or trauma, or by patients in intensive care units with multiple intravenous lines in the arms and with endotracheal intubation.[18] Intact auditory attention, memory skill, adequate spelling, and message production capability using eye blink, eye gaze, head nod, or other motoric movements are necessary.

This communication board works by an indirect selection method. The patient is presented with letter choices so that he/she can signal either positive or negative responses. The directions for using this type of communication board are as follows:

1. The assistant begins by slowly naming the vowels.
2. The patient indicates with eye blink or head nod when the row that contains the letter wanted is named.
3. The assistant repeats the vowel again and slowly names each letter in the row selected by the patient.

Figure 1. User-friendly communication board for nonverbal, severely physically disabled individual. The alphabet is arranged in normal sequence with vowels at the beginning of each row. Ten blank spaces are for ten numbers or other personal choices, i.e., words or brief functional messages.

Ⓐ	B	C	D	1	2
Ⓔ	F	G	H	3	4
Ⓘ	J	K	L	M	N
Ⓞ	P	Q	R	S	T
Ⓤ	V	W	X	Y	Z
5	6	7	8	9	0

Reproduced from Wu, Y., and J.A. Voda, "User-friendly communication board for nonverbal, severely physically disabled individuals," *Arch Phys Med Rehabil* 66:827–828, 1985, with the permission of the Archives of Physical Medicine and Rehabilitation.

4. The patient indicates again when the letter wanted has been named.
5. This process is continued in the same manner until the message has been spelled out or the words can be guessed.

Elastic Stockinette for Controlling Distal Edema

Edema in the legs is one of the common problems of disabled individuals. Custom-made Jobst stockings provide proper gradient pressure and can achieve good results. Another simple procedure using elastic stockinettes to control leg edema has been tried at this Center (the Rehabilitation Institute of Chicago—RIC) with success (data to be published). Various lengths of elastic stockinettes with a cut at the heel for pressure relief are applied according to the pressure needed (Figure 2). One can begin with a layer of calf-high stockinette and two or three layers of ankle-high stockinettes. The distal circulation should be observed carefully before more layers of elastic

Figure 2. Application of layers of elastic stockinettes for controlling limb edema.

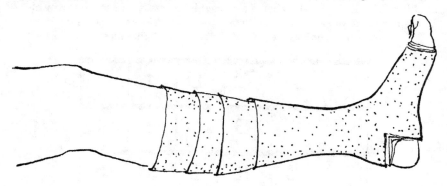

stockinettes are added. The elastic stockinettes are not too tight to apply and the desired pressure can be obtained by adding more layers of elastic stockinettes to the affected area. The sizes and layers of elastic stockinettes are determined by the degree of edema and the circumference of the limb to be treated.

RIC-Wu (Touchless) Catheter and Wu Reusable Catheter

With a regular rubber catheter kept in a sterile plastic tube, it is possible to perform urinary catheterization without directly touching the catheter with ungloved hands. This is the principal feature of both the RIC-Wu (Touchless) Disposable Catheter[16] (internationally patented, distributed by C.R. Bard Co., U.S.A.*) and the Wu Reusable Catheter[14] (patented but open to manufacture with permission). The RIC-Wu Catheter has been used widely for sterile intermittent catheterization in spinal cord-injured patients[12] (Figure 3). Being disposable, the RIC-Wu Catheter is not economical for long-term, frequent use. The Wu Reusable Catheter (Figures 4 and 5) was tested clinically but has not been manufactured. Since this catheter can be resterilized with a simple and effective procedure using povidone iodine or hydrogen peroxide solution, it may be advantageous in developing countries where disposable devices are not affordable. Clinical evaluation of long-term use of the Wu Reusable Catheter in a larger population remains to be done.

Wheelchair for Use in Developing Countries

David Constantine, a C4–5 quadriplegic, and Simon Gue jointly designed a wheelchair for use in developing countries (personal communication). The

---

*Address of this and other manufacturers mentioned in this chapter may be found in the Appendix, p. 333.

Figure 3. Design and use of RIC-Wu Catheter. To use the catheter kit, the top chamber is first opened (a), lubricant is deposited on the catheter guide (b), and then the top chamber is applied over glans penis after cleansing preparation of the urethral meatus and glans (c). The inner catheter tube is then grasped from outside the bag and pushed into the bladder.

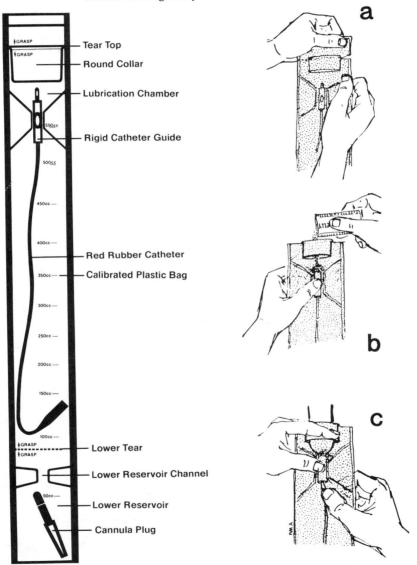

Tear Top
Round Collar
Lubrication Chamber
Rigid Catheter Guide
Red Rubber Catheter
Calibrated Plastic Bag
Lower Tear
Lower Reservoir Channel
Lower Reservoir
Cannula Plug

a
b
c

Reprinted from Wu, Y., "Total bladder care for the spinal cord injured patient," *Ann Acad Med, Singapore* 12:387–399, 1983, with the kind permission of the Annals of the Academy of Medicine, Singapore.

Figure 4. Design of Wu Reusable Catheter: To assemble the catheter, the first straight rubber catheter is cut at its tapering section next to the wide end to form the connector (A); the long end is discarded. The cut opening of the connector must be slightly larger than the shaft of the second catheter (B) so that the tip of the second catheter can pass through. Two holes in the tapered section of the second catheter (B) aid in rinsing and sterilization, and permit exit of air trapped in the Penrose latex tube (one inch in flat diameter). Contact rubber cement is used to fasten the connector (A) and the second catheter (B) to each end of the Penrose latex tube, as shown by the stippled areas (D). End-to-end assembly (E) permits retention of the catheter in sterile condition after resterilization with hydrogen peroxide or povidone iodine solution.

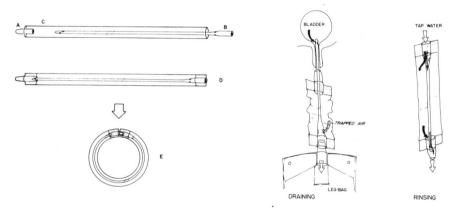

Reproduced from Wu, Y., B.B. Hamilton, M.A. Boying, and J.B. Nanninga, "Reusable catheter for long-term sterile intermittent catheterization," *Arch Phys Med Rehabil* 62:39–42, 1981, with the permission of the Archives of Physical Medicine and Rehabilitation.

Figure 5. Position of hands for catheterization with Wu Reusable Catheter.

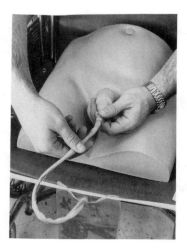

design won first prize in the 1989 design competition at the Royal College of Art, London. The project team, following a six-week feasibility tour of India and Bangladesh in December 1989, is preparing production plans in India and other developing countries. The design is not patented. Potential manufacturers are welcome to contact the developers* for design details. Versatility was an important consideration in their design. The chair can be converted from a regular chair to a chair for shower or toilet use (Figure 6). Its simple design lends itself to easy construction. More importantly, the creation of this stylish, "good-looking" chair improves the user's life rather than catering to his or her disability.

Low-Cost Beds for Prevention of Pressure Sores

James Reswick, of the National Institute on Disability and Rehabilitation Research, Washington, D.C., developed an unusual bed to prevent pressure sores (personal communication). A prototype device was made for clinical trial in India in 1988 using multiple layers of equal-arm levers to support 3/16-inch-thick wooden disks, cut from dowels 1-1/4 inches in diameter. The wooden disks were held by diagonal nylon cords to form a net-like bed surface (Figure 7A). This is a labor-intensive product that uses local materials and may be suitable for a region where labor cost is low. Detailed information is available from the developer.†

Another interesting low-cost bed is made of wooden rods covered by a canvas and is being used in some areas in India (Figure 7B). Detailed information on this design is not available to the author. It appears that pressure relief is achieved either by having the canvas over the rods pulled slightly by the staff or having the rods rotated intermittently by the patient. The author does not currently have information on the effectiveness during actual application of either of these two beds.

ORTHOTICS

Many advances in orthotics are reflections of new materials (i.e., graphite composite) and modular components. Besides common applications to assist movement, resist or restrict joint motion, realign damaged joints, or simulate the results of proposed reconstructive surgery, orthoses are being used to reduce hypertonicity in spastic limbs in patients with cerebral palsy or head trauma. Functional electrical stimulation of gait muscles combined with an orthosis for standing or ambulation is being studied in spinal cord-injured patients.

---

*Information is available from David Constantine, 62 Saltram Crescent Maida Vale, London W9, England; telephone 01 960 1754; fax 01 225 1487.

†Contact J.B. Reswick, National Institute on Disability and Rehabilitation Research, U.S. Department of Education, 400 Maryland Ave., S.W., Washington, D.C. 20202-2572.

Figure 6. Low-cost, stylish, and award-winning wheelchair designed by David Constantine of London for developing countries.

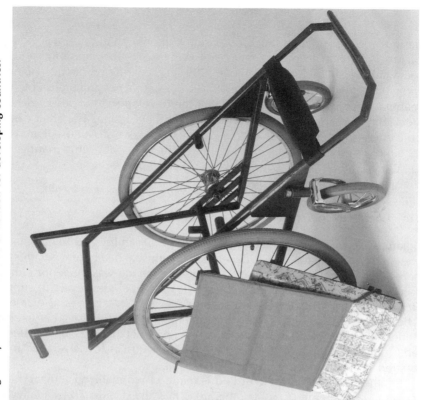

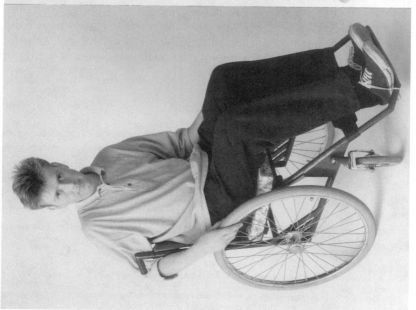

Photographs courtesy of D. Constantine and S. Gue.

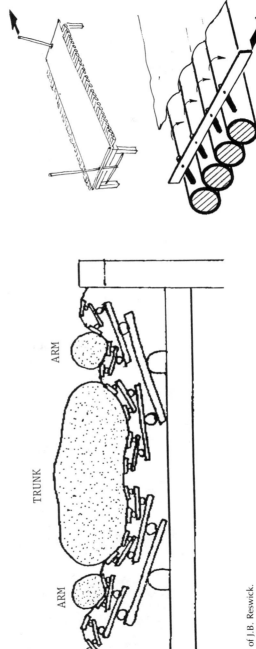

Figure 7. A. Low-cost lever bed, designed by James B. Reswick, Sc.D., for prevention of pressure sores. The disks are connected by nylon ropes to form the bed surface, which is easily contoured to the body shape. The wooden disks are supported from below by three layers of equal-arm lever assemblies. B. Low-cost bed made of round wooden rods covered by a canvas or heavy sheath. The bed surface is not contoured to the body shape. Pressure relief is easily achieved by pulling the canvas slightly with the handle or rotating the rods.

ARM

TRUNK

ARM

A

Courtesy of J.B. Reswick.

313

Plastic Ankle-Foot Orthosis with Flexible Joint

One design often used at the Rehabilitation Institute of Chicago is the plastic articulated ankle-foot orthosis (AFO) with the Gillette flexible ankle joint (Figure 8). This type of orthosis can be fabricated initially with a rigid ankle joint for control of both dorsiflexion and plantar flexion as well as knee stabilization. Once converted to an articulated ankle-foot orthosis, a wedge over the heel cord is used to control the genu recurvatum. The posterior wedge can also be replaced with a strap for control of excessive dorsiflexion.

Boston Orthoses for Scoliosis and Back Pain

A well-structured exercise program in combination with the use of the Milwaukee brace has successfully treated many patients with mild scoliosis since pioneering work by W. Blount and A. Schmidt. In the early 1970s the Boston brace was designed, using prefabricated plastic (polypropylene) pelvic girdles in 16 different sizes that fit 95% of the patients with nonoperative scoliosis. Static correction of the curve is achieved by direct stress via the orthosis, and dynamic correction is accomplished by exercise while in the orthosis.[4] This system can be fit more rapidly because of prefabrication and

Figure 8. Plastic ankle-foot orthosis can be converted from rigid to articulated ankle.

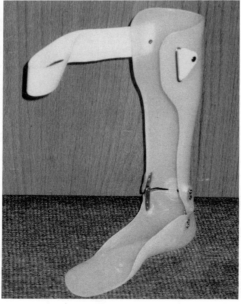

causes fewer skin problems due to total contact construction. Necessary local pressure is achieved by padding added inside the Boston brace. If needed, a cervical extension can be attached for chin support. A similar concept was later used for treating patients with back disorders. The low-profile Boston Overlap Brace (BOB) is a prefabricated low-profile orthosis made of flexible low-density polyethylene thermoplastic with an optional foam liner (Figure 9). Combining an exercise program with the application of this orthosis is essential for good outcome.[8]

LSU Reciprocating Gait Orthosis

The concept and design of the reciprocating orthosis was developed by Wally Motloch in 1967 at the Ontario Crippled Children's Center in Toronto. The idea was brought to the United States of America when Roy Douglas moved to Louisiana State University (LSU) in 1977. Since then, the LSU Reciprocating Gait Orthosis (Figure 10) has been used by patients with spina bifida, cerebral palsy, and paraplegia. It is designed to combine the left and right orthoses with Bowden cables so that the force from one orthosis is transmitted to the other. Flexion of one hip joint tends to force the other hip joint into extension, thus providing coordinated motion between the legs and making possible a "reciprocating" gait. Detailed information on construction and components is available from Durr-Fillauer Medical, Inc.

Figure 9. Prefabricated Boston Overlap Brace for back disorders.

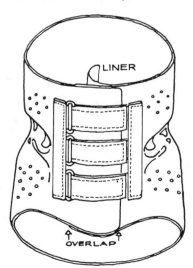

Reproduced from "B.O.B.—The Boston Overlap Brace Manual,"
with the permission of O & P Systems, Inc., Avon, MA.

Figure 10. LSU Reciprocating Orthosis. Cables cross from anterior or posterior lever on one hip to the same lever on opposite hip to promote compensatory motion.

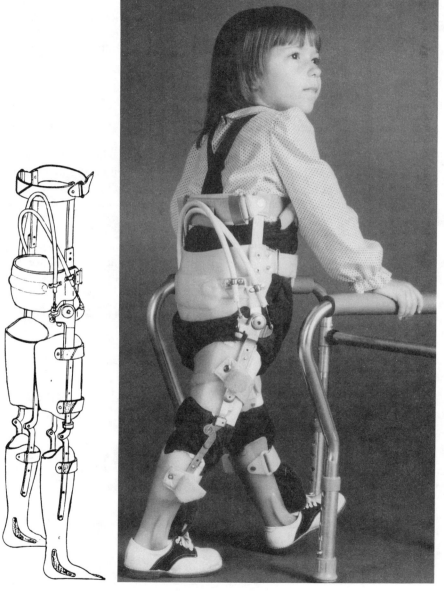

Reproduced from ''The LSU Reciprocating Gait Orthosis—A Pictorial Description and Application Manual,'' with the permission of Durr-Fillauer Medical, Inc., Chattanooga, TN.

PROSTHETICS

In the past decade many advances have been introduced in the field of prosthetics. The most significant impacts derive from the evolution of new above-knee socket designs and the development of energy-storing feet. New materials and procedures also have been adapted for patient care to improve functional outcome, reduce complications, or facilitate prosthetic service.

Removable Rigid Dressing

Immediate postsurgical fitting (IPSF), as first reported by Berlemont in France (1961) and pioneered by E. Burgess in this country in the late 1960s,[2] established the concept of preprosthetic stump management with a rigid dressing. This approach was simplified in the Removable Rigid Dressing, which consists of a below-the-knee plaster cast suspended in place by stockinette attached to a supracondylar plastic cuff (Figure 11).[15] The cast is made with graded pressure relievers over bony prominences, using cotton spacers which are discarded after the cast is set (Figures 12 and 13).[17] Since the cast is removable, the staff can observe wound healing, check skin response to weight-bearing exercise, and add stump socks to facilitate stump shrinkage. The amount and duration of weight-bearing exercise, in the wheelchair (Figure 14) or on an automobile jack used as a temporary weight-bearing pylon, can be adjusted according to the condition of wound healing. If a pressure sore is observed, the pressure area of the cast can be softened from the outside with a hammer and then pushed out from the inside for localized pressure relief.

Energy-Storing Prosthetic Foot

An energy-storing foot is a new concept in the prosthetic field. These new prosthetic feet are able to store energy during mid-stance to heel-off and to release the stored energy at push-off. To some extent, the energy-storing foot functions like a rubber ball, while the traditional SACH foot works like a clay ball. When both balls are dropped to the ground, the rubber ball bounces back with its absorbed impact energy, but the clay ball simply deforms and stays on the ground. The energy-storing foot allows young traumatic amputees to participate in sports. Four types of energy-storing feet are available in the United States: Seattle Foot, Flex-Foot, Carbon Copy II, and Quantum Foot.[7]

With support from the Veterans Administration and in collaboration with engineers from Boeing Company, the Prosthetic Research Study in Seattle, Washington, developed the Seattle Foot, which became commercially available in 1985 (Figure 15). The recent addition of the Seattle Ankle/Shank unit to the Seattle Foot has produced a significant increase in the range of energy storing and release during the gait cycle. For geriatric patients, Seattle Light Foot is frequently used.

Figure 11. Components of the Removable Rigid Dressing and application on the below-knee residual limb.

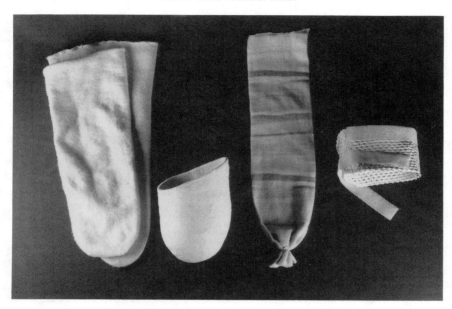

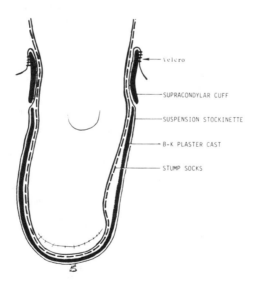

13. Making and application of the Removable Rigid Dressing.

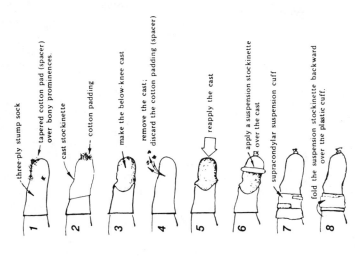

1. three-ply stump sock

tapered cotton pad (spacer) over bony prominences.

2. cast stockinette

cotton padding

3. make the below-knee cast

4. remove the cast; discard the cotton padding (spacer)

5. reapply the cast

6. apply a suspension stockinette over the cast

7. supracondylar suspension cuff

8. fold the suspension stockinette backward over the plastic cuff.

Reproduced from Wu, Y., H.J. Krick, and J.A. Sankey, *Proceedings, Rehabilitation Engineering Society of North America, 8th Annual Conference*, Memphis, TN, 1985. Used with permission.

Figure 12. Cotton pads are used as spacers for pressure relief and are discarded after the cast is set.

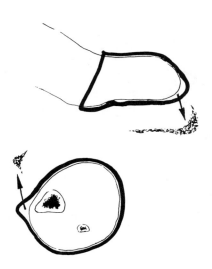

First published in Wu, Y., and H.J. Krick, "Removable rigid dressing for below-knee amputees," *Clin Prosthet Orthot* 11:33–44, 1987.

Figure 14. Progressive weight-bearing in the wheelchair.

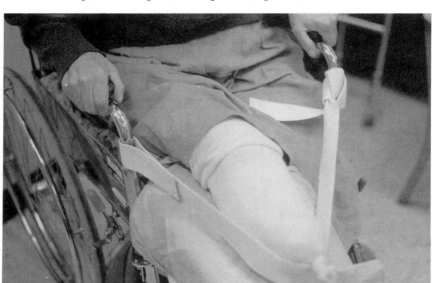

First published in Wu, Y., and H.J. Krick, "Removable rigid dressing for below-knee amputees," *Clin Prosthet Orthot* 11:33–44, 1987.

Figure 15. Seattle Foot.

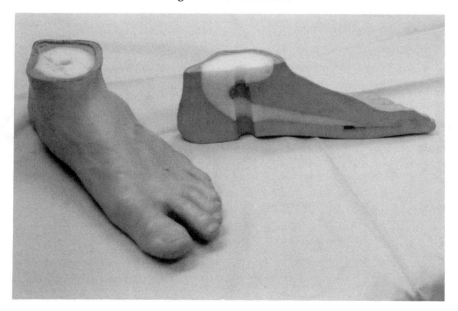

At the same time the Seattle Foot was being developed, Van Phillips, an amputee prosthetist, created a graphite composite energy-storing foot, Flex-Foot, that combines the foot and shank into a springing unit (Figure 16). Being light in weight and stronger in a relatively long segment of a prosthesis, it provides excellent resiliency and reduces distal weight distribution. It is custom made for individual body weight and activity level. High cost limits its wide use. The present world record in the 100-meter dash for below-knee amputees (11.7 seconds) is held by Dennis Oehler using a below-the-knee Flex-Foot prosthesis.

In 1986, Carbon Copy II was introduced. It has a reinforced Kevlar/nylon design for a rigid ankle block and dual flexible deflection plates to provide two-stage resistance at heel-off and toe-off. The newest energy foot to come onto the market is the Quantum Foot distributed in the United States by Hosmer Dorrance Co. of California (Figure 17). Its structural components comprise a sole spring, a secondary spring, and an ankle base. The sole spring is designed to simulate the normal heel-to-toe walking action, while the secondary spring gives extra stored energy for more active pursuits. Since the springs are not as wide as in the Flex-Foot it offers a greater range of rotation, inversion, and eversion. It is covered with ready-made cosmetic finishing.

Sauerbruck Trimodular Physiological Prosthesis

This prosthesis was designed and manufactured in Argentina.[1] During the past 10 years, a total of 2,610 above-knee prostheses, 2,090 below-knee prostheses, and 192 hip-disarticulation prostheses have been manufactured in that country. The friction control mechanism for the above-knee prosthesis consists of two metal bands in the back of the knee bolt. The friction control assembly grasps the knee bolt during extension to limit terminal swing impact and, owing to decompression of the rubber washer, loosens during flexion. The shin is trimodular in construction and made of seamless steel tubes. The telescoping tubes allow adjustment of prosthetic length. The ankle has an alignment device made of two spheroidal disks, a concave one and a convex one. A slot allows the disks to slide relative to each other for the correction of dorsiflexion and plantar flexion as needed.

Jaipur Foot

This prosthetic foot was developed in Jaipur, India, for amputees who customarily do not wear shoes and who walk on rugged terrain and through the mud.[10] It also allows squatting and sitting cross-legged on the floor. It has an acceptable cosmetic appearance and is made of waterproof latex rubber material (Figure 18). Its biomechanical features are somewhat different from those of the traditional SACH foot. Unlike the SACH foot, which

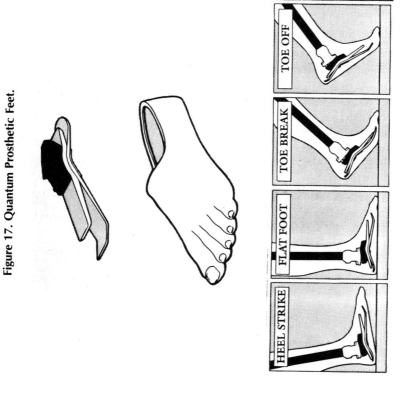

Figure 17. Quantum Prosthetic Feet.

HEEL STRIKE   FLAT FOOT   TOE BREAK   TOE OFF

Used with the permission of Hosmer Dorrance Corporation, Campbell, CA.

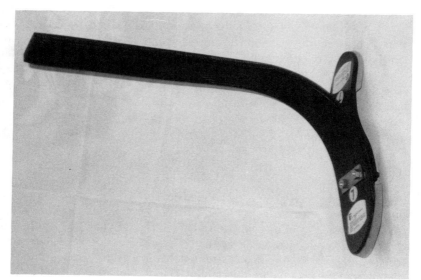

Figure 16. Flex-Foot prosthesis.

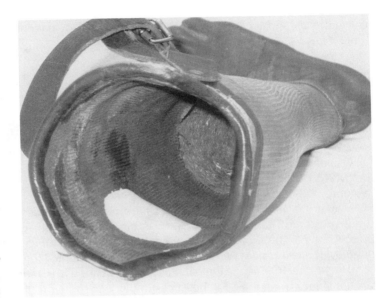

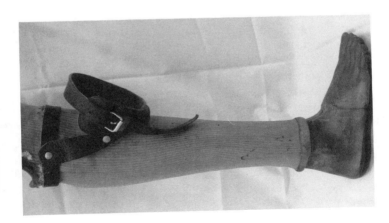

18. Jaipur foot and leg with open-ended aluminum socket. The ankle-foot is flexible to permit squatting. Its dorsal surface of soft, resilient, lightweight cushion compound is of lighter color for cosmesis. The dark sole is made of tread compound to provide toughness and durability.

has a solid keel, the Jaipur foot does not have a keel in the center. Therefore, it works more or less like a pylon with a soft cushion heel and flexible forefoot. It has a greater range of dorsiflexion, thus allowing the wearer to squat and to walk on uneven surfaces. The latex rubber foot and aluminum shank also permit patients to work in rice fields barefoot. The set-up for mass production is not expensive. With minimal modifications, and using local materials and technologies, it can be suitable for patients in remote country sites.

Scotchcast-PVC Below-Knee Prosthesis

In an ideal prosthetic management program for below-knee amputees, maximal stump shrinkage is achieved in the Removable Rigid Dressing before a preparatory or definitive prosthesis is made. The Scotchcast below-knee preparatory prosthesis can be useful in a busy rehabilitation center. This system uses a water-activated fiberglass casting tape (Scotchcast casting tape by 3M Co. for fracture immobilization) for direct socket fabrication on the stump, which then follows unique alignment steps to join the socket to a polyvinyl chloride (PVC) pylon-foot-shoe unit.[13] Using this approach, a skillful prosthetist can fabricate a preparatory prosthesis in less than two hours. Although these materials may not be readily available in developing countries, the technique used in this system may be adapted for local needs.

The technique for making the patellar tendon-bearing (PTB) socket directly over the stump using the Scotchcast casting tape is similar to that using the Removable Rigid Dressing, except that more pressure relief is provided over the distal tibial end and the trim line of the socket. Patches of cotton padding over the bony prominences, especially the distal end of the tibia, are used as a "spacer" to provide graded pressure relief (Figure 19). During the casting, the five-ply wool stump sock will adhere to the casting tape and is used as a soft interface between the skin and the socket.

Once the socket is made, the patient is asked to wear two or three tube socks and try out the socket on a padded automobile jack. This is to determine the height, preflexion, and medial-lateral tilting of the socket, as well as the comfort of socket fitting (Figure 20).

Alignment of the socket and the pylon-foot unit is somewhat different from the standard approach, yet follows the same biomechanical principles (Figure 21). A supracondylar strap and sometimes a waist belt (Figure 22) are used for suspension. Realignment of the prosthesis can be done by adding a wedge in the shoe. This system has served below-knee amputees well as a preparatory prosthesis.

New Above-the-Knee Socket Design: Ischium Containment

One of the major advances in prosthetic technology is the reevaluation of above-the-knee socket designs. For about four decades, the traditional

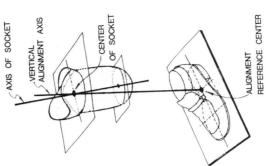

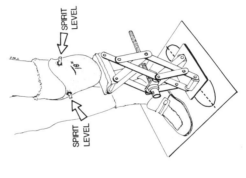

20. **Left: The position (axis and height) of PTB socket in space during full weight-bearing by the patient must be determined. The anterior and lateral spirit levels are used to maintain the mediolateral tilt and flexion of the socket. The height of the socket is monitored by a mark (18 inches) from the ground. Right: Relationship between the socket and pylon-foot-shoe unit to be used in the alignment.**

Figures 19 and 20 reproduced from Wu, Y., M.D. Brncick, H.J. Krick, T.D. Putnam, and J.S. Stratigos, "Scotchcast PVC interim prosthesis for below-knee amputee" (technical note), *Bull Prosthet Res*, BPR 10–36:40–45, 1981; used with permission.

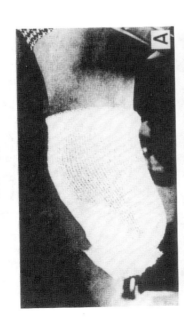

Figure 19. Application of cotton padding (A) for pressure relief during casting of the Scotchcast PTB socket (B).

Figure 21. Steps of alignment: A. Place the "Alignment Reference Center" of shoe print into the vertical alignment axis (plumb line).
B. Adjust the axis of the socket according to the levels, and the height according to the mark 18 inches from work table top.
C. Bring the "center" of PTB socket into alignment axis (pointed by the plumb line) and adjust rotation of prosthetic foot.
D. Match plyon-foot-shoe unit to the shoe print on the cardboard.
E. Soften and mold the four bars, held by double side mounting tapes, onto the socket.

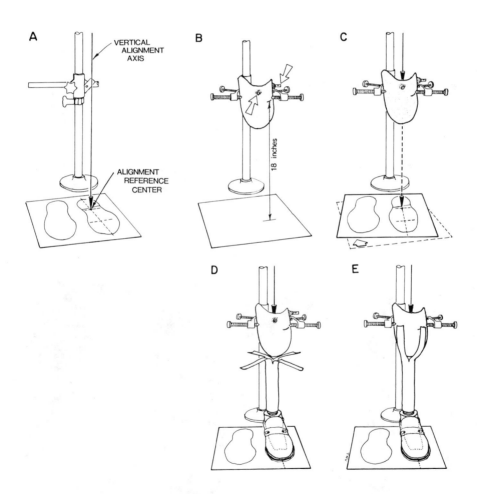

Reproduced from Wu, Y., M.D. Brncick, H.J. Krick, T.D. Putnam, and J.S. Stratigos, "Scotchcast PVC interim prosthesis for below-knee amputee" (technical note), *Bull Prosthet Res*, BPR 10–36:40–45, 1981; used with permission.

Figure 22. Gait training using Scotchcast-PVC prosthesis.

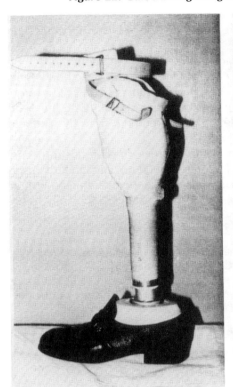
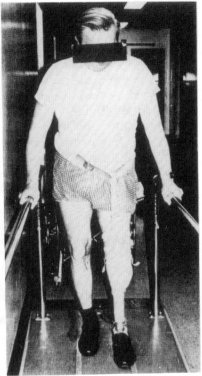

Reproduced from Wu, Y., M.D. Brncick, H.J. Krick, T.D. Putnam, and J.S. Stratigos, "Scotchcast PVC interim prosthesis for below-knee amputee" (technical note), *Bull Prosthet Res*, BPR 10–36:40–45, 1981; used with permission.

quadrilateral socket was considered the standard. Then, in the mid-1970s, Ivan Long noticed frequent abduction of the femur in the above-the-knee socket in x-ray studies. He attempted to reduce the diameter between the medial and lateral walls and placed the socket in an adducted position during prosthetic alignment.[5] By doing so, the ischium was incidentally contained in the medial wall of the socket. The idea was further expanded by John Sabolich[9] and others and led to significant improvement in the overall functional outcome of above-knee amputees. The ischium containment socket had several advantages over previous quadrilateral socket design:

1. The primary weight-bearing area during the stance phase is increased from only the tip of the ischial tuberosity in the quadrilateral socket to include

the medial surface of the ischial tuberosity as well. The change from a flat surface to a wider, contoured surface increases the weight-bearing area and reduces unit weight-bearing pressure; thus, the stance phase becomes more comfortable.

2. Since the weight-bearing surface is extended medially in the ischium containment socket, the fulcrum is closer to the midline of the body. Since the lever arm from the center of gravity to the fulcrum is smaller, less torque is generated by body weight during the stance phase than with the quadrilateral socket (Figure 23). Thus, less effort is required from the abductor muscles to counterbalance the torque.

3. As the hip abductor muscles act to balance the torque from body weight during the stance phase, the femur is abducted, which in turn pushes the socket laterally (Figure 24). This is why lateral gapping frequently occurs in the traditional quadrilateral socket during mid-stance, especially in ger-

Figure 23. Shifting of the fulcrum medially reduces the torque generated by body weight during the stance phase. Change from a flat surface in quadrilateral socket (left) to a wider and contoured surface in the ischium containment socket (right) increases the weight-bearing area and reduces unit pressure during the stance phase.

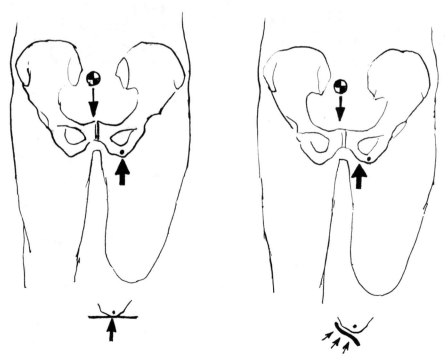

Figure 24. In the quadrilateral socket, contraction of the abductor muscles (b) to counteract the torque from body weight (a) leads to abduction of the femur (c), which in turn pushes the prosthetic socket laterally, as evidenced by lateral gapping (d) during the stance phase. Lateral gapping is prevented by either a strong medial musculature (e) or a high medial wall in the ischium containment socket, the so-called "bony lock" (f).

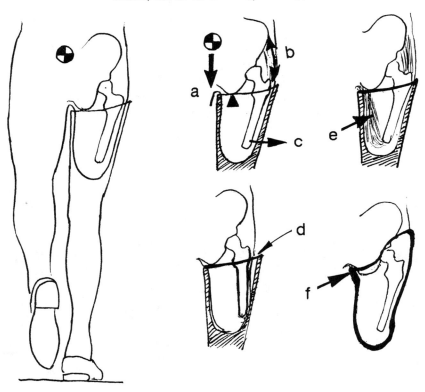

iatric patients with weak medial musculature, and also why a pelvic band is often needed. On the other hand, in the ischium containment socket, lateral movement of the prosthetic socket is limited by a high medial wall, the so-called "bony lock" (Figure 24). This works on a principle similar to our previous practice of adding a soft wedge on the posterior-medial corner of the quadrilateral socket, both to improve fitting comfort by providing a wider contoured weight-bearing surface and to reduce lateral gapping by containment of the ischial tuberosity.

4. Placing the femur in an adducted position in the socket allows the hip abductors to be kept in the advantageous stretched position for more effective contraction.[6]

Many terminologies have been used in the past five years to describe new socket designs, including the narrow M-L (medial-lateral diameter) socket, normal shape–normal alignment (NSNA), controlled adducted trochanter/controlled alignment method (CAT/CAM), naturally shaped sockets, and so on. The Workshop on Above-Knee Socket Design, sponsored by the International Society for Prosthetics and Orthotics and held in 1987 in Miami, and the follow-up meeting among U.S. Prosthetic Educators, recommended use of the terminology ischial-ramal containment (IRC) or ischium containment (IC) socket in order to differentiate the distinctive features of the new socket designs from earlier quadrilateral designs[11] (Figure 25).

Besides the change in socket shape—from the quadrilateral contour with a shorter anterior-posterior diameter to the ischium containment socket with narrower medial-lateral diameter and a higher medial trim line—there has also been a change from a solid socket to a partial flexible socket or an

Figure 25. New ischium containment socket (left, posterior view). The socket has an inner flexible socket (shown held by hand) and an outer rigid frame (right, lateral view).

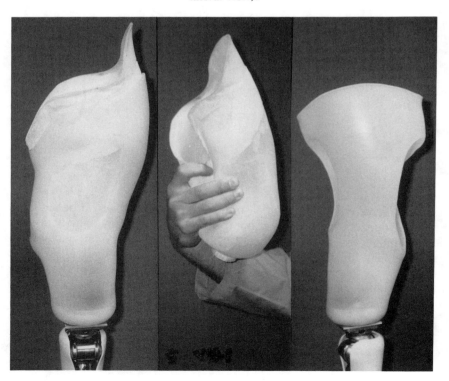

inner flexible socket within an outer rigid frame. Flexibility and lightness of weight have greatly improved comfort and wearing tolerance. The inner socket is removable from the outer rigid frame and can be easily replaced with a new one to accommodate stump shrinkage.

Other Advances in Prosthetics

Many more new technical improvements are being worked out or developed. The Utah Elbow (by Motion Control Co.) is one of the high-tech products that allow proportional myoelectric control of the elbow and terminal device (often an Otto Bock hand) alternatively. The Utah Arm, a high-cost modular system, is used for patients with amputation above the elbow or higher. The Boston Elbow (by Liberty Mutual Insurance Co.) is significantly less costly than the Utah Elbow; it has similar function but weighs more. Hush Elbow (by Hosmer Corp.) costs less, but is used mostly for switch control at this time. Further advancement, in a physiological sense, will be the application of extended physiological proprioceptive (EPP) control to an

Figure 26. Silicone suction suspension below-knee socket.

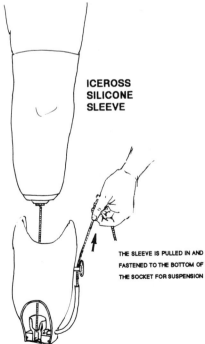

ICEROSS
SILICONE
SLEEVE

THE SLEEVE IS PULLED IN AND
FASTENED TO THE BOTTOM OF
THE SOCKET FOR SUSPENSION

externally powered upper limb prosthesis. This will eventually allow the patient not only to proportionally control movement but also to receive feedback through his/her body proprioception.

The computer-aided-design/computer-aided-manufacture system (CAD/CAM) for fabrication of a below-the-knee prosthesis, developed in England and Canada, is being tested at three centers in the United States. Full clinical application of the system may be possible in a few years.

A silicone suction suspension (3S system) socket for below-the-knee prostheses (Figure 26), initially introduced by Oessurr Kristinsson of Iceland, is now being used more widely.[3] The Icelandic Roll-On Suction Socket (ICEROSS, available from Cascade Orthopedic Supply, Inc.) provides an excellent interface between the skin and the rigid socket as well as an excellent suction suspension system for the below-knee prosthesis.

REFERENCES

1. Angarami GR, Samaria CE. An efficient low cost prosthetic structural system. *J Prosthet Orthot.* 1989;1:86–91. Information available from: Gerardo R. Angarami, C.P., Director, Orthopedia Alemana, Montevideo 865, Buenos Aires, Argentina.
2. Burgess EM, Romano RL. The management of lower extremity amputees using immediate postsurgical prostheses. *Clin Orthop.* 1968;57:137–146.
3. Fillauer CE, Pritham CH, Fillauer KD. Evolution and development of the silicone suction socket (3S) for below-knee prostheses. *J Prosthet Orthot.* 1989;1:92–104.
4. Hall J, Miller ME, Schumann W, Stanish W. A refined concept in the orthotic management of scoliosis. *Orthot Prosthet.* 1975;29:7–13.
5. Long IA. Normal shape–normal alignment (NSNA) above-knee prosthesis. *Clin Prosthet Orthot.* 1985;9:9–14.
6. Lehneis HR. Beyond the quadrilateral [editorial]. *Clin Prosthet Orthot.* 1985;9:6–8.
7. Michael J. Energy storing feet: a clinical comparison. *Clin Prosthet Orthot.* 1987;11:154–168.
8. Micaheli LJ. The use of the modified Boston brace system (BOB) for back pain: clinical indications. *Orthot Prosthet.* 1985;39:41–46.
9. Sabolich J. Contoured adducted trochanteric-controlled alignment method (CAT-CAM): introduction and basic principles. *Clin Prosthet Orthot.* 1985;9:15–26.
10. Sethi PK, Udawat MP, Kasliwal SC, Chandra R. Vulcanized rubber foot for lower limb amputees. *Prosthet Orthot Int.* 1978;2:125–136. Information available from: Dr. P.K. Sethi, Rehabilitation Research and Regional Limb Fitting Centre, S.M.D. Medical College and Hospital, Jaipur 302004, India.
11. Schuch CM. Report from the international workshop on above-knee fitting and alignment techniques. *Clin Prosthet Orthot.* 1988;12:81–98.
12. Wu Y. Total bladder care for the spinal cord injured patient. *Ann Acad Med Singapore.* 1983;12:387–399.
13. Wu Y, Brncick MD, Krick HJ, Putnam TD, Stratigos JS. Scotchcast PVC interim prosthesis for below-knee amputee [Technical note]. *Bull Prosthet Res.* 1981;BPR10–36(Fall):40–45.
14. Wu Y, Hamilton BB, Boyink MA, Nanninga JB. Reusable catheter for long-term sterile intermittent catheterization. *Arch Phys Med Rehabil.* 1981;62:39–42.
15. Wu Y, Keagy RD, Krick HJ, Stratigos JS, Betts HB. An innovative removable rigid dressing technique for below-the-knee amputation. *J Bone Joint Surg [Am].* 1979;61A:724–729.
16. Wu Y, King RB, Hamilton BB, Betts HB. RIC-Wu catheter kit: new device for an old problem. *Arch Phys Med Rehabil.* 1980;61:455–459.
17. Wu Y, Krick HJ. Removable rigid dressing for below-knee amputees. *Clin Prosthet Orthot.* 1987;11:33–44.
18. Wu Y, Voda JA. User-friendly communication board for non-verbal, severely physically disabled individuals. *Arch Phys Med Rehabil.* 1985;66:827–828.

APPENDIX: SUPPLIERS AND MANUFACTURERS

Bard Home Health Division, C.R. Bard Inc., 111 Spring Street, Murray Hill, NJ 07974. *(RIC-Wu (Touchless) Disposable Catheter)*

Cascade Orthopedic Supply, Inc., P.O. Box 649, Chester, CA 96020. Telephone: (800) 824-4175; in California, (800) 822-8190. *(Icelandic Roll-on Suction Socket)*

Durr-Fillauer Medical, Inc., 2710 Amnicola Highway, Chattanooga, TN 37406. Telephone: (615) 624-0946, (800) 251-6398. Telex: 558422. *(LSU Reciprocating Gait Orthosis)*

Flex-Foot Inc., 14 Hughes, B-201, Irvine, CA 92714. Telephone: (800) 233-6263. Fax: (714) 582-0821. *(Flex-Foot)*

Hosmer Dorrance Corporation, 561 Division Street, P.O. Box 37, Campbell, CA 95008. Telephone: (408) 379-5151. *(Quantum Foot)*

Ohio Willow Wood Company, 15441 Scioto Darby Road, P.O. Box 192, Mount Sterling, OH 43134. *(Carbon Copy II Foot)*

O&P Systems, Inc., 20 Ledin Drive, Avon, MA 02322. Telephone: (800) 262-2235. *(Boston Overlap Brace)*

Model and Instrument Development, 861 Poplar Place South, Seattle, WA 98144. Telephone: (206) 325-0715, (800) 248-MIND. Fax: (206) 322-6463. *(Seattle Foot)*

Chapter 17

ADVANCES IN BURN REHABILITATION

Elizabeth A. Rivers and Steven V. Fisher

In this chapter considerable space is devoted to describing advances in classification and the pathology and surgical treatment of burns. This background is needed to understand burn rehabilitation treatment. The overlapping stages of healing and varied treatment modalities create a unique opportunity for concurrent contributions of rehabilitation and surgical team members, with the goal being that the patient recover the best possible function and cosmesis. There have been major advances in surgical and medical burn treatment that have a direct impact on burn rehabilitation, having changed the scope, duration, modalities, and outcome of rehabilitation therapy.

CLASSIFICATION OF BURNS

Burn severity is classified according to the patient's age, the agent causing cell damage, the percentage of cutaneous surface injured, the depth of tissue destruction, the body areas injured, and types of associated injury or illness. The depth and percentage of tissue destruction from an injuring agent vary widely depending on duration and intensity of the agent. Therefore, the mechanism of burn should be immediately documented.

Body Surface Area

The procedure for estimating the body surface affected has not changed in the last 50 years. For small burns, a rough estimate of the injured area can be made using the patient's palm print (excluding the fingers), which is approximately 1% of the body surface area. For larger burns in the adult, the "rule of nines" can be used; that is, the head, each arm, front of chest, back of chest, abdomen, buttocks, front of leg, and back of leg are each 9% of the body. The Lund and Browder[12] chart provides a more accurate estimate. Adjustments must be made for the additional epithelial surface covering the child's relatively large head.

334

Depth

Most wounds are of mixed depth, and even experienced surgeons have difficulty accurately determining the depth by appearance at the time of injury.[2] The nomenclature of depth of burn has been changed to more clearly depict the injury. Superficial partial thickness burns are allowed to heal spontaneously. In the last 10 years, deep dermal burns, formerly called second-degree burns, have been tangentially excised by the third day and split-thickness grafted to decrease pain, speed healing, and improve the final epithelial quality. If they are allowed to regenerate from epithelial remnants at the base of sweat and oil glands and hair follicles, the wounds scar heavily. Full thickness burns, formerly called third-degree burns, are devoid of epithelial remnants and can only re-epithelialize from the periphery. Preferably, these areas are grafted or primarily closed if of a significant size.

ADVANCES IN NUTRITION AND ANTIBIOTIC THERAPY

Understanding of the nutritional requirements after a serious burn injury has changed drastically in recent years. With reduced catabolism, the patients have more muscle mass with which to exercise and participate in their rehabilitation. Physiological and biochemical alterations include increased energy expenditure, increased coenzyme needs, and enhanced total body nitrogen loss. Energy expenditure and protein requirements can be determined by using a variety of formulas.[11,16] These formulas may overestimate calorie needs by as much as 60%. However, when used in conjunction with indirect calorimetry a more exact measure of energy expenditure is achieved.[5] Precise macronutrient requirements are not clear. One common formula used to calculate adult energy needs is the following: calorie need = (25 kcal x kg actual weight) + (40 kcal x % total body surface area (TBSA) burned). The protein need = (1 gram x kg actual weight) + (3 grams x % TBSA burned). Although formulas vary considerably, current knowledge favors a high protein, high carbohydrate regimen with conservative amounts of fat, preferably less than 15%. Micronutrient requirements have also been increased, especially for vitamins A and C and for zinc, which have been found to be necessary cofactors in a variety of enzyme systems.[8] Micronutrient needs for the adult are minerals and vitamins in accordance with the recommended daily allowance, plus supplementation with 1 g of vitamin C, 10,000 IU of vitamin A, and 220 mg of zinc sulfate.

Nutritional therapy plays an important role in promoting optimal conditions for wound healing. Nutritional therapy can be achieved using an oral diet, tube feedings, or total parenteral nutrition. An oral diet alone is used for patients who have less severe burns and are able to eat a high-calorie, high-protein diet. When patients are unable to consume at least 75% of their caloric needs by an oral diet, nocturnal or continuous tube feedings are provided. Recently developed small, nonirritating nasogastric enteral tubes with thin guide wires to aid in proper placement improve patient tolerance of these feedings. If patients are unable to tolerate enteral nutrition for more than two to three days, total parenteral nutrition is given, tailored to macro- and micronutrient recommendations. Useful parameters to assess nutritional outcome include monitoring compliance with dietary goals, nitrogen balance, and weight change.[15]

Better understanding of antibiotic metabolism in burned individuals and proper dosing of antibiotics have minimized sepsis and decreased mortality. Consequently, as patients survive more severe burns, their potential to suffer greater disability increases if they do not receive rehabilitation.

ACUTE AND SUBACUTE REHABILITATION CARE

Techniques of Wound Care

In the last 10 years scores of topical antimicrobial agents and wound dressings have been developed. However, meticulous wound hygiene remains the primary defense against bacterial colonization, dermal destruction, and subsequent sepsis. In the meantime there has been no resolution to the controversy regarding the relative benefits of immersion compared to spray cleansing. It is important for each individual working with the patient to see the wounds unwrapped to understand better the extent and depth of injury, the involvement of joints, and the extent of contracture.

Numerous biological dressings have been developed in the past 10 years. Pigskin, or synthetic equivalents such as Duoderm, Opsite, Tegaderm, N-ter-face, Tegapore, Biobrane, or Second Skin, protect the wound from air, cover raw nerve endings, and make the wound nearly pain free. These dressings, if adherent, provide an ideal bacteria-free environment for wound healing. However, these dressings can only promote healing in a viable bed, i.e., one in which adequate uninfected dermal tissue is present. The wound must have dead epithelium (blisters) removed and must have a moist, pink, sensitive surface. Mottled red and white or nonpainful areas denote full thickness burns, which will not heal under biological dressings.

When the biological dressing does not adhere to the wound, an antibacterial ointment or creme such as Silvadine or Bacitracin is utilized. Silvadine is generally recommended for larger area burns. The therapist provides the local wound care after removal of the wound dressing. Cleansing and debridement are followed by exercise, both active and passive, with terminal stretch as prescribed, after which the wound is redressed. When gauze bandages are used and have become adherent to the wound bed, it is particularly advantageous to do the exercises with the dressings removed in order to reduce pain.

Surgical Management

With improved intraoperative monitoring capabilities, increased experience, and improved skill of surgeons in the last 15 years, tangential excision and grafting of the burn wound has become a standard of care. The resultant more rapid closure of wounds reduces hospital stays and morbidity, improves skin durability, and reduces the need for reconstructive surgery. This single development has radically changed the rehabilitation approach to burn injury. Those interested in greater detail regarding surgical management are referred to Heimbach and Engrav's text.[9]

REHABILITATION GOALS FOR THE BURNED PATIENT

Overall Rehabilitation Management

The basic goals of exercise, positioning, edema control, and orthotics—which are similar in all phases of burn healing—will be addressed before the specific techniques of burn rehabilitation at the acute, subacute, and maturation phases of wound healing are discussed. The goals of exercise are to stretch healing skin, improve circulation to the healing tissues, maintain full range of joint motion, promote motor skills and coordination, preserve functional independence, maintain strength and endurance, decrease pain, reduce depression, and return control to the patient. The goals of positioning are to prevent contractures, reduce edema, protect vulnerable or exposed tendons, and facilitate favorable wound care. The goals of edema control are to improve wound healing, decrease pain, decrease scar deposition, and improve range of motion. Orthotics share the same goals as therapeutic positioning in the acute and subacute stages. In addition, orthotics immobilize a body part after grafting, protect exposed tendons, support joints in peripheral neuropathies, and maintain the functional position in unresponsive patients. In the stage of maturation the goals are expanded to include reduction of contractures, restoration of lost function, and reduction and mobilization of hypertrophic scars.

For the sake of discussion, rehabilitation management is divided into three overlapping phases. The first phase of recovery begins with the burn incident. It continues through the epithelial healing in partial thickness injury or through debridement in full thickness tissue destruction. Superficial burns that heal in two weeks mature in this phase. The second phase of burn recovery is immobilization during the grafting period. This period begins with a skin graft and continues until that graft has vascularized. The third or final recovery phase begins when stable epithelium covers either the healed partial thickness injury or the grafted wound. This period of wound maturation continues for up to two years.

Rehabilitation Techniques during the Acute Phase of Burn Healing

Exercise

Ambulation and active range of motion exercises are the most important rehabilitation modalities immediately after the injury. During this early rehabilitation phase, supervised active range of motion orients the patient toward recovering mobility. Transferring to a chair and walking, as well as slow, fully active movement, will speed healing by reducing edema and will improve the patient's confidence. Use of the Invacare wheeled walker equipped with an overhead bar provides upper extremity elevation and hand grasp (see Figure 1). An ambulation program is instituted and progress recorded. Multiple repetitions are painful and unnecessary, as is heavy resistance at this stage of recovery. However, if the injured tissue is maintained in one position for a prolonged time, the collagen fibers will begin to contract, scar tissue will grow, and contractures will rapidly develop. For the uncooperative or comatose patient, the involved joints are moved passively through the maximum possible range for two or more repetitions twice daily.

Positioning

Positioning is defined as the proper arrangement of body parts. Burn patients have the potential to develop contractures; supervised positioning attempts to limit this complication. The patient often assumes a flexed, adducted position in an attempt to withdraw from pain. An extended position is no more painful, but moving to that position is uncomfortable. Exercise is possible only four hours per day, and extended positioning must be utilized for most of the remainder of the day. The most effective and least expensive positioning occurs when the patient voluntarily maintains antigravity positioning with pillows, foam wedges, or bedside tables. Commercially available arm troughs that mount to the bed or overhead suspension slings help to provide a more adjustable elevated position (Figure 2). Custom-fitted thermoplastic orthoses are more expensive and need to be checked frequently for pressure areas. Elevated positions aid in reduction of edema, which in turn reduces pain and decreases scar formation. Positioning never replaces active range of motion, and, therefore, the previously mentioned exercises must be performed twice daily for a minimum of two repetitions to avoid contractures. Figure 3 demonstrates the optimal positioning for the recumbent patient.[10]

Orthoses

It is beyond the scope of this chapter to discuss all orthotic devices used. For more information the reader is directed to several other excellent

Figure 1. Invacare wheeled walker, equipped with overhead bar.

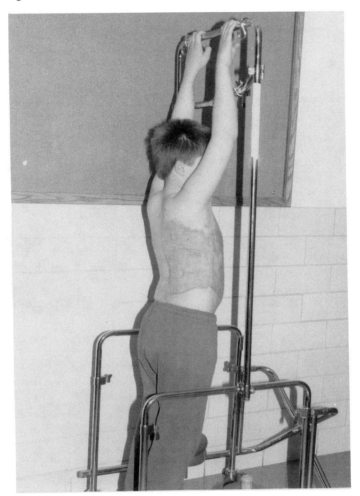

sources.[3,13,18,25] Orthotics is an extension of positioning. Orthoses also provide protection to the tissue and reduce edema. These devices should be removed several times a day for active exercise and assessment of the healing wounds. Night splinting is indicated when the patient requires assisted positioning during sleep. Temporary biological or other wound dressings do not contraindicate the use of a properly fitted orthosis. Low temperature thermoplastic materials are easily fabricated and refitted. In the burned hand, a resting wrist-finger-thumb orthosis is used for positioning when the patient is unconscious or uncooperative. Antigravity elevation is universally used for reduction of edema, and orthoses are designed as an adjunct. In addition,

Figure 2. Overhead suspension slings, using orthopedic bed frame and counter-balanced pulley system.

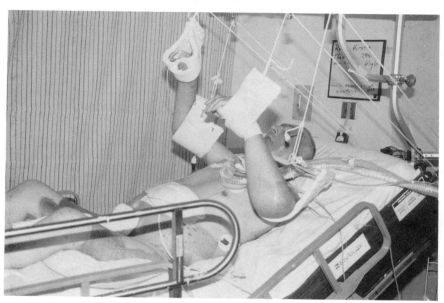

for the hand a continuous passive motion machine may be helpful to decrease swelling.[4] Protection is given by a finger extension trough, secured with a pressure distributing bandage, if the proximal interphalangeal joints or dorsal hoods are exposed. Other structures of the hand that may need protection during inactive periods are the tendons in the carpal tunnel, the oblique retinacular ligament, and the deep finger flexors. Similarly, in the lower extremities the anterior tibialis and Achilles tendons, if exposed, may need protection during rest and orthotic support during activity or exercise. Proper fitting of the ankle-foot orthosis is important to ensure relief from pressure for the peroneal nerve.

When the bottoms of feet are burned, double depth, adapted footwear protects the foot by reducing pressure, which decreases pain during walking. The foam ankle-foot orthosis overcomes the weight of bedding and supports the ankle in the neutral position.

In the case of a circumoral burn, the microstomia correction orthosis should be judiciously used for exercise and for positioning (see below).

Control of edema for a burn of the lower extremity is most effectively provided by figure of eight elastic bandages, wrapped with a gradient pressure from distal to proximal. Early, when activity is mild, these bandages stay in place adequately to support the lymphatics and improve venous return, without interfering with topical antimicrobials or bandages. Fingers,

Figure 3. Anti-contracture positioning. The patient is lying supine and is shown from a ventral view.

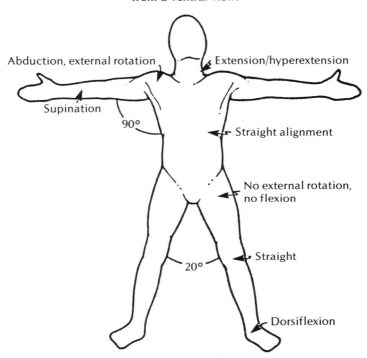

Abduction, external rotation

Extension/hyperextension

Supination

90°

Straight alignment

No external rotation, no flexion

Straight

20°

Dorsiflexion

Based on Figure 1 (p. 8) in Helm, P.A., C.G. Kevorkian, M. Lushbaugh, G. Pullium, M.D. Head, G.F. Cromes, "Burn injury: rehabilitation management in 1982," *Arch Phys Med Rehabil* 63:6–16, 1982. Reprinted with the permission of the Archives of Physical Medicine and Rehabilitation.

hands, arms, trunk, and buttocks may be bandaged using an elastic bandage of the appropriate width. These bandages have the advantage of preventing purple discoloration, tingling, burning, pain, blistering, and irritation from exposure to cold or trauma. However, when the patient is very active, slippage is a problem and these wraps become serial tourniquets. At this time, the use of cotton and rubber tubular bandages, such as Tubigrip, or custom fabricated or individually measured commercial garments has begun.

Rehabilitation Techniques during the Immobilization Phase of Burn Healing

During the phase of autografting, exercise is discontinued over the grafted area plus one joint distal and one joint proximal to the graft. Otherwise, the management discussed for the acute phase pertains. When the graft is on a lower extremity, ambulation is not resumed until the skin is stable. Earlier ambulation is possible when the leg is supported with an Unna dressing and elastic wrap. Orthotics or positioning or both are used to maintain the grafted area in optimal position. Tangential excision and early grafting have resulted in better and more rapid graft healing, which allows for earlier resumption of exercise and functional activity.

In the last decade plastic and reconstructive surgical techniques have advanced significantly. These advances include free-flap wound coverage, tissue expansion techniques, advances in pedicle grafts, graft placement in cosmetic units, and more frequent use of scalp as a donor site. With the rapid, satisfactory wound closure permitted by these techniques, outcome from rehabilitation is expedited and therefore is more cost effective, and disability is reduced. Some of these techniques require longer immobilization of the grafted area than the usual time needed for a split thickness skin graft. The rehabilitation staff must collaborate with the plastic surgeon to preserve functional ability while the wound is healing. The patient may require extra care in positioning and management of tissue pressure utilizing high technology "flotation" mattresses and beds, such as Clinitron, Kinaire, and Roho. Water beds also distribute pressure to reduce decubiti; however, the patient experiences increased perspiration, which heightens the risk of maceration.

Rehabilitation Techniques during the Maturation Phase of Burn Healing

The recovery process takes place during a continuum of several years. Throughout this period, the frequent changes in a patient's condition require a process of ongoing evaluation and appropriate adjustments in the therapy program.[7]

Exercise

Full active range of motion returns most quickly when minimal inflammatory processes occur, when grafts are on dermal remnants, and when the patient continues hourly elevated active motion during waking hours. *Daily half-hour periods of painful, aggressive stretching by a therapist to achieve elongated connective tissue by itself will be ineffective.* With reminders, the patient can move through the extremes of motion, which will prevent loss of joint function and will better nourish cartilage and surrounding soft tissue. The object of exercise is to speed healing by improving circulation, decreasing edema, and decreasing inflammatory response. Reciprocal pulleys, two-handed calisthenics, slow bicycling, and dowel exercises are the safest methods of providing self-directed, passive, assisted motion early after the injury. The therapist, as coach, provides many choices and written graded programs which break activity down into small component parts so that improvement can be documented. Active motion and gentle terminal stretch are continued despite open tendons, with the exception of open dorsal hood mechanisms over the proximal interphalangeal (PIP) joint. If the dorsal hood is destroyed, the PIP joint is rested in extension until skin coverage is complete. Otherwise, it is kept in extension until it heals or until a reconstructive surgeon recommends an alternate position.

The neck, axilla, elbow, wrist, thumb, ankle, and hip are particularly vulnerable to contracture from unsupervised assumption of a flexed posture. Cocontraction of muscles in anticipation of pain slowly exacerbates progressive joint contractures.

Gentle terminal stretch by the therapist helps the patient understand that the joint will slowly move further after his active motion (Figure 4A). Also, as the patient avoids taking the joint off stretch, discomfort decreases. Each patient can learn to do his own terminal stretch with his other hand or with environmental surfaces, such as stretching the heel cord by wall push-offs with the heels flat on the floor. Prolonged, gentle manual or mechanical stretching is needed to reduce severe contractures. The entire length of the scar band must be elongated by combined stretching of the joints involved. Microscopic tears in the connective tissue will increase the inflammatory process and will slow ultimate healing. Therefore, the force must be gentle, but progress daily as tolerance increases, and it frequently must be accompanied by an orthosis that preserves the increased range of motion (Figure 4B).

Patients with large body surface area burns (>50%) or who are immobile for prolonged periods are likely to develop heterotopic ossification.[23] When suspected, x-rays or bone scan should be performed and treatment changed accordingly.

Manual resistive, progressive, or progressive resistive exercises done daily help the patient regain strength and endurance. Automated machines such as the Baltimore Therapeutic Equipment Work Simulator (BTE), Cybex, Stair Master, rowing machines, or stationary bicycles provide graphic feedback regarding progress, thereby offering encouragement and motivation to the patient as well as objective performance measures to the physician and therapist. When automated equipment is not available, traditional weight lifting equipment, such as that found in any physical therapy gym, can provide feedback as the weights and repetitions are increased. Outpatient treatments have the additional benefit of establishing a pattern of leaving the protective home environment every day. Early return to part-time work increases social contacts and may improve self-esteem as strength and endurance increase.

Figure 4. Management of foot contractures.
A. Active range of motion with terminal stretch of toes. Therapist gently continues stretching toes into plantar flexion after patient achieves maximal active motion.

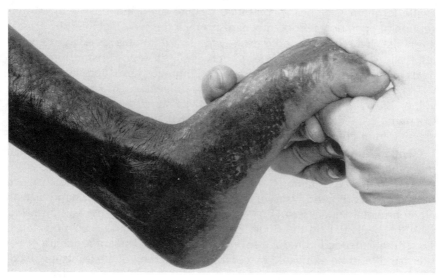

B. Serial cast of foot. Maximal benefits of prolonged stretch maintained with plaster cast worn overnight.

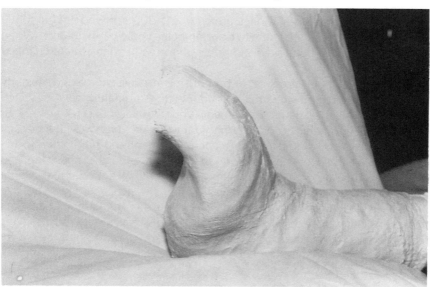

Figure 4 (continued).
C. Examples of inserts for added pressure. Hypertrophic scars in concave or irregular areas respond to silicone or felt inserts.

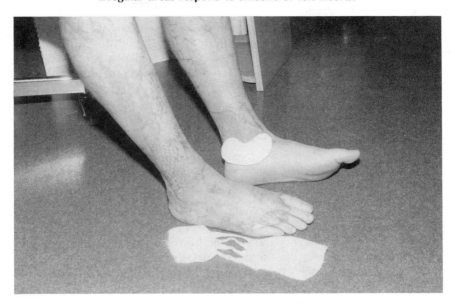

D. Elastic garment over inserts. Note metatarsal bar insole to flex toes and additional dorsal silicone conformer insert.

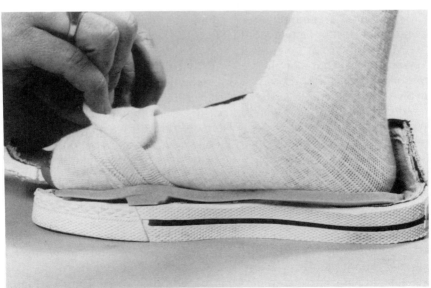

Positioning

Positioning is used as a method of prolonged stretching for contracted tissue. Patients are encouraged to independently assume positions that stretch contractures when resting between exercise sessions. For example, a patient who has an axillary contracture would sit with his arms forward flexed on an elevating table or abducted over the back of a couch. Elevated positioning assists venous return, which diminishes painful blisters. A wide variety of newer arm supports and foot braces that attach to or are incorporated into the hospital bed are commercially available. Especially in this phase of wound healing, positioning cannot replace but merely supplements active exercise or gentle prolonged stretching of contracted soft tissue and epithelium.

Orthoses

A wide variety of new orthotic materials and designs are available to assist patients in regaining functional mobility of contracted joints. The general principles of orthotic management of the burn patient are mentioned, and the more recent advances in orthotics will be discussed in some detail.

Orthoses allow painless maintenance of exercise gains and are greatly appreciated by the patient. The splint blocks undesirable motion and encourages active motion away from the restrictive orthosis. The patient controls the speed and number of repetitions of stretch. The tissue becomes warm and moist under the total contact orthosis. Skin softened in this way is more comfortable to stretch (Figure 5).

Microstomia, a commonly seen contracture following facial burns, responds to correction appliances that may be dynamic[2] or static[1] (Figure 6). The MPA, which has been available since 1975, was the first adjustable contracture-prevention appliance. It is difficult to fit this appliance with a transparent facial orthosis, which is commonly needed for facial burns that involve the oral area. Rivers et al.[19] suggest use of an acrylic splint formed in a dental laboratory to a dentist's positive cast of the patient's teeth. This splint preserves dental alignment when the patient is wearing a transparent orthosis or an elastic hood with a silicone insert for scar control. Commercially available cheek retractors used by dentists are a safe and inexpensive appliance for exercise and contracture stretching.

Rivers[21] described a transparent orthosis for the face and neck that has proven very successful for management of hypertrophic scarring (Figure 6C). The four-step fabrication process,[20] which includes taking a negative facial impression, forming a positive plaster cast, fabricating a transparent plastic total contact orthosis, and fitting the orthosis, is time consuming. In the properly fitting orthosis, the scar tissue is flattened against the underlying skeletal structure, thereby minimizing hypertrophic scars. The facial con-

Figure 5. Management of elbow contracture.

A. Elbow contracture with hypertrophic scar which developed despite use of elastic garments.

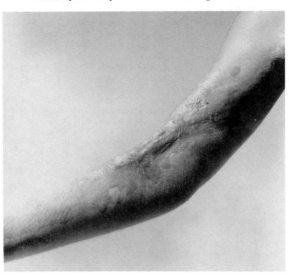

B. Drop-out total contact elbow orthosis, secured wrist to elbow, leaving arm free for extension.

C. Results after a few days of using the orthosis at night.

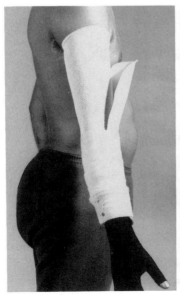
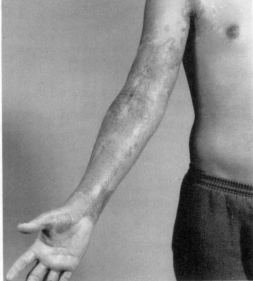

Figure 6. Management of facial burns with hypertrophic scars.

A.

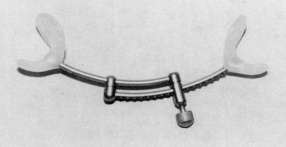

B.

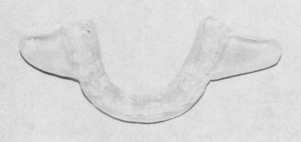

Figure 6 (continued).

C. Application of MacFarlane orthosis (see arrows). Clear facial orthosis and neck orthosis compress facial scars and elongate neck contractures. Brightly colored elastic head band used to secure facial orthosis appeals to children.

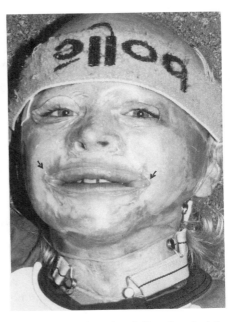

D. Syringe case or tube used for prolonged passive stretch, twice daily, when facial orthosis is removed. Note that neck orthosis is worn during stretch.

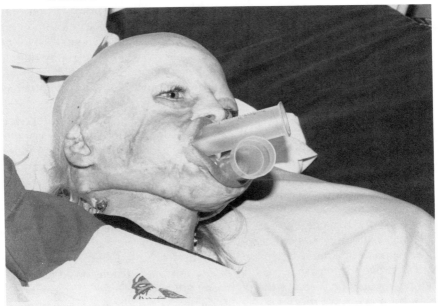

tours are well preserved. An elastic hood, worn with a silicone insert, will also control facial scars. The patient must be observed for complications of sleep apnea[22] or mandibular retraction.[21]

The patient will need nasal conformer inserts if scars develop inside the nostril. Corneal domes are temporarily needed for protection and humidity when the patient is unable to close the eyelid either because of coma or because the skin of the lid is contracted. A microstomia stretching orthosis is used to correct microstomia and to preserve dental alignment when the scar is over the upper teeth. When any of these are prescribed, the patient will need two sets of face orthoses to accommodate them. The patient benefits from written instructions, especially when many splint combinations are used. The face orthosis must also fit with the neck splint when both are needed at the same time.

In a 10-year study,[6] the need for reconstructive procedures declined with the increased use of transparent and molded polyvinyl chloride neck orthoses. Initially, a soft foam neck splint is an adequate reminder to extend the neck. When numerous bulky, unnecessarily strong scars appear, the foam will compress, allowing neck flexion, scar growth, and contraction during wound maturation. A vinyl tubing splint has slightly greater stability, allows exercise, and toughens skin. A hard plastic splint will be needed 23 hours a day to preserve body contours. The anterior border of the mandible should be free, allowing neck rotation and preventing mandibular retraction.

A commercially available figure-of-eight clavicle strap is an effective, simple method to support and compress the anterior and posterior axillary folds. When the tissue is durable enough not to blister from friction, the strap may be worn at all times. Children respond better to custom-fitted single-arm strapping, which does not rub over the back of the neck. Use of total contact axillary splints when the patient is inactive, preferably during sleep, decreases the pain of stretching severely contracted axillary tissue and speeds return of full active motion. Care must be exercised to avoid nerve compression when the axillary orthosis is worn for prolonged, uninterrupted periods of time. Soft inserts or overlays of silicone, Hollister odor absorbent dressings, felt, or similar materials improve total contact of the orthosis, thereby minimizing scarring. In the last decade numerous product improvements have assisted in orthotic fit. These include varying densities of foam, adhesive-backed materials, hypoallergenic solid silicone elastomers, and silicone expanding elastomers which mold in place to the involved areas.

Scars of the antecubital or olecranon areas are challenging owing to the difficulty of compressing the tissue adequately without causing blisters during motion or decubiti when the patient is at rest. A plaster drop-out orthosis will improve supination as well as elbow flexion or extension, depending on the application. Later, a thermoplastic orthosis, secured wrist to elbow, may be used as a "drop-out" splint (Figure 5). Splints must be removed daily for active exercise, especially when the inflammatory process is active. Newer "continuous passive motion machines" provide continuous movement through the pain-free range at night or for prescribed periods during the day (Figure 7). They also provide supination, and some machines include shoulder motion.

Edema control combined with active exercise is the most effective way to prevent wrist, hand, and finger contractures. "Boxer" wraps with Elset or one-inch elastic or self-adhesive bandages are inexpensive compressive techniques. A disadvantage of this wrap in the comatose or uncooperative patient is the tendency to bring the hand into a posture of metacarpophalangeal hyperextension. However, the utilization of newer fabrics such as

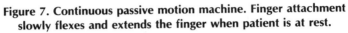

Figure 7. Continuous passive motion machine. Finger attachment slowly flexes and extends the finger when patient is at rest.

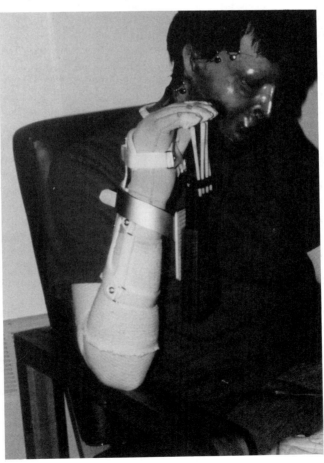

antron nylon, spandex, polyester, and lycra in commercially available gloves such as Isotoners has improved early external support for the burned hand. A severe dorsal and volar burn usually needs stretching in both flexion and extension. Early use of serial casting to manage hand and wrist contractures has become a more common therapeutic measure in the last decade. The advantages of serial plaster splints are low cost, increased patient compliance, and prevention of slippage. The cast may be removed, and its removal is followed by prolonged stretching and then active exercise and strengthening for several hours. The cast is then reapplied, stretching the tissue away from the tightest residual contractures. Used as an early adjunct to active motion or to a continuous passive motion machine, plaster serial casting will prevent many contractures and decrease pain. The cast is usually fitted over wrinkle-free elastic gloves or tightly wrapped Webril. This avoids edema of parts not included in the cast. Newer silicone elastomer has been used for total contact stretching. Disadvantages include blisters, maceration, and difficulty in keeping the elastomer odor free.

When commercial garments are not available, but a sewing machine, serger, and lycra fabric are, the garment may be fabricated. The patient's body part is traced onto the fabric with the grain straight. A ball point needle and a stretch stitch are needed to prevent damage to the elastic threads. After sewing along the tracing, the garment is cut out with a narrow selvage. The garment is worn with the seam to the outside to protect fragile epithelium. Adaptations can be made using inserts, tucks, or darts as needed.

Contractures such as cupping, tight index finger/thumb web space contracture, and thenar eminence/hypothenar eminence contracture may be modified by hand-based orthotics. The contractures are often stretched out with a cast and later maintained by a total contact thermoplastic splint. Otoform K or other silicone elastomers, thermoplastic, felt, Betapile, Webril, lamb's wool, Tubiton, or any soft material may successfully stretch the thumb web and interdigital spaces. The splints are usually applied between two pairs of Isotoner gloves when the tissue is fragile. These spacers may be attached to a button on the Tubigrip sleeve, avoiding a tight wrist band which produces distal edema and also irritates the base of the thumb. Single-finger trough splints of silicone or thermoplastic are helpful in stretching flexion contractures or protecting unstable proximal or distal interphalangeal joints. They are often worn with night casts or splints.

If scoliosis or other trunk contractures resistant to active exercise develop, a spinal orthosis may be indicated. Hip orthoses are rarely needed, but when they are, spica serial casting is effective in increasing hip motion.

Knee contractures are seldom noted when early ambulation is instituted. However, they can be treated similarly to elbow contractures. Toe extension contractures develop in growing children if the scar tissue is dense and cutaneous decussations are relatively small. During the day, sheepskin-lined, high-top tennis or orthopedic shoes (Figure 4D) flex the toes. A steel shank prevents an upward metatarsophalangeal hyperextended and curled-toe position. This shoe needs a rocker bottom to move from foot flat to toe-off. When the foot resists stretching and is serial casted (Figure 4B) into ankle dorsiflexion and toe flexion, a temporary lift on the opposite shoe will prevent hip and knee strain during ambulation. Usually, the cast is applied for one to four weeks at a time and its use is continued until active motion is maintained. Active children need a fiberglass cast reinforcement for durability. If healed tissue on the sole of the foot remains fragile, a varied-density soft orthotic insert (Figure 4C), made to a plaster foot model by an orthotist, is the most satisfactory solution. The patient may need several inserts to keep the tissue dry and comfortable. Taking time each day to change the orthotic insert, stocking, and shoe will help to prevent skin breakdown and subsequent forced rest and immobility, and may prevent pain or prolonged time off from work.

External Vascular Support and Tissue Compression

Elevated positioning combined with external vascular support usually provides adequate control of swelling. However, for the severe circumferential burn, lymphedema may become progressively worse as the patient increases time spent standing. Numerous companies have introduced both off-the-shelf and custom-fitted garments for external vascular support and burn scar compression. Off-the-shelf items such as Tubigrip shaped support bandages, cotton and rubber cylinders, and vests and Bioconcepts premade gloves, digisleeves, or stockings are less expensive, and the authors believe that in the vast majority of cases they are as effective as custom-fitted garments. For relief of severe, unresponsive chronic edema that is not controlled by support stockings or the traditional pneumatic pumps such as Jobst, the newer type Wright linear compression pump is effective.

PAIN MANAGEMENT

Burn wound treatment and exercise are painful. Despite mythology to the contrary, studies confirm that hurting is experienced by everyone, be they infants, toddlers, or senior citizens, male or female, since all have similar physiological transmission of pain stimuli. Each group has different needs regarding monitoring of the effect of medications, different rates of metabolizing medications, and differing abilities to describe their pain. Marvin[14] proposes that as myths about narcotic addiction are dispelled among health care workers and as newer drugs are developed, use of patient-controlled analgesia or long-acting oral narcotics to control pain will increase. The last decade has brought the realization that unless a patient was chemically dependent before being burned, addiction from the liberal use of narcotics during the acute phase of burn care is unlikely to occur. The patient must be gradually weaned from potent narcotics prior to discharge from the hospital.[24]

For the superficial burn, which is only painful for one to three days, ibuprofen or acetaminophen provides adequate analgesia. For outpatient treatment of the superficial partial thickness burn, which is painful for 5 to 14 days, acetaminophen with codeine or oxycodone provides adequate analgesia for wound care, exercise, and sleep. Deep partial thickness burns are very painful throughout the healing process, and methadone, slow-release oral morphine, or "pain cocktails" provide a baseline of pain control.[17] Improved analgesia aids in comfortable exercise and self-care, promoting patient collaboration and successful rehabilitation. The recently developed drugs oxazepam and midazolam provide amnesia of the acute pain of dressing changes and stretching exercise, thereby reducing the anticipatory anxiety for future procedures.

In the past 10 years there has been an increased willingness to supplement narcotic pain relief with behavioral interventions such as hypnosis, visualization, or relaxation. These interventions relieve depression and feelings of anger, fear, loneliness, or helplessness that bring pain acutely to the patient's awareness. Patients benefit from sharing personal experiences of pain relief in a trauma group, led by a professional trained in group behavioral interventions. When a patient requests sleeping and pain pills, careful physician inquiry will sometimes reveal that antidepressants, anti-inflammatories, or antihistamines are indicated.

Interventions for itching are based on the etiology. Patients are relieved to learn that posthealing pruritus decreases spontaneously in 12 months. As wound healing progresses, alternating antihistamine medications such as diphenhydramine hydrochloride (25 mg to 100 mg every four hours) with cyproheptadine hydrochloride (4 mg) may be necessary to prevent scratching. As soon as practical, doses of itch medications should be reduced during waking hours to improve alertness and ability to exercise. Keeping the skin moist, maintaining external vascular support, and using TENS units, vibrators, and behavioral interventions such as Benson's relaxation response or hypnosis remain the primary treatment modalities for postburn pruritus.

An innovation in pediatric postburn care has been the development of Burn Camp experiences for children. Burn Camps are usually a week-long, supervised, outdoor group adventure for children aged 7 to 17. Wearing support garments or splints and doing stretching exercise is easier in this relaxed environment with the support of peers and counselors (Figure 8). As the children mature, many camps invite them to become junior counselors. Campers have time for exploring nature, participating in sports activities, making new friends, and socializing with therapists, nurses, and physicians in a relaxed environment. The teasing and stares experienced at school or in other public areas do not happen at camp. Sharing experiences with other burned kids can help heal the child's emotional pain. Camp

Figure 8. Tire swing at Burn Camp. Burn exercises can be enjoyable. Note clear facial orthosis and elastic support garment on arm.

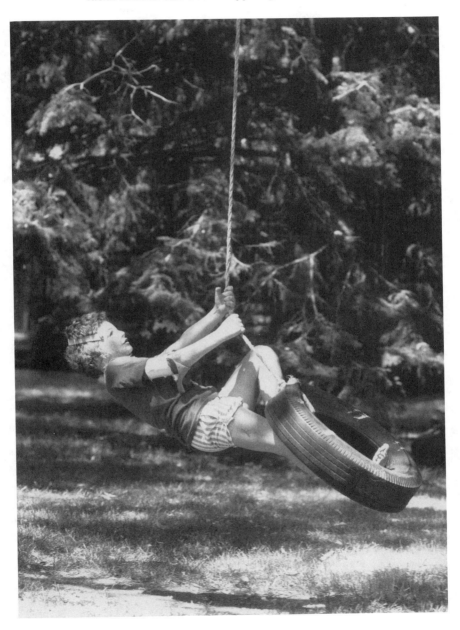

participation improves a burned child's self-esteem and confidence while redefining the injury and reducing the intensity of the traumatic experience.

VOCATIONAL MANAGEMENT

Evidence accumulated during the last decade indicates that, in the United States, if an injured employee does not return to work within the first 12 months after injury, he will never return to work. Employers have shown an increased willingness to accommodate the injured worker. Rehabilitation professionals must consider on-the-job exposure to heat, cold, irritants, ultraviolet light, vapors, and chemicals when planning early re-entry to the work force. Some employers prefer that the employee successfully participate in a work readiness assessment, work capacity, or work hardening program before returning to previous responsibilities. The authors realize that return to work is dependent on cultural and socioeconomic forces that vary from country to country.

Acknowledgment.   The authors wish to thank Donna Powell, R.D., for her assistance in the preparation of the nutrition section.

REFERENCES

1. Carlow DL, Conine TA, Stevenson-Moore P. Static orthoses for the management of microstomia. *J Rehabil Res Dev.* 1987;24(3):35–42.
2. Conine TA, Carlow DL, Stevenson-Moore P. Dynamic orthoses for the management of microstomia. *J Rehabil Res Dev.* 1987;24(3):43–48.
3. Covey MH, Prestigiacomo MJ, Engrav LH. Management of face burns. In: Campbell MK, Covey MH, eds. *Topics in acute care and trauma rehabilitation.* Frederick, MD: Aspen; 1987:40–49. (Monograph series vol 1, no 4).
4. Covey, MH. Application of CPM devices with burn patients. *J Burn Care Rehabil.* 1988;9(5):496–497.
5. Cunningham JJ, Hegarty MT, Meara PA, et al. Measured and predicted calorie requirements of adults during recovery from severe burn trauma. *Am J Clin Nutr.* 1989;49:404–408.
6. Feldman AE, MacMillan BG. Burn injury in children: declining need for reconstructive surgery as related to use of neck orthoses. *Arch Phys Med Rehabil.* 1980;61:441–449.
7. Giuliani CA, Perry GA. Factors to consider in the rehabilitation aspect of burn care. *Phys Ther.* 1985;65(5):619–623.
8. Gottschlich MM. Acute thermal injury. In: Lang CE, ed. *Nutrition support in critical care.* Rockville, MD: Aspen; 1987:159–181.
9. Heimbach DM, Engrav LH. *Surgical management of the burn wound.* New York: Raven Press; 1984.
10. Helm PA, Kevorkian CG, Lushbaugh M, Pullium G, Head MD, Cromes GF. Burn injury: rehabilitation management in 1982. *Arch Phys Med Rehabil.* 1982;63(1):6–16.
11. Hildreth MA, Herdon DN, Desai MH, et al. Reassessing caloric requirements in pediatric patients. *J Burn Care Rehabil.* 1988;2:616–618.
12. Lund CC, Browder NC. The estimation of areas of burns. *Surg Gynecol Obstet.* 1944;79:352.
13. Mackin EJ. Prevention of complications in hand therapy. *Hand Clin* 1986;2(2):429–447.
14. Marvin JA. Pain management. In: Campbell MK, Covey MH, eds. *Topics in acute care and trauma rehabilitation.* Frederick, MD: Aspen; 1987:23. (Monograph series vol 1, no 4).

15. Murphy M, Bell SJ. Assessment of nutritional status in burn patients. *J Burn Care Rehabil.* 1988;9:432–433.
16. O'Neil CE, Hustler D, Hildreth MA. Basic nutritional guidelines for pediatric burn patients. *J Burn Care Rehabil.* 1989;10:278–284.
17. Perry S, Heidrich G. Management of pain during debridement: a survey of US burn units. *Pain.* 1982;13(3):267–280.
18. Pullium GF. Splinting and positioning. In: Fisher SV, Helm PA, eds. *Comprehensive rehabilitation of burns.* Baltimore: Williams & Wilkins; 1984:64–95.
19. Rivers E, Collin T, Solem LD, Ahrenholz D, Fisher S, Macfarlane J. Use of a custom maxillary night splint with lateral projections in the treatment of microstomia. *Proceedings of the American Burn Association's annual meeting.* Orlando, FL; 1985.
20. Rivers EA. Management of hypertrophic scars. In: Fisher SV, Helm PA, eds. *Comprehensive rehabilitation of burns.* Baltimore: Williams & Wilkins; 1984:177–217.
21. Rivers EA. Rehabilitation management of the burn patient. In: Eisenberg MG, Grzesiak RC, eds. *Advances in clinical rehabilitation,* vol 1. New York: Springer; 1987:177–214.
22. Robertson CF, Zuker R, Dabrowski B, Levinson H. Obstructive sleep apnea: a complication of burns to the head and neck in children. *J Burn Care Rehabil.* 1985;6:353–357.
23. Teperman PS, Hilbert L, Peters WJ, Pritzker KPH. Heterotopic ossification in burns. *J Burn Care Rehabil.* 1984;5:283–287.
24. Thompson TL, Steele BF. The psychological aspects of pain. In: Simmons RC, ed. *Understanding human behavior in health and illness.* 3rd ed. Baltimore: Williams & Wilkins; 1985:60–67.
25. Wright PC. Fundamentals of acute burn care and physical therapy management. *Phys Ther.* 1984;64:1217–1231.

Chapter 18

REHABILITATION OF PATIENTS WITH RHEUMATIC DISEASES

Lynn H. Gerber

ASSESSMENT OF THE PATIENT

The development of an appropriate treatment and rehabilitation program for any rheumatic disease is dependent upon a sound evaluation. Traditionally, rheumatologists have focused their attention on examinations of joints, from which they gleaned information about pain and articular swelling as well as the ability to generate a strong grasp[2] and walk a measured course in a specified period of time. Other standard measures include goniometry, muscle testing, and descriptions of deformity.

Recently, rheumatologists have acknowledged the need to learn more about function among these patients who experience chronic, unpredictable, and debilitating disease. Function is defined broadly and includes indicators of physical performance as well as psychological, social, and vocational activities.

A number of functional assessments specifically for this patient population have been developed recently. The assessments have been standardized, follow a questionnaire format, are quantifiable, and have been validated. A summary of their pertinent characteristics is provided in Table 1, which is adapted from Liang.[26] These assessment instruments[8,14,23,29,35] are useful for measuring multi-dimensional aspects of the impact of the disease, including activities of daily living (ADL), pain, affect, fatigue, and financial impact, among others. They should be used to assist in identifying functional problems, planning treatment, and evaluating treatment efficacy in persons with rheumatic disease. One such recommended assessment is presented in the appendix to this chapter.[8]

TREATMENT

In general, treatment for patients with rheumatic diseases must be comprehensive and tailored to the needs of individual patients. Typically, these patients have pain, stiffness, decreased mobility, decreased stamina, and

Table 1. Functional assessments.

Instrument	Reliability	Validity	Measurement precision	Type of assessment
Jette[23]	+	+	good	ADL—scored for pain, difficulty, dependence
AIMS[29]	+	+	good	Function (disability?)
HAQ[14]	+	+	good	Function (disability?)
Convery[8]	+	+	good	ADL

fatigue, and experience interrupted sleep patterns and, often, loss of independence in self-care and other ADL. These losses and the unpredictable nature of inflammatory disease present difficulties to patients and caregivers that can lead to depression and loss of self-esteem. Multidisciplinary interventions are needed to help achieve a good functional outcome.

Nonpharmacological techniques for managing the above-listed symptoms include the following modalities: heat and cold, rest and exercise, electricity, splinting and traction, and adaptive equipment and education. The rationale behind the use of many of the treatments and their application to patients with rheumatic disease has been documented.

Heat and Cold

Heat modalities have been described as effective in relieving pain, increasing range of motion, and lowering intra-articular temperature when the heat modality used was superficial. These observations have established the basis for prescribing heat prior to treating a patient with a stretching program to increase range of motion (ROM). However, some evidence suggests that use of heat for treating a crystal-induced arthritis may cause increased volume of joint fluid and number of white blood cells.[11]

Clinically, heat is recommended for relief of joint pain and joint stiffness. Heat should be superficial when joint inflammation is acute, but deep heat may be used when the process is chronic or subacute.[13] Methods of superficial heat delivery typically used in arthritis are hot packs, heating pads, whirlpool, and paraffin. Deep heating methods include diathermy and ultrasound.

Cold therapy has also been used successfully in treating arthritis patients. Some, in fact, prefer it to heat. Cold is a good analgesic, decreases muscle spasm, and helps control joint edema. Cold packs have been shown to be as effective as hot packs in promoting ROM, and as good or better in relieving pain and joint stiffness. Cold should not be used in patients with Raynaud's phenomenon, cryoglobulinemia, or cold-induced urticaria.

Electricity

Electricity has been used in the treatment of muscle spasm and contracture for two decades.[12] The results of well-designed, controlled trials to determine efficacy are not available, but clinical improvement in muscle spasm has been reported when faradic electrical stimulation was used. The application of transcutaneous electrical nerve stimulation (TENS) to rheumatoid joints[28] and in the treatment of rheumatoid neuropathy[39] has been reported to be a useful adjunct for pain relief. Electrical stimulation has also been used for maintaining muscle bulk and strength in the face of denervation,[39] but this application is still open to question. However, exercise plus faradic electrical stimulation was superior to exercise alone in preserving resting muscle strength and bulk of muscle in patients postmeniscectomy.[17]

Rest

Patients with rheumatoid arthritis are generally fatigued; in addition, they have stiff, swollen, and often painful joints. Historically, acute flares of inflammatory arthritis were treated with bed rest and significant reduction in physical activity. This method of treatment, while it has been demonstrated to reduce inflammation without significant loss of range of motion,[1] does result in muscle atrophy and in demineralization of bone. Hence, the amount of time spent in bed should probably not exceed two weeks. It remains unclear whether it is the physiology of rest, independent of the addition of splints, that results in an observed diminution of swelling. One study suggested that simply admitting patients with arthritis to a hospital for a course of rehabilitation improved their arthritis and increased their functional level.[37] This benefit persisted, resulting in sustained improvement in function even one year after hospital discharge.

A controlled trial during which patients were taught to rest in order to avoid fatigue during physically active periods resulted in an increased ability to remain physically active.[16]

Exercise

The general benefits of exercise are acknowledged to be increased strength and greater mobility, improvement in endurance, and an enhanced sense of well-being. Exercise can be prescribed safely for persons with arthritis, but the technique should be tailored to the level of disease activity and the nature of the problem. For example, spondylarthropathies are associated with contractures and bony ankylosis; hence, when exercise is initiated early in the course of the disease, a heat and stretching program is most likely to increase ROM. Both active and passive stretching may be used.[7] For management of acute crystal-induced arthritis (e.g., gout or pseudogout), passive exercise has been associated with increases in joint effusion and the intra-articular white cell count. Hence, only moderate active ROM should be pursued.

Isometric exercise is the most commonly prescribed form of exercise because it is well tolerated and is associated with the lowest intra-articular pressures.[22] Isometric exercise can be done using a six-second isometric contraction daily at two-thirds maximal effort. A brief isometric contraction of this sort has been shown to be as effective in increasing muscular strength as an isotonic program.[27]

Isotonic exercise may be used in the treatment of arthritic patients whose arthritis is not in a significant flare. Programs that utilize a regime of lifting the maximum possible amount of weight are not recommended for arthritics. Variations have been devised in which low weights and low numbers of repetitions are used.[5] In addition, isotonic regimens for arthritics frequently are modified to decrease the arc through which weight is lifted.

Isokinetic exercise is not commonly used therapeutically for arthritics. However, those with mild osteoarthritis or nonactive rheumatoid arthritis who have stable joints might benefit from this form of exercise, using medium velocity and limited range of motion. Isokinetic exercise offers no advantage in muscle strengthening over isotonic or isometric exercise.[10] Isokinetic dynamometers have been used to quantify strength in arthritics, and their application has been reported to have no adverse effects on joints.[20]

Exercise for arthritis is often performed in water. This medium can be used for assisting ROM exercise, for strengthening, and for increasing endurance. Aquatic therapy is often the best kind during postoperative care. Water is an analgesic milieu, providing local and systemic relaxation. The water temperature should be 88–90°F and activity should be limited to brief periods of time (20–30 min); lap swimming should not be permitted. Exercise in this environment may produce syncope or cardiac failure.

The use of aquatic training for patients with rheumatoid arthritis has been demonstrated to improve fitness and to increase muscular strength.[9] Patients with inflammatory and degenerative arthropathies are generally deconditioned, which is a factor contributing to their fatigue. Programs designed to improve strength and fitness have been effective in also improving the patient's cardiovascular functioning and sense of well-being.[18,32,34] Bicycle ergometry has been used frequently in this population, and the evidence indicates that it does not result in articular damage or premature degenerative change.[10] Patients with rheumatoid arthritis should be carefully monitored for signs of excessive exercise, such as pain after exercise persisting for more than a few hours; increased joint pain and/or swelling; unusual fatigue, lasting even until the next day; and weakness. Reduction in frequency or intensity or change in type of exercise is recommended if any signs of overexercise are noted.

See Table 2 for recommended exercises for the various arthritides.

Table 2. Exercise recommendations for specific rheumatic diseases.

Type of disease	Isometric strengthening	Isotonic strengthening[a]	Active ROM	Passive ROM	Electrical stimulation	Endurance training[b]
Osteoarthritis stages	+/−	+	+	−	−	+ walk, swim
RA:						
Acute phase	+	−	+	−	−	−
Subacute	+	+/−	+	−	−	+
Inactive	+	+	+	−	−	+
JRA	+	+	+	−	−	+
Ankylosing spondylitis	+	−	+	+ & positive	−	+
Seronegative arthritis (see RA)						
PSS	+	+/−	+	+	−	−
Polymyositis:						
Acute	+/−	−	+	−	−	−
Subacute	+	+	+	−	−	+
Systemic lupus	+	+	+	−	−	+
Vasculitis with neuropathy	+	−	+	+	+	−

[a]Low weight, short arc, few repetitions. Isokinetic exercise may have limited application.
[b]Low-impact endurance training is appropriate: swimming, walking, stationary bicycle.

Splinting

Orthotic devices and casts are used to immobilize a painful body part, mobilize a stiff joint (as in postoperative extension on trigger splints), support a body part in a functional position, or maintain alignment so as to reduce deformity and preserve function.

Plaster knee casts have been demonstrated to be effective in stretching out contractures and in reducing pain and swelling without significant loss of ROM.[31] Equally beneficial, and quite safe to use, are wrist splints. Historically, these were made of plaster and designed to support the wrist in a neutral position while permitting relatively free motion of the fingers. Finger ring splints to control swan-neck and boutonnière deformities are also used. Newer materials, such as low-temperature heat-moldable plastics, have made custom fitting much easier. These splints are useful in reducing swelling and improving grip strength.[15]

A large body of clinical experience exists regarding the use of a variety of types of splints for support, immobilization, and assistance in function, but few trials have been performed to prove their efficacy. An illustration of the most frequently prescribed splints and their indications for patients with arthritis is presented in Figure 1.

Foot and ankle problems are prevalent among arthritics. They affect the

Figure 1. Commonly used hand splints.

Anatomical Site	Problem	Splint
Wrist	Swelling Pain Carpal tunnel	Functional wrist splint " " " " " "
Hand	Swelling Pain	Resting hand splint " " "
	Swan neck | Boutonnière |	Finger ring splint
Thumb	Carpometacarpal pain Metacarpophalangeal pain Metacarpophalangeal instability	Thumb post splint " " " " " "

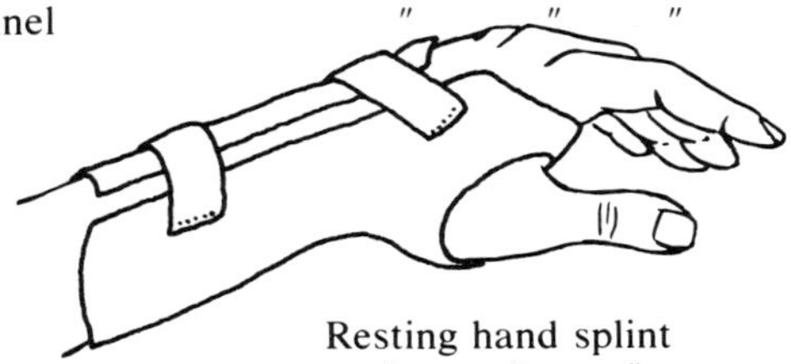

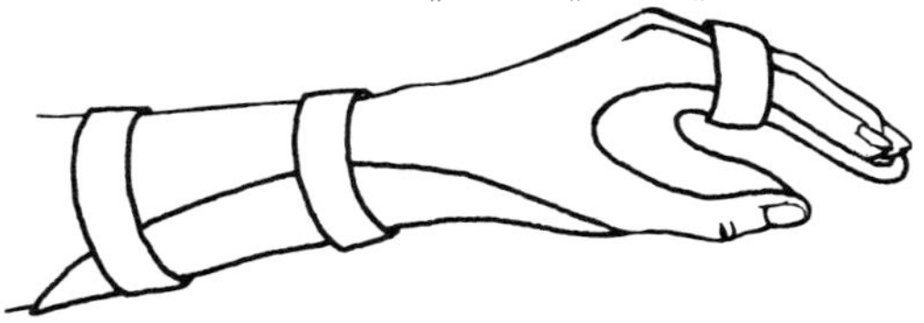

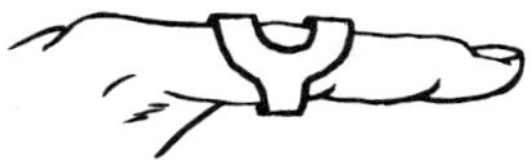

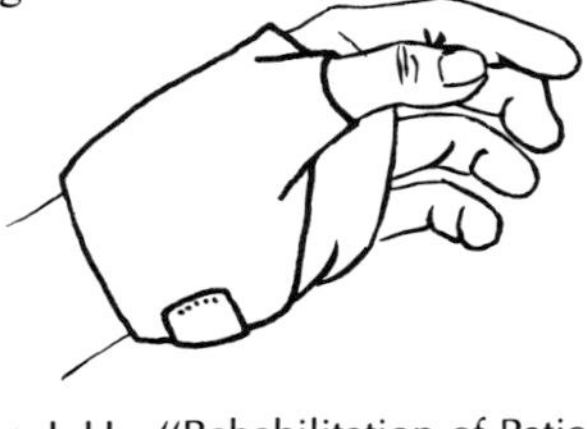

Reproduced from Gerber, L.H., "Rehabilitation of Patients with Rheumatic Disease," in Kelley, W.N., E.D. Harris, S. Ruddy, and C.D. Sledge (eds.), *Textbook of Rheumatology* (Philadelphia: W.B. Saunders, 1989), with the permission of the publisher.

forefoot as a result of metatarsophalangeal subluxation and cocktoe deformities, and also the hindfoot, especially the subtalar joint. Shoe modifications and insoles have been used effectively to relieve pain by unloading or immobilizing a painful area; to balance the foot and provide a more stable walking surface with better floor contact; and to provide assistance in simulating a more natural, energy-efficient gait. Typically, shoes should be made of soft material (canvas or leather), with a wide forefoot and deep toe box in order to accommodate the foot. The sole should be composed of crepe or other soft material that can help absorb ground reaction forces. The heel height should not exceed two inches. Corrective insoles are most effective when custom molded; however, a metatarsal pad placed proximal to the MTPs may be adequate to relieve metatarsalgia. The use of a scaphoid pad may reduce the amount of pronation and relieve stress on the tarsal navicular. An external metatarsal bar may also help relieve metatarsalgia. Rigid high-temperature plastics (subortholene and polypropylene) can be used to immobilize portions of the foot, such as the subtalar joint. The University of California–Berkeley (UCBL) or National Institutes of Health hindfoot orthosis is commonly recommended for hindfoot problems.[21] Patients with difficulty transferring body weight over the forefoot can benefit from a rocker sole, which provides a half-inch addition to the sole proximal to the metatarsal heads that facilitates roll-off of the forefoot. This sole modification is particularly useful in postoperative patients following metatarsal head resection. Examples of shoe inserts are presented in Figures 2 and 3.

Orthoses are commonly used to relieve neck pain. When the pain originates from degenerative disc disease, a soft cervical collar, in conjunction with pain management and possibly traction, is the usual prescription. Degenerative disc disease is common in arthritis patients, whether they have inflammatory or degenerative disease. Cervical spine subluxation at C1–2 is less common than disc disease, but it is a more serious problem whose inappropriate management may produce cord compression or death. Management of C1–2 subluxation of more than 8 mm should include orthopedic evaluation and use of a rigid collar, that is, a SOMI or a two-post Thomas collar. This is necessary to reduce the amount of forward flexion to a minimum. These collars provide a greater degree of protection from high impact than either a soft or Philadelphia collar.[24]

Knee braces are commonly used to manage instability or patellar dysfunction in cases of degenerative arthritis. However, they are rarely used on patients with rheumatoid arthritis.

Traction and Massage

Mobilization techniques include use of massage as well as a motorized traction apparatus. Treatment of this kind is recommended for relief of pain,

**Figure 2. Shoe inserts. Top: University of California–
Berkeley (UCBL) polyethylene insert.
Bottom: (L to R) pelite; plastazote; two combination
insoles of plastazote and leather or Spenco; Spenco.**

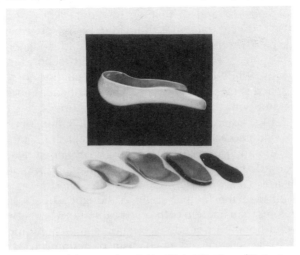

Reproduced from Gerber, L.H., "Rehabilitation of Patients
with Rheumatic Disease," in Kelley, W.N., E.D. Harris, S.
Ruddy, and C.D. Sledge (eds.), Textbook of Rheumatology
(Philadelphia: W.B. Saunders, 1989), with the permission of
the publisher.

Figure 3. Hindfoot orthosis made of subortholene.

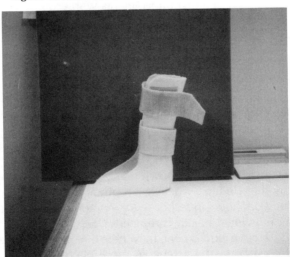

Reproduced from Gerber, L.H., "Rehabilitation of Patients
with Rheumatic Disease," in Kelley, W.N., E.D. Harris, S.
Ruddy, and C.D. Sledge (eds.), Textbook of Rheumatology
(Philadelphia: W.B. Saunders, 1989), with the permission of
the publisher.

especially that resulting from nerve root compression in the cervical spine. Traction has been shown to be effective in immobilizing individuals who are in need of bed rest and in helping to reduce knee and hip flexion contractures.[19,36] Cervical traction is thought to be most useful clinically for reducing neck pain, improving functional (pain-induced) lordosis, or relieving radicular pain.[36] Twenty-five pounds of distraction force is needed to reduce lordosis, while the amount of force needed to increase cervical intervertebral space is 60 pounds. Traction is usually administered with the patient supine and with the neck in flexion. The use of this treatment for patients with C1–2 instability is contraindicated. Often, the instability is painless and is *not* associated with neurological signs or symptoms. Therefore, lateral flexion and extension views must be obtained. Neck symptoms are usually secondary to degenerative changes that are present in the lower cervical levels (C4–C7).

Traction applied to the lumbar spine is thought to be less effective in reducing symptoms than traction of the cervical spine. There is little evidence that even several hundred pounds of traction significantly increases intervertebral disc space. Hence, its mechanism of action must be other than production of discal distraction.

Massage is considered to be a form of manual traction. Its efficacy is probably attributable to its impact on local blood and lymph flow and its usefulness as a relaxation technique. It assists in musculotendinous stretching. Although its effectiveness has not been documented, massage remains a frequently prescribed treatment for patients with arthritic conditions.

Adaptive Equipment and Education

An estimated 30 million persons in the United States are affected by musculoskeletal disorders. Many of these people have work-related disability (especially low-back pain), and many are unable to continue working as a result of their arthritic condition. Several studies of the economic impact of this inability to work have indicated that people with chronic inflammatory disease are often impoverished.[25] Outcome from arthritis is frequently related to educational level.[30] The ability to continue working may be similarly influenced, because it has been shown that patients with some control over the type of work they do (i.e., whether it is physically demanding), and who are able to alter work hours in response to symptoms, can continue working while pursuing individual health care needs.

The use of adaptive equipment may help an individual remain more functional. This equipment can enable more energy-efficient movement, extend reach, provide support, or lessen the weight on painful lower extremity joints. Environmental adaptation can make a significant difference for some individuals, who would find work, school, or living routines impossible without them. Further, these adaptations may provide a safer environment for patients, especially in the bathroom. Elevated chairs, bathroom safety seats, and wall-mounted bars can increase functional independence.

It has only recently been shown that patients with rheumatic diseases have swallowing disorders. In the recent past, these problems were attributed to esophageal dysmotility, but data suggest that the disorder is more likely associated with pharyngeal dysfunction. The swallowing difficulty is frequently compounded by weakness in the flexor and extensor muscles of the neck, making therapeutic head positioning difficult. Head flexion and lateralization are often necessary to compensate for a weak posterior pharynx. Patients with polymyositis are at greatest risk for dysphagia and aspiration. When rheumatoid arthritis and scleroderma patients have dysphagia, it is most likely due to cervical spine arthritis in the former and esophageal dysmotility in the latter. The symptoms are different in the two groups. The rheumatoid patient may complain of a sticking sensation in the throat, while the scleroderma patient complains of food being stuck behind the sternum. Treatment consists of providing recommendations about proper food consistency (e.g., pureed) and the need to chew well before swallowing.

SPECIAL CONSIDERATIONS

Postoperative Rehabilitation

Postoperative rehabilitation for persons undergoing joint replacement is usually prescribed by orthopedic surgeons whose established routines are based on mechanical and physiological principles; programs are then modified to take account of individual patient capabilities. In general, after total hip arthroplasty (THA), the following precautions are taken: hip abduction is prohibited; internal hip rotation is prohibited; and hip flexion to more than 90° is initially discouraged. At first, partial weight-bearing is permitted while walking with crutches (three-point gait); full weight-bearing is permitted by six weeks. Exercise programs are designed to maintain (or increase) range of joint motion and to increase strength, especially in hip abductors, extensors, flexors, and quadriceps. Attention must be given to establishing leg length equality, as well as to restoring abductor strength. Isometric quad strengthening and gluteal setting begin on the first postoperative day, with isotonic exercises commencing as early as day 10.[33] Porous coated prostheses require six weeks of protected ambulation.

Rehabilitation following total knee arthroplasty (TKA) varies with the type of arthroplasty used. Most TKA uses only partially constrained knees which permit 90–100° knee flexion. ROM exercises to insure full extension and 90° of flexion are begun immediately. Weight-bearing is limited initially to partial (about 25 pounds) using a three-point gait, and is then advanced to full weight-bearing by 10–12 weeks. Porous coated prostheses require protected weight-bearing for six weeks. Isometric exercise may be started on postoperative day one and isotonic on day seven; the few pounds of resistance used initially may be increased when the wound heals. Hydrotherapy is useful in aiding the progress of exercise. A four-foot-deep therapeutic pool with an access ramp, heated to 90°F, can facilitate ROM activity and provide early buoyancy assistance for ambulation.

Rehabilitation of Children

Children with rheumatic disease have unique rehabilitation needs. Changes occur quickly, and if joint position and strength are not maintained, significant harm can ensue in a brief period of time. The result may be a contracted, atrophic, nonfunctional limb.

Rest is an important cornerstone for treating inflammatory arthritis. Complete bed rest is occasionally required when there is systemic illness or carditis. During the period of bed rest, active or active-assisted ROM exercise should be carried out at least daily. Posture should be prone, when possible, in order to avoid hip and knee flexion contractures. Splinting of wrists may be needed to preserve a functional hand position. Strengthening exercises should be performed to tolerance, consisting of cold or other therapy to reduce pain and inflammation, followed by isometric exercises. As the child's general medical condition improves, hydrotherapy or an aerobic program may be added.

Most importantly, contractures should be prevented. If they occur, traction to reduce hip or knee contractures, serial casting for knee and elbow, or heat and stretch with adjunctive wrist, ankle, and knee splinting (especially at night) should be used.[3,4]

Since children depend so much on others for their care, parents or other care-givers must be in agreement with treatment goals and must be committed to supervising or participating in the treatment. If they are not, children will not receive needed therapies.

Rehabilitation of Nonarticular Rheumatism

Ligaments, tendons, fasciae, and bursae may be involved in inflammatory processes that cause pain, erythema, abnormal patterns of motion, and possibly disability. Control of symptoms is the primary treatment goal, with modalities of heat and cold used to control pain; a program designed to restore strength and ROM or maintain them is carried out simultaneously. Fibrositis, a syndrome characterized by (a) shoulder girdle pain, (b) trigger points characteristically in the trapezius, serratus anterior, olecranon, femoral condyles, and other anatomical loci, and (c) sleep disturbances,[38] often responds to local injections of lidocaine, massage, and stretching techniques. These patients are not physically fit, and so strengthening as well as conditioning exercises are beneficial.[6]

Recreational Activities

Arthritis patients should be encouraged to pursue appropriate recreational activity to improve stamina, enhance their sense of well-being, and provide social integration. Recreational activity should be preceded by programs designed to increase the strength of larger antigravity muscles in the upper and lower extremities and to restore functional ROM if this is lacking. Typically, swimming, walking, cycling, and boating are recommended activities. Contact sports are discouraged and high-impact sports are not recommended for patients with joint effusion, instability, or active myositis. Patients who have received total joint replacements should be cautioned against performing contact sports or high-impact sports as well as those that require sudden rotatory movements (tennis, basketball).

REFERENCES

1. Alexander GJM, Hortas C, Bacon PA. Bed rest, activity and the inflammation of rheumatoid arthritis. *Br J Rheumatol.* 1983;22:134–140.
2. An KN, Chao EYS, Askew U. Hand strength measurement instruments. *Arch Phys Med Rehabil.* 1980;6:366–368.
3. Ansell BM. Rehabilitation in juvenile chronic arthritis. *Clin Rheum Dis.* 1981;7:469–484.
4. Ansell BM. The hand in juvenile arthritis. *Clin Rheum Dis.* 1984;10:657–672.
5. Atha J. Strengthening muscles. In: Miller DI, ed. *Exerc Sport Sci Rev.* 1981;9:146–152.
6. Bennett RM, Clark S, Goldberg L, et al. Aerobic fitness in patients with fibrositis: a controlled study of respiratory gas exchange in ^{133}xenon clearance for exercising muscle. *Arthritis Rheum.* 1989;32:454–461.
7. Bulstrode SJ, Barefoot J, Harrison RA, et al. The role of passive stretching in the treatment of ankylosing spondylitis. *Br J Rheumatol.* 1987;26:40–42.
8. Convery MR, Minteer MA, Amiel D, Connett KL. Polyarticular disability: a functional assessment. *Arch Phys Med Rehabil.* 1977;58:494–499.
9. Danneskiold-Samsoe B, Lyngberg K, Rsium T, et al. The effect of water exercise therapy given to patients with rheumatoid arthritis. *Scand J Rehabil Med.* 1987;19:31–35.
10. DeLateur BJ, Lehmann JF, Warren CG, et al. Comparison of effectiveness of isokinetic and isotonic exercise in quadriceps strengthening. *Arch Phys Med Rehabil.* 1982;53:60–64.
11. Dorwart BB, Hansell JR, Schumacher HR Jr. Effects of cold and heat on urate crystal-induced synovitis in the dog. *Arthritis Rheum.* 1974;17:563–571.
12. Duncan ME. Transcutaneous nerve stimulation in rheumatoid neuropathy. *Rheumatol Rehabil.* 1982;21:187.
13. Fiebil A, Fast A. Deep heating of joints: a reconsideration. *Arch Phys Med Rehabil.* 1976;57:513.
14. Fries JF, Spitz P, Kraines RG, Holman HR. Measurement of patient outcome in arthritis. *Arthritis Rheum.* 1980;23:137–145.
15. Gault SJ, Spyker JM. Beneficial effect of immobilization of joints in rheumatoid and related arthritides: a splint study using sequential analysis. *Arthritis Rheum.* 1969;12:34–44.
16. Gerber LH, Furst G, Shulman B, et al. Patient education program to teach energy conservation behaviors to patients with rheumatoid arthritis: a pilot study. *Arch Phys Med Rehabil.* 1987;68:442–445.

17. Gould N, Donnermeyer D, Gammon GG, et al. Transcutaneous muscle stimulation to retard disuse atrophy after open meniscectomy. *Clin Orthop.* 1983;178:190–197.
18. Harkcom TM, Lampman RM, Banweel BF, et al. Therapeutic value of graded aerobic exercise training in rheumatoid arthritis. *Arthritis Rheum.* 1985;28:32–39.
19. Hinterbuchner C. Traction. In: Rogoff JB, ed. *Manipulation, traction and massage.* Baltimore: Williams & Wilkins; 1980:184–210.
20. Hsieh LF, Didenko B, Schumacher HR, et al. Isokinetic and isometric testing of the knee musculature in patients with rheumatoid arthritis with mild knee involvement. *Arch Phys Med Rehabil.* 1988;68:294–297.
21. Hunt GC, Fromherz WA, Gerber LH, Hurwitz SR. Hindfoot pain treated by a leg-hindfoot orthosis: a case report. *Phys Ther.* 1987;67:1384–1388.
22. Jayson MIV, Rubenstein D, Dixon AS. Intra-articular pressure in rheumatoid geodes. *Ann Rheum Dis.* 1970;29:496.
23. Jette AM. Functional status index: reliability of a chronic disease evaluation instrument. *Arch Phys Med Rehabil.* 1980;61:395–401.
24. Johnson RM, Hart D, Simmons EF, et al. Cervical orthoses. *J Bone Joint Surg [Am].* 1977;59A:332–339.
25. Kramer J, Yellen E, Epstein W. Social and economic impacts of four musculoskeletal conditions. *Arthritis Rheum.* 1983;26(7):901–907.
26. Liang MH, Jette AM. Measuring functional ability in chronic arthritis: a critical review. *Arthritis Rheum.* 1981;24:80–86.
27. Liberson WT. Brief isometric exercises. In: Basmajian J, ed. *Therapeutic exercise.* 4th ed. Baltimore: Williams & Wilkins; 1984.
28. Mannheimer C, Lard S, Carlsson CA. The effect of transcutaneous electrical nerve stimulation (TENS) on joint pain in patients with rheumatoid arthritis. *Scand J Rheumatol.* 1978;7:13.
29. Meenan RF, Gertman PM, Mason JH. Measuring health status in arthritis: the arthritis impact measurement scales. *Arthritis Rheum.* 1980;23:146–152.
30. Mitchell J, Burkhauser RV, Pincus T. The importance of age, education, and comorbidity in polyarthritis. *Arthritis Rheum.* 1988;31:348–358.
31. Nicholas JJ, Ziegler G. Cylinder splints: their use in the treatment of arthritis of the knee. *Arch Phys Med Rehabil.* 1977;58:264–267.
32. Nordemar R. Physical training in rheumatoid arthritis: a controlled long-term study; II, functional capacity and general attitudes. *Scand J Rheumatol.* 1981;10:25–30.
33. Opitz JL. Total joint arthroplasty: principles and guidelines for postoperative physiatric management. *Mayo Clin Proc.* 1979;54:602–612.
34. Panusch RS, Brown DG. Exercise in arthritis. *Sports Med.* 1987;4:54–64.
35. Pincus T, Summey JA, Soraci SA Jr, Wallston KA, Hummon RP. Assessment of patient satisfaction in activities of daily living using a modified Stanford Health Assessment Questionnaire. *Arthritis Rheum.* 1983;26:1346–1353.
36. Rogoff JB. Motorized intermittent traction. In: Rogoff JB, ed. *Manipulation, traction and massage.* Baltimore: Williams & Wilkins; 1980:211–216.
37. Spiegel JS, Spiegel TM, Ward NB, et al. Rehabilitation for rheumatoid arthritis patients: a controlled trial. *Arthritis Rheum.* 1986;29:628.
38. Wolfe F, Hawley DJ, Cathey MA, et al. Fibrositis: symptom frequency and criteria for diagnosis. *J Rheumatol.* 1985;12:1159–1163.
39. Zislis JM. Hydrotherapy. In: Krusen FH, Kottke FJ, Elwood PM. *Handbook of physical medicine and rehabilitation.* 2nd ed. Philadelphia: WB Saunders; 1971:346–362.

General Bibliography

Much of the material presented was derived from the following sources:

1. Gerber L. Rehabilitation of patients with rheumatic diseases. In: Kelley WN, Harris ED, Ruddy S, Sledge CB, eds. *Textbook of rheumatology.* Philadelphia: WB Saunders; 1989.
2. Hicks JE, Nicholas JJ, Swezey RS, eds. *Handbook of rehabilitative rheumatology.* Boston: American Rheumatism Association; 1988.

APPENDIX: PATIENT ASSESSMENT QUESTIONNAIRE[8]

Activities and Lifestyle Index

The questions below concern your daily activities. The few minutes you spend answering these questions can provide a more complete picture of how a medical condition may affect your life, adding to information from standard medical tests such as blood tests and x-rays. Please try to answer each question, even if you do not think it is related to you or any condition you may have. Please answer exactly as you think or feel, as there are no right and wrong answers.

Please check (√) the ONE best answer for your abilities.

YOUR NAME
TODAY'S DATE   TIME OF DAY   A.M. / P.M.

AT THIS MOMENT, are you able to:	Without ANY Difficulty	With SOME Difficulty	With MUCH Difficulty	UNABLE To Do
a. Dress yourself, including tying shoelaces and doing buttons?	_____	_____	_____	_____
b. Get in and out of bed?	_____	_____	_____	_____
c. Lift a full cup or glass to your mouth?	_____	_____	_____	_____
d. Walk outdoors on flat ground?	_____	_____	_____	_____
e. Wash and dry your entire body?	_____	_____	_____	_____
f. Bend down to pick up clothing from the floor?	_____	_____	_____	_____
g. Turn regular faucets on and off?	_____	_____	_____	_____
h. Get in and out of a car?	_____	_____	_____	_____

How SATISFIED Are You With Your Ability To:	VERY Satisfied	SOMEWHAT Satisfied	SOMEWHAT Dissatisfied	VERY Dissatisfied
a. Dress yourself, including tying shoelaces and doing buttons?	_____	_____	_____	_____
b. Get in and out of bed?	_____	_____	_____	_____
c. Lift a full cup or glass to your mouth?	_____	_____	_____	_____
d. Walk outdoors on flat ground?	_____	_____	_____	_____
e. Wash and dry your entire body?	_____	_____	_____	_____
f. Bend down to pick up clothing from the floor?	_____	_____	_____	_____
g. Turn regular faucets on and off?	_____	_____	_____	_____
h. Get in and out of a car?	_____	_____	_____	_____

• **How do you feel TODAY compared to most days during the past week?**
Please check (√) only one.
____ Much better **today** than most days
____ Better **today** than most days
____ The same **today** as most days
____ Worse **today** than most days
____ Much worse **today** than most days

• **Which of the following best describes you TODAY?**
Please check (√) only one.
____ I can do everything I want to do.
____ I can do most of the things I want to do, but have some limitations.
____ I can do some, but not all, of the things I want to do, and I have many limitations.
____ I can do hardly any of the things I want to do.

How Often Is It Painful For You To:	Never	Sometimes	Most Of The Time	Always
a. Dress yourself, including tying shoelaces and doing buttons?				
b. Get in and out of bed?				
c. Lift a full cup or glass to your mouth?				
d. Walk outdoors on flat ground?				
e. Wash and dry your entire body?				
f. Bend down to pick up clothing from the floor?				
g. Turn regular faucets on and off?				
h. Get in and out of a car?				

• **How Much Pain Have You Had Because Of Your Condition IN THE PAST WEEK?**

Place a mark on the line below to indicate how severe your pain has been:

NO PAIN ├───┤ PAIN AS BAD AS IT COULD BE

This section is concerned with your attitudes toward how you see yourself dealing with your condition. Each item is a belief with which you may: 1) STRONGLY DISAGREE, 2) DISAGREE, 3) DO NOT AGREE OR DISAGREE, 4) AGREE, or 5) STRONGLY AGREE. Circle the number beside each statement that best describes how you feel about the statement. Since these questions are a measure of your personal beliefs, there are no right or wrong answers.

	STRONGLY DISAGREE	DISAGREE	DO NOT AGREE OR DISAGREE	AGREE	STRONGLY AGREE
1. My condition is controlling my life.	1	2	3	4	5
2. Managing my condition is largely my own responsibility.	1	2	3	4	5
3. I can reduce my pain by staying calm and relaxed.	1	2	3	4	5
4. Too often, my pain just seems to hit me from out of the blue.	1	2	3	4	5
5. If I do all the right things, I can successfully manage my condition.	1	2	3	4	5
6. I can do a lot of things myself to cope with my condition.	1	2	3	4	5
7. When it comes to managing my condition, I feel I can only do what my doctor tells me to do.	1	2	3	4	5
8. When I manage my personal life well, my condition does not flare up as much.	1	2	3	4	5
9. I have considerable ability to control my pain.	1	2	3	4	5
10. I would feel helpless if I couldn't rely on other people for help with my condition.	1	2	3	4	5
11. Usually, I can tell when my condition will flare up.	1	2	3	4	5
12. No matter what I do, or how hard I try, I just can't seem to get relief from my pain.	1	2	3	4	5
13. I am coping effectively with my condition.	1	2	3	4	5
14. It seems as though fate and other factors beyond my control affect my condition.	1	2	3	4	5
15. I want to learn as much as I can about my condition.	1	2	3	4	5

Chapter 19

MANAGEMENT OF ACUTE AND CHRONIC PAIN

Nicolas E. Walsh, Daniel Dumitru, John C. King, and Somayaji Ramamurthy

GENERAL OVERVIEW

Pain is purely subjective, difficult to define, and often difficult to describe or interpret. It is currently defined as an unpleasant sensory and emotional response to a stimulus associated with actual or potential tissue damage.[5,25] However, pain has never been shown to be a simple function of the amount of physical injury; it is extensively influenced by anxiety, depression, expectation, and other psychological variables. It is a multifaceted experience, an interweaving of the physical characteristics of the stimulus with the motivational, affective, and cognitive functions of the individual. The result is behavior based upon an interpretation of the event, influenced by present and past experiences.

Acute pain is a biological symptom of an apparent nociceptive stimulus, such as tissue damage due to disease or trauma. The pain may be highly localized and may radiate. It is generally sharp and lasts only as long as the tissue pathology itself persists. Acute pain is generally self-limiting, and as the nociceptive stimulus lessens, the pain decreases. Acute pain usually lasts less than three months.[23] If it is not effectively treated, it may progress to a chronic form.

Chronic pain is a disease process. It is defined as pain lasting longer than the usual course of an acute disease or injury, and hence differs significantly from acute pain. The pain may be associated with chronic pathology or may persist after recovery from a disease or injury. As with acute pain, treatable chronic pain due to organic disease is managed by effectively treating the underlying disorder. Chronic pain is often poorly localized and tends to be dull, aching, and constant. The associated signs of autonomic nervous system response may be absent, and the patient may appear exhausted, listless, depressed, and withdrawn.

Proper management of pain requires an understanding of its complexity and a knowledge of the non-neurological factors that determine its individual

Table 1. Differentiating features of acute and chronic pain.

Acute pain	Chronic pain
Pain is a biological symptom	Pain is a disease
Short duration	Long duration (at least 6 months)

Therapy:
  Narcotics indicated
  Surgery very effective
	Therapy:
	  Multimodal
	  Narcotics, non-narcotics, analgesics, antidepressants
	  Surgery less effective
	  Active patient participation essential

Pain with anxiety	Pain with depression
Pathology predicts outcome	Psychological factors most predictive of outcome
Diagnosis relatively easy	Diagnosis relatively complex
Goal = complete recovery	Goal = functional recovery

expression (Table 1). Treatment of pain with physical modalities is as ancient as the history of man, but the use of interdisciplinary rehabilitation techniques has gained acceptance only within the last few decades.

Pain is the most frequent complaint of patients seeking medical attention. It is also the most common disease symptom and the primary reason people consume medication. Individuals complaining of pain should be examined to discover the anatomical location of pain, derangement of mechanical structures, and underlying pathological conditions. A careful history and physical examination are important to reach a diagnosis. Laboratory tests and x-rays may be necessary, but can have limited diagnostic value.

The spine and extremities contain innumerable pain-sensitive nerve endings, i.e., nerve endings which when adequately stimulated initiate streams of nerve impulses which are interpreted as pain when they come to consciousness. Certain tissues contain especially high concentrations of pain-sensitive nerve endings: nerves, blood vessels, muscles, ligaments, joints, and especially the periosteum. Pain may result from irritation, injury, inflammation, or infection of any of these tissues.[17] Conditions causing pain in the torso and extremities are those of neurogenic, musculoskeletal, referred, and autonomic origin (Table 2).

PAIN OF NEUROGENIC ORIGIN

Neurogenic pain in the back and extremities is commonly due to spinal cord/nerve root compression, neuritis, peripheral nerve compression, peripheral neuropathy, or spinal cord injury.

Table 2. Common origins and types of torso and extremity pain.

Neurogenic Pain	*Musculoskeletal Pain*
Spinal cord compression	Degenerative joint disease
Nerve root compression	Tendonitis and bursitis
Neuritis	Cervical spondylosis
Peripheral nerve compression	Degenerative disk disease
Peripheral neuropathy	Rheumatoid arthritis
Torticollis	Fracture
Herpetic neuralgia	Neoplasm
Myelopathy	Osteomyelitis
Neoplasm	Acute strain
Meningitis	Myofascial pain
Neuroma	Fibromyalgia
Referred Pain	*Autonomic Dysreflexic Pain*
Cardiac	Reflex sympathetic dystrophy
Neoplasm	Causalgia
Myofascial pain	
Viscera	

Pain due to Spinal Cord/Nerve Root Compression

Compression at the cervical level characteristically produces spinal and radicular signs in the upper limbs, associated with long tract signs in the lower extremities. Compression at the lumbar level characteristically produces radicular signs in the lower limbs. There is loss of power and bulk in affected muscles of the shoulder/pelvic girdle and extremity.

Management. A careful history and a physical examination are essential for effective physiological treatment of pain. The examination should ascertain the extent of the pathology and the mechanism of pain. In the acute injury, radiographs should be carefully reviewed for fracture, subluxation, or dislocation. Once fracture or dislocation has been ruled out, most patients should be treated conservatively. The specific management of intraspinal nerve root or cord compression depends on the suspected diagnosis, severity of symptoms, and the extent of neurological involvement.

Patients who should be treated conservatively are those with acute localized pain in the spinal or paraspinal region with or without peripheral radicular radiation. These individuals do not have neurological deficits indicative of spinal cord or severe nerve root compression. The most likely diagnosis is an acute intervertebral disk protrusion, and, with time, complete recovery can usually be anticipated.

Conservative management of acute disk herniation most commonly consists of rest and the use of an orthosis to minimize spinal movements. It can be beneficial to keep the muscles relaxed during the acute stage, for which cyclobenzaprine and diazepam may be useful. Nonsteroidal anti-inflammatory drugs (NSAIDs), in addition to decreasing the inflammation, are likely to reduce the pain and swelling. Muscle spasm associated with acute disk herniation may also be reduced by ice massage or spray of a vapocoolant such as ethyl chloride or fluorimethane. Cervical traction may be applied in the hospital or at home. Intermittent cervical traction is utilized to distract the posterior elements of the spinal column and may relieve pressure on impinged nerve roots. Traction is applied for 15–20 minutes per treatment, with a heating modality (usually hot pack) used prior to the treatment to promote relaxation of the neck muscles. Intermittent cervical traction usually starts on normal adult females at 10–20 pounds and normal adult males at 15–25 pounds. The amount of traction is increased 2–5 pounds every treatment or every other treatment until the desired therapeutic range of 35–50 pounds is reached. The force of the traction should pull the neck into mild anterior flexion. Treatments are normally carried out a minimum of three times a week for a period of two to three weeks. Home traction programs utilize constant weight and normally start with five pounds, increasing by one to five pounds daily or every other day. Most patients show response between 20 and 30 pounds, although some patients require as much as 35–50 pounds. In both intermittent and static traction the patient is ideally in the supine position. A great deal of caution should be used with cervical traction in patients with displaced cervical vertebrae, lytic lesions of the cervical spine, rheumatoid arthritis, or severe stenotic disease of the carotid or vertebral arteries. Heat followed by gentle limbering movements of the spine and extremity may also reduce pain and muscle spasm.

If symptoms persist despite conservative treatment, an epidural steroid injection should be considered. Methyl prednisolone (Depo-Medrol) 80 mg or triamcinolone 25–50 mg is injected at the level of the disk herniation. Improvement is likely to be seen in 24–48 hours. If there is improvement, no further epidural injections are given. If improvement is partial or negligible after 10–14 days, a second injection of steroid is given. Two to five milliliters of 1% lidocaine or 0.5% bupivacaine may be injected before or during steroid injection to confirm the correct placement of the drugs in the epidural space. If two injections of steroid placed epidurally do not produce any significant improvement, further injections are unlikely to be useful. Alternately, there is no rationale for giving a series of injections if the patient is pain free after the first injection. If neurological deficits and pain continue or worsen despite appropriate conservative treatment, surgical treatment should be considered.

Acute pain can be accompanied by signs of moderate sensory or motor deficit in a root distribution. Such signs are represented by some loss of strength, paresthesia, and mild sensory impairment or loss of muscle stretch reflexes. If these signs worsen or do not subside after a trial of conservative treatment, the patient should be hospitalized to ensure immobilization and rest and for further diagnostic investigations. Epidural steroids or chemonucleolysis have been used at this stage to halt the progress of the nerve compression.

Even if the patient's symptoms completely subside with any of the modalities, he or she should be given appropriate exercises to stretch and strengthen the muscles. Instruction in appropriate body mechanics and continued observation are required to evaluate the precipitating factors and prevent recurrence.

Surgical decompression is indicated for patients showing signs of spinal cord compression. It is also advisable for nerve root compression with intractable or severe progressive pain or signs of severe neurological deficit. If there are no contraindications to surgery, myelography/CT scan/MRI should be performed to establish a diagnosis and determine the site and extent of compression. If indicated, operative treatment should soon follow.

Patients in whom spinal cord compression develops rapidly require prompt investigation and surgical decompression. Impaired bladder or rectal control constitutes an emergency. Diagnostic investigations usually include plain films of the spine and an emergency myelogram/CT scan/MRI. In the course of these investigations, patients should be kept fasting to allow the immediate institution of anesthesia if surgical intervention is required.

The physical therapy treatment plan depends on past medical intervention, extent of the lesion, and stage of recovery. During the acute stage, the patient may be treated with bed rest and immobilization. Ice massage and transcutaneous electrical nerve stimulation (TENS) may also be utilized. Ice massage is applied for an average of 5–10 minutes, depending upon the size of the area to be treated. Routinely, the area is approximately 50–100 square centimeters and is draped with towels on all sides. The ice is moved rapidly over this area, resulting in a cold burning sensation that is usually uncomfortable for about one minute. The area will then become numb, at which time deep massage utilizing the ice may begin, continuing for 8–15 minutes. Cold should be used with caution over areas of reduced sensation or poor circulation. In addition, ice massage should be avoided in patients with sensitivity to cold, as in Raynaud's phenomenon, cryoglobulinemia, paroxysmal cold hemoglobinuria, or marked pain to cold. Cold reduces pain, relaxes muscles, and minimizes spasticity. In addition, the immune response in local edema is reduced, as are regional blood flow, collagen extensibility, and metabolic rate.

TENS units usually have variable current amplitude, pulse width, and pulse rate. The pulse rate should be preset between 70–150 pulses per second, pulse width should be less than 130 microseconds, and amplitude should be set at a level between first sensation and that which can no longer be tolerated by the patient. It is routine to allow the patient to vary the amplitude to a comfortable level. Electrode placement is highly variable; however, an initial placement with the electrodes in a crisscross pattern over the area of pain often proves most optimal. TENS units are absolutely contraindicated for use over demand cardiac pacemakers, the carotid sinus, phrenic nerve pacemakers, implantable pumps, or a pregnant uterus, or when the patient is on electronic life-support equipment.

In the subacute period, the patient is started on an exercise program suited to the level and direction of the protrusion. Aggressive physical therapy may begin in the chronic stage; if the patient is still using a cervical collar for pain relief, wearing time is gradually reduced. The cervical collar is fitted with the neck in slight flexion and usually prescribed for 7–14 days. Immobilization beyond the early acute stage will increase muscle weakness, promote poor postural habits, and lead to tightening of soft tissue structures. Such contractures may become a source of significant pain. Therapeutic intervention includes flexion-extension-rotation, strengthening, and mobilization exercises.

Pain due to Neuritis

Brachial Plexalgia

The brachial plexus may be injured by traction, penetrating wounds, or compression. Acute nontraumatic brachial plexus neuropathy is a disorder of unknown cause. Antecedent needle injections into shoulder muscles, intercurrent infections, and an allergic basis have been suggested as possible etiologic factors. Typically this disorder begins with aching pain in the lateral aspect of the shoulder or, less often, in the region of the elbow or arm. Muscle weakness develops within a few hours or days, and atrophy follows; sensory loss is usually minimal and is restricted to a small patch in the cutaneous distribution of the axillar nerve. The upper brachial plexus is affected more commonly than the lower, and therefore the weakness and atrophy are more often located in the region of the shoulder. In mild cases, improvement begins in a few weeks and clinical recovery is complete within months. More characteristically, improvement does not begin for several months and may not be complete for years. Nevertheless, eventual complete or almost complete recovery is likely. Rarely, as one side improves, the other brachial plexus becomes affected. Careful EMG examination may reveal more extensive involvement of nerves than was expected from the clinical examination. The cerebrospinal fluid is usually normal. There is no known treatment.

Herpetic Neuralgia

Herpes zoster (shingles) is a reactivation of latent varicella (chickenpox) virus. The viral inflammation of the dorsal nerve root and ganglion causes cutaneous vesicle formation, which is often accompanied by pain in a radicular distribution. This pain may vary from a light burning sensation to a deep visceral pain and can be intermittent or constant. During the acute stage, NSAIDs and sympathetic blocks provide excellent pain relief. The majority of patients recover from the acute episode in about two weeks without sequelae. In patients under 40, it is uncommon for any pain to continue after the vesicles heal. In approximately 30% of patients over 40, the pain may last for months or years, and 50% or more of patients over 60 are likely to develop post-herpetic neuralgia.

Management. Multiple reports indicate that post-herpetic neuralgia may be prevented if the patient is treated with a sympathetic block within one month of onset.[27] Post-herpetic neuralgia is, thus, a preventable syndrome, but a difficult problem to treat once established. A significant number of patients will experience pain relief with sympathetic blocks. If the syndrome is allowed to progress untreated for three months to a year, its management becomes more difficult.[29]

The most effective treatment for the management of established post-herpetic neuralgia is the use of a tricyclic antidepressant such as amitriptyline (Elavil) in small doses.[26] Most patients obtain pain relief with 25 mg to 75 mg administered at bedtime. If the patient does not get complete pain relief with administration of tricyclics alone, fluphenazine (Prolixin) may be added, beginning with 1 mg at bedtime and progressing as needed to a maximum dosage of 1 mg three times a day. Anticonvulsants, such as Dilantin, have also been administered with varying results.[36] Success in achieving pain relief using subcutaneous infiltration of local anesthetic and triamcinolone (two injections per week for two weeks) has been reported.[7] TENS is beneficial in some patients, particularly when other techniques have given partial relief. Peripheral nerve blocks and destructive neurosurgical procedures have not proven useful in treating established post-herpetic neuralgia.

Pain due to Entrapment of Peripheral Nerves

The peripheral nerve trunks of the limbs are particularly prone to compression and entrapment, although any nerve passing over a rigid promontory or through a bony canal or tight fascial plane is vulnerable. A common example is carpal tunnel syndrome in patients who use their wrists excessively in activities such as knitting or typing. Sites of compression for the median nerve include the pronator teres muscle and the carpal tunnel ligament; for the ulnar nerve, the elbow, wrist, pisohamate tunnel, palm, and metacarpal heads; and for the radial nerve, the axilla, posterior aspect of the humerus, the supinator muscle, and the radial aspect of the distal forearm. The most common entrapment neuropathies of the upper extremity are carpal tunnel syndrome, ulnar nerve palsy, and neuroma/scar pain.

Median Nerve

In carpal tunnel syndrome, the median nerve is compressed as it passes through the canal formed by the carpal bones and ligament. Some cases are idiopathic, and in these cases surgeons report a flattening of the median nerve just distal to the crease of the wrist and either thickening of the ligament or, more commonly, noninflammatory thickening of the flexor tendons. The median nerve may be compressed within the carpal tunnel by a ganglion or by degenerative joint and synovial changes from rheumatoid arthritis, myxedema, or acromegaly. It should be noted that any underlying process that causes soft tissue swelling (endocrine disorders, pregnancy, collagen vascular disease, or others) is likely to make patients more susceptible to compression and nerve entrapment.

Carpal tunnel syndrome principally affects women. Pricking numbness and pain in the fingers and hands, occurring especially during the night and relieved by changing the position of the hands (shaking them), are characteristic. It is uncommon for patients to localize the numbness to the exact cutaneous distribution of the median nerve. Furthermore, the aching discomfort that may accompany the numbness can extend up the arm. Atrophy of the muscles innervated by the median nerve (for example, the thenar muscles) is a late sign. In many cases it is possible to reproduce the painful numbness by holding the wrist in extreme flexion (Phalen's sign). Also, a burst of digital tingling may occur when the skin over the nerve at the wrist is percussed (Tinel's sign). There may be sensory loss in the distribution of the median nerve, although more frequently none is detected.

Management. Since carpal tunnel syndrome may be brought on by an excess of gardening, ironing, sewing, crocheting, or similar activity, improvement may follow the discontinuation of these activities. Immobilization of the wrist with a volar splint of the forearm and hand may give relief. Injections of corticosteroid preparations beneath the carpal ligament sometimes help. Treatment for an associated disease (myxedema, rheumatoid arthritis, acromegaly) may result in an improvement. However, in most instances the treatment of choice is surgical resection of the carpal ligament, which usually provides almost immediate relief.

Ulnar Nerve

The ulnar nerve may be injured at the elbow, especially in persons with a shallow ulnar groove, those who rest their weight on the elbows excessively, or those who are cachectic and immobilized. Contrary to the findings in carpal tunnel syndrome, muscle weakness and atrophy characteristically predominate over sensory symptoms and signs, possibly because the ulnar nerve at the elbow has relatively fewer sensory fibers than the median nerve at the wrist. The patient notices atrophy of the first dorsal interosseous muscle or difficulty in performing fine manipulations. There may be numbness of the small finger, the ulnar half of the proximal and middle phalanges of the ring finger, and the ulnar border of the hand.

Management.   Treatment consists of preventing further injury. A doughnut-shaped cushion for the elbow may be helpful. Mobilizing and transplanting the nerve to a position in front of the medial epicondyle may prevent further progression of the disorder.

Neuroma/Scar Pain

Surgery may result in a neuroma or entrapment of branches of the nerve by scar tissue, which may produce disabling pain. Intraneural fibrosis or entrapment restricts the nerve and can reduce vascularity at the site of injury. The regenerating end becomes sensitive to pressure and other manipulation. Neuromas should be considered when numbness or burning is in the distribution of a specific nerve and when pain is produced by neuroma palpation. Diagnosis may be established if infiltrating the scar or neuroma with local anesthetic results in complete pain relief.[28]

Management.   Repeat injection of local anesthetic may produce significant pain relief, especially if followed by appropriate physical therapy. The treatment course usually involves ultrasound followed by stretching or deep massage of the scar. This multimodal therapy has provided permanent or extended pain relief (longer than six months) in many patients. When the local anesthetics do not provide prolonged relief, other interventions should be considered. Cryoanalgesia using a cryoprobe to freeze the neuroma for one minute at $-20°C$ has been used with success. The advantage of using a cryoprobe is that it provides a physical method of blocking the nerve without producing further neuromas or neuritis. Neurolytic agents such as phenol or alcohol have also been used to relieve neuroma and scar pain. However, incomplete blockage with these anesthetics can result in neuritis, producing severe pain.[30] Neurolytic techniques should be used only after repeated injections of local anesthetics produce consistent pain relief proportional to the local anesthetics' duration of action. Historically, surgical revision of the scar was often considered, but it is not very effective unless significant nerve entrapment is present and the scar can be stretched out. Electrical stimulation of the peripheral nerve proximal to the site of injury has been reported to be effective.[39]

Cancer Pain

Pain is one of the greatest fears and a major source of morbidity for patients with cancer. Cancer pain is the result of tumor intrusion into normal tissue, causing irritation of pain-transmitting nerve endings by traction or compression. These pain-transmitting nerve terminals are especially abundant in periosteum, perineurium, endosteum (variably), fascia, ligaments, and capsules of organs. Relief from the mechanical stimulation of these endings relieves pain. Cancer cells themselves do not initiate pain except by these mechanical means. Therefore, for relief of pain, attention should be devoted to identifying and relieving the mechanical cause. Clinical experience suggests that if the mechanical irritation cannot be relieved adequately by therapeutic stretching, massage, exercise, orthotics, and thermotherapy, as appropriate to the situation, relief from cancer pain may require a multi-disciplinary approach including multiple modalities, appropriate analgesic drugs, neurosurgical and anesthetic procedures, psychological intervention, and supportive care. Nonnarcotic, narcotic, and adjuvant analgesic drugs are the primary therapy for patients with cancer pain. Anesthetic, physiatric, behavioral, and occasionally neurosurgical approaches are commonly used with pharmacological intervention. Noninvasive measures in the treatment of cancer pain generally have a low risk of complications, are less costly than surgical interventions, and produce minimal serious side effects. These modalities may be used singly for mild pain and are normally used in combination with drug therapy for moderate or severe pain. Commonly used noninvasive measures include cutaneous stimulation, thermal modalities, and behavioral intervention.[4] Narcotic analgesics are the main drugs of choice for relief of truly intractable pain due to cancer. This combination of treatment is estimated to provide adequate pain relief in at least 90% of cancer patients with pain.[9,20]

The World Health Organization has recommended a systematic approach to the selection of pharmacological agents for treating patients with cancer pain (Table 3).[41] Their protocol is based on the premise that doctors and health care professionals should have the knowledge to use a few simple drugs well. A three-step analgesic ladder is the scheme used for analgesic selection and is summarized as follows: (1) Those patients who have mild to moderate pain should be initially treated with a nonopioid analgesic such as aspirin or one of the other nonsteroidal anti-inflammatory drugs and an adjuvant analgesic if indicated. (2) Patients who have moderate to severe pain or are not able to achieve adequate relief with step 1 should be started on a weak oral opioid, such as codeine, along with a nonopioid and an adjuvant analgesic if indicated. (3) Patients who have very severe pain or do not achieve adequate relief on the step 2 regime should be treated with a potent opioid such as morphine, with or without a nonopioid, or with an adjuvant analgesic if indicated.

Narcotic analgesics are the drug of choice for relief of intractable pain due to cancer.[2] All clinically useful narcotics produce similar side effects in equianalgesic doses. Of the side effects reported, the most common are respiratory depression, constipation, nausea, and vomiting. There are sig-

Table 3. Clinical classification of cancer pain intensity.

Intensity	Fail to respond to:	Relieved by:
'Mild' 1–3		Non-narcotic analgesics; Acetaminophen NSAIDs (ASA, ibuprofen, naproxen, tolmetin, sulindac)
'Moderate' 4–6	Non-narcotic analgesics	Weak narcotic analgesics:[a] Codeine Oxycodone Combination with ASA/ acetaminophen
'Severe' 7–10[b]	Weak narcotic analgesics	Potent narcotic analgesics Morphine Hydromorphone Meperidine Methadone

[a]Although narcotics vary in potency, they are equal in efficacy; that is, by increasing the dose of a less potent narcotic one can achieve the same analgesic effect produced by the more potent narcotic.
[b]The use of a combination of non-narcotic and narcotic drugs results in improved pain relief without increasing narcotic doses.
Note: NSAID = nonsteroidal anti-inflammatory drug; ASA = acetylsalicylic acid.

nificant differences in their action time, equianalgesic dose, and parenteral/oral ratio (Table 4). Dependence and addiction have not been major problems in patients who receive appropriately dosed narcotic analgesics for chronic severe cancer pain.[25] The patient does not suffer psychological dependence or the acute cravings of the classical drug addict. Variations in doses are indicated as the disease progresses or remits, but a continual increase in the dose due to tolerance is seldom required.[15]

Morphine is the prototype of the narcotic drugs. It is prescribed by many clinicians. Pain relief is often obtained by titrating the dose to the patient's needs. Previously, the major limitation of morphine was an observed duration of action of four hours or less. Sustained-release oral morphine (MS Contin/Roxanal SR) has been used successfully with 12- and 8-hour dosing schedules in patients with advanced cancer.[20]

There is no pharmacological rationale or empirical evidence for administering narcotic elixirs, such as Brompton's cocktail, in the management of cancer pain.[38] The analgesic drug cocktail neither decreases toxicity nor potentiates pain relief.

Medications for cancer pain should be administered orally on a regular basis, with the interval between doses based on the duration of the analgesic effect for the patient. The object is to titrate the level of analgesic to an optimal dose that prevents the recurrence of pain. It is recommended to give medications orally whenever possible because this method facilitates ambulatory care, allows greater independence, and does not represent he-

Table 4. Narcotic medications.

Drug	Equianalgesic dosage (mg)[a]				Action times			
	IM	PO	IV	Rectal	Half-life (h)	Duration (h)	Onset (min)	Peak (min)
Butorphanol (Stadol)	2		1			3–4	10	30–60
Codeine	130	200			3	4–6	15–30	60–120
Fentanyl (Innovar)	0.1					1–2	5–15	30
Hydromorphone (Dilaudid)	1.5	7.5	1			2–4	15–30	30–90
Levorphanol (Levo-Dromoran)	2	4	1			4–5	60	60–90
Meperidine (Demerol)	75	300	50		3–4	2–4	10–15	30–60
Methadone (Dolophine)	10	20[b]	5			6–8	10–15	60–120
Morphine	10	30[b]	5			2–4	20	30–90
Sustained release oral morphine	10	30[b]				8–12		
Nalbuphine (Nubain)	10		5			3–6	10–15	30–60
Oxycodone hydrochloride (Numorpham)	15	30				4–5	10–15	30–60
Oxymorphone hydrochloride (Numorpham)	1		0.5	10		4–5	5–10	30–90
Pentazocine (Talwin)	60	180			2–3	2–3	10–15	30–60
Propoxyphene (Darvon)		300				4–6	15–60	120–180

[a]Equal in analgesia to 10 mg of morphine administered subcutaneously or intramuscularly.
[b]For chronic dosing only. For single dosing use 60 mg.
Note: IM = intramuscular; PO = oral; IV = intravenous.

roic intervention to the patient. In general, it is better for the initial dosage of medication to be too high rather than too low. Starting suboptimally and titrating upward results in the patient experiencing anxiety due to a lack of adequate analgesia. The "as needed," or PRN, schedule **does not** have a place in the control of chronic cancer pain. The PRN schedule results in operant conditioning, craving, a sense of dependence, and anxiety about the drug wearing off. In cancer pain management, the drugs with a longer duration of action are usually preferred. It is important to remember that patients usually accept two to three tablets per administration in conjunction with additional medications. More than four tablets per administration are generally not acceptable. An alternative is to increase the potency of the tablet. There is considerable patient-to-patient variation with respect to an effective analgesic dosage. It is important to remember that the maximum or recommended dosages of narcotic medications were derived mainly from postoperative parenteral single-dose studies and are not applicable to administration by mouth in the long-term treatment of pain in advanced cancer. Dependency and respiratory depression should not be feared since they are rarely a problem. The most serious side effects (i.e., constipation and nausea) should be prevented or treated. The pharmacological mechanism that makes oral narcotic drug therapy superior to parenteral administration is that the plasma level of the analgesic is maintained above the concentration necessary for analgesia over a longer period of time.

Adjuvant analgesic agents include several different categories of drugs, such as anticonvulsant agents, phenothiazines, butyrophenones, tricyclic antidepressants, antihistamines, amphetamines, steroids, and L-dopa. The effect of analgesic drugs is augmented by various adjuvants that act on mood. Such drugs may be used to increase the efficacy and reduce the dose of narcotic analgesics.[4,19] These medications produce pain analgesia in certain forms of cancer pain by mechanisms that are not clearly established but do not directly involve the opiate receptor system. While the analgesic effects of these drugs have been suggested in some controlled clinical trials, most usage is based on anecdotal data or clinical surveys.

In situations suggesting the need for neurolytic block, the patient's limb function must be evaluated. When the limb is functional and/or sensate, the use of a neurolytic block is not indicated to resolve the pain, as the sequelae include dysfunction or deafferentation pain. It is suggested that epidural narcotics be utilized as an alternative. Neurolytic blocks are not normally recommended for the management of nonmalignant pain.

During cancer patients' hospitalization, outpatient treatment, and everyday activities, it is essential that they maintain their functional skills, strength, and mobility. Progressive immobilization is an insidious aspect of this disease and is often iatrogenic. While radiation or chemotherapy may render a patient unable to perform activities one day, it is important that the patient consistently be evaluated and involved in active physical, occupational, corrective, and recreational therapy programs. The physiatrist may offer numerous means of combatting immobility and its morbidity.

Pain due to Peripheral Neuropathies

The most common painful neuropathies are the subacute sensory/motor neuropathies. The three most common of this group are diabetic neuropathy (distal symmetric neuropathy and diabetic amyotrophy), toxic neuropathies of heavy metals and industrial solvents, and nutritionally related neuropathies of alcohol, isoniazid, and vitamin deficiencies. Up to 60% of patients with diabetes eventually develop pain and paresthesias due to distal symmetrical neuropathy. While the symptoms are usually minimal, in some patients they are severe. Typically, the individual complains of burning or aching in the distal lower extremities. Diabetic ophthalmoplegia, acute mononeuropathy, and asymmetric mononeuritis multiplex are characterized by focal pain which may be severe. Pain due to alcoholic neuropathy and other nutritionally related neuropathies is often characterized by tingling dysesthesias or a burning sensation of the feet. This neuropathy is most likely caused by nutritional deficiencies. Similar pain may occur in association with eccentric diets and malnutrition. Diseases with ascending motor paralysis, such as Guillain-Barré syndrome, porphyria, and poliomyelitis, are associated with muscular-type pain.

Management.   Management of pain associated with these disorders is begun by treating the underlying disease. This requires removing offending toxins, treating heavy metal poisoning with kelating agents, correcting vitamin deficiencies, or maintaining control of diabetes.

There have been few placebo-controlled, double-blind, crossover studies concerning the effectiveness of medications in alleviating the pain of peripheral neuropathy. The pilot studies suggest that amitriptyline[22] and carbamazepine[14] are effective therapy for painful neuropathy. Pain due to alcoholic neuropathy is resolved after abstinence from alcohol, return to proper diet, and vitamin replacement. Symptoms may be alleviated by methylated lotions. Pain due to polyarteritis may resolve after corticosteroid treatment, whereas pain due to cryoglobulinemia may be relieved with plasmapheresis. Discomfort due to brachial neuritis and other self-limiting conditions resolves spontaneously in weeks to months, whereas pain secondary to diabetic neuropathies rarely disappears completely. Drugs that induce painful peripheral neuropathies include isoniazid (Laniazid) and hydralazine (Hydralyn), which cause a decrease in tissue levels of pyridoxal phosphate; and nitrofurantoin (Furadantin), which has neurotoxic effects. Pain in patients with ascending motor paralysis appears to be best relieved by narcotics.[31] The chronic relapsing polyneuropathies of porphyria, polyarteritis, and idiopathic polyneuritis may be reduced with plasmapheresis.

The patient with chronic painful peripheral neuropathy has many of the problems associated with chronic pain, including depression, inactivity, disuse syndrome, and significant alteration of lifestyle. Psychological intervention and physical therapy are important aspects of treatment for these patients. Conventional physical therapy modalities, TENS, and general conditioning programs are often helpful, as are psychological programs and other nonpharmacological methods of pain control.

Pain due to Central Nervous System Diseases

Pain may result from diseases of the central nervous system and altered central nervous system receptor fields following peripheral nerve injury.

Multiple Sclerosis

Multiple sclerosis is a chronic remitting and relapsing disease characterized by multiple foci of demyelination that are distributed randomly in the white matter of the central nervous system. Patients may present initially with paroxysmal lancinating and intense burning pain primarily affecting the face, shoulder region, or pelvic girdle. These painful paresthesias have been reported in 13–64% of patients with multiple sclerosis.[18] Pain of this nature has shown limited response to tricyclic antidepressants, carbamazepine (Tegretol), and phenytoin (Dilantin).

Thalamic Pain/Stroke Pain

Pain resulting from central lesions within the thalamus is often described as an agonizing burning pain on the side contralateral to that of the thalamic lesion. Overreaction to minimal cutaneous stimulation and aggravation by emotional stress and fatigue are characteristic findings. Sensory alteration is variable in these patients, and motor weakness is minimal. Information on thalamic pain syndrome is limited; multiple treatment regimes have been recommended on the basis of anecdotal reports.[21]

Lesions of central spinal thalamic tracts may result in pain distributed to the level of the tract involved. Any section of the spinal cord involving the spinal thalamic tract results in loss of pain and temperature perception on the contralateral side at a level below the injury. Tract pain is similar to thalamic pain, but is often less intense. The pain may be described as burning, pulling, or swelling.

Torticollis

Torticollis is a severe state of contraction of the sternocleidomastoid muscle. It is usually unilateral (but occasionally bilateral) and produces a tilting of the head to the affected side, with flexion of the neck and deviation of the head.

Management. The diverse variety of therapeutic approaches for torticollis underscores the lack of knowledge of its etiology. Surgical approaches have been advocated most often and include cervical rhizotomy, thalamotomy, dorsal column stimulation, and excision of the sternocleidomastoid muscle, all of which produce varying degrees of disability and generally a poor therapeutic result. Psychological approaches such as psychotherapy, hypnosis, behavior modification, and biofeedback have been advocated. Drug therapy with amantidine, haloperidol, and apomorphine have usually given poor and unreliable results. Thus, despite much investigation, spasmodic torticollis remains an essentially intractable and disabling condition of unknown or multiple causes.

Block of the spinal accessory nerve is helpful in evaluating the contribution of the trapezius and sternocleidomastoid muscles to torticollis. Frequently, other neck muscles are also involved, and a cervical plexus block may be necessary to relieve all the muscle spasm. Once the muscles are relaxed, the degree of fibrotic and bony changes may be evaluated. If the block of the accessory nerve results in significant improvement, repeated blocks followed by physical therapy to stretch affected muscles and strengthen the opposing muscles are likely to be helpful. The physical therapy program for torticollis is similar to that discussed in the section on pain of musculoskeletal origin in this chapter. Neurolytic block of the accessory nerve may be necessary to provide long-term relief. Psychological factors should be considered and treated concomitantly.

The physical therapy approach to a patient with the diagnosis of torticollis consists of postural activities, with maintenance of cervical function as the primary goal. Modalities incorporated in the treatment are ultrasound alone or in combination with electrical stimulation, vigorous soft tissue massage, manual stretching, passive to resistive range of motion exercises, relaxation techniques including biofeedback, and cervical mobilization. Patients should also be given a home program to ensure continuation of treatment and optimal achievement of goals.

Phantom Limb Pain

Phantom limb pain involves an amputated or totally denervated portion of the body. It has been suggested that the etiology of phantom limb pain is related to deafferentation of neurons and their spontaneous and evoked hyperexcitability. The pain is described as a continuous cramping, aching, or burning sensation with occasional superimposed electriclike exacerbations. Recent studies suggest that between 50% and 80% of amputees have phantom limb sensation and 5% to 15% have phantom limb pain.[33] The current data do not suggest a predisposition for phantom limb pain related to type of amputation or premorbid characteristics.

Management. Multiple modalities, adjuvant medications, and anesthetic and surgical procedures have been used in the treatment of phantom limb pain, with varying long-term success. Although at least 68 methods of treating phantom limb syndromes have been identified, successful treatment of persistent types is not commonly reported.[16,34] Transcutaneous nerve stimulation, tricyclic antidepressants, anticonvulsants, and chlorpromazine have each been used with varying success, as have chemical sympathectomy and neurosurgical procedures. Treatments yielding a temporary decrease in pain include analgesics, anesthetic procedures, residual limb desensitization, physical modalities, and sedative/hypnotic medication. One survey reported that treatments reducing residual limb problems also resulted in decreased phantom pain.[35] Therapeutic regimens have had less than a 30% long-term efficacy.

Phantom limb pain is reported more frequently in patients with residual limb pain. In the early evaluation of phantom limb pain, it is important to rule out residual limb pain due to a neuroma as the etiology of the pain complaints. Residual limb pain is present at the site of the extremity amputation. This sharp, often jabbing, pain is usually aggravated by pressure or by infection in the residual limb. Pain is often elicited by tapping over a neuroma in a transected nerve. The increased sensitivity of sprouts from cut peripheral nerves to noradrenaline and adrenaline may partially explain why emotional states such as stress or anxiety occasionally provoke attacks of phantom limb pain.

Pain due to Spinal Cord Injury

The precise etiology underlying pain in spinal cord injuries is not known, but recent evidence suggests that trauma-induced alterations of the pain pathways are primarily involved.[42] Hypersensitivity of the structures in the ascending pathway may play a role. Studies indicate that 50% of all spinal cord-injured patients have pain that is mild to moderate in severity; approximately 20% experience severe pain.[40] Patients describe their pain as having one or more of the following components: burning sensation in body parts below the injury, deep aching sensation over and around the site of injury, and radicular pain with lancinating characteristics. Burning pain in spinal cord-injured patients may be a variation of deafferentated pain and may result from loss of inhibitory or augmentation of excitatory influences. The most effective treatments for this type of pain include tricyclic antidepressants and neuroaugmentive techniques.[6]

Spinal fracture site pain results from an alteration of body mechanics, causing pain-sensitive structures to be stretched or compressed. This mechanical pain may be the result of vertebral endplate fractures, annulus fibrosus tears, or internal disk herniation following a spinal fracture.[24] Fracture site pain or mechanical pain is often exacerbated by activity. NSAIDs, trigger point injections, TENS, cognitive/behavioral techniques, and adjuvant medication may be helpful. Orthotics may also be used to decrease the mechanical stress and alleviate the underlying etiology.[8]

Radicular pain in these patients may be secondary to compression of nerve roots by a herniated nucleus pulposus, fracture fragment, or dislocated vertebra, or may be the result of traumatic arachnoiditis. This type of pain is most effectively treated with anticonvulsants, with TENS as a useful adjuvant.

PAIN OF MUSCULOSKELETAL ORIGIN

Musculoskeletal pain is often localized in specific areas of the torso and extremities as a result of the characteristics of the specific structures.

Pain due to Myofascial Pain Syndrome

Myofascial pain syndrome is commonly seen among patients being evaluated and treated for acute and chronic pain. It is characterized by pain originating from small circumscribed areas of local hyperirritability and myofascial structures, resulting in local and referred pain. The pain is aggravated by stretching the affected area, cooling, and compression, which often gives rise to a characteristic pattern of referred pain.[37] Although the exact pathophysiology of the trigger point phenomenon has not been identified, myofascial pain syndromes appear to be initiated by trauma, tension, inflammation, and other factors. The trigger point acts as a source of chronic nociception. The resultant muscle dysfunction and altered mechanics lead to the referred pain and associated phenomena. Myofascial pain may be of primary or secondary origin; hence, underlying factors must be evaluated.

This syndrome is much more common than radiculopathy or the other causes of spinal and extremity pain. However, before attributing a patient's symptoms to myofascial pain syndrome, it is extremely important to rule out other primary problems such as radiculopathy, disk disease, malignancies of the vertebrae, and referred pain stemming from visceral disease. Myofascial pain syndromes are characterized by the absence of neurological signs and the presence of trigger points. Typically, patients complain of neck or back pain, often radiating to the arm or leg. It may be associated with pain referred to different parts of the body. Trigger points may occur in any muscle or muscle group. They are commonly found in muscle groups that are routinely overstressed or those that do not undergo full contraction and relaxation cycles. In the upper body, the trigger points are often located in the sternocleidomastoid muscle, producing pain in the face, behind the eye, and in the neck; in the splenius capitis muscle, producing pain in the top of the head, suboccipital region, and the upper part of the neck; in the levator scapulae muscle, producing pain in the neck and shoulder region; and in the posterior cervical region, over the trapezius muscle. In the lower body they are located in the gluteus group, resulting in pain in the buttock, posterior leg, and calf; in the tensor fasciae latae, resulting in pain in the lateral leg; in the quadratus lumborum, resulting in pain in the paraspinals and buttock; and in the gastrocnemius muscles, resulting in pain in the calf and foot. The location of the trigger points in the individual muscles is fairly constant and is important to know. With experience, it is easy to locate these points and to feel subtle changes such as nodules, knots, or bands in the involved muscle. If an injection of local anesthetic relieves the pain, diagnosis of myofascial pain is confirmed.

Management. Trigger points are best located by deep palpation of the affected muscle, which elicits the pain both locally and in a referred zone. Trigger points are usually a sharply circumscribed spot of exquisite tenderness. When they are present, passive or active stretching of the affected muscle routinely increases pain. The muscle in the immediate vicinity of the trigger point is often described as ropy, tense, or having a palpable band. Compared with normal muscle under equivalent pressure, the trigger point region displays isolated bands and increased tenderness and produces referred pain. The most reliable method of treating trigger points consists of routine, regular stretching to restore the normal resting length of the muscle. Methods to interrupt the pain cycle include injection or needle stimulation of the hypersensitive trigger points.[19]

Injection and stretching of the involved muscle is very effective treatment of myofascial pain in the acute stage. The muscle is injected with a local anesthetic and steroid. The choice of local anesthetic is not crucial, since injection of saline or any local anesthetic produces equally good results. It is important to reproduce the patient's pain by injecting right into the band or the nodule. Injection of a short-acting local anesthetic such as 1% lidocaine or mepivacaine is less painful than injection of 0.5% bupivacaine. Physicians prefer to use mixtures containing either 0.5% bupivacaine and 2% lidocaine or 0.5% bupivacaine and 0.5% etidocaine. After the injection, the patient is advised to keep the muscle in a relaxed state for four days. If this is not done, muscle spasms are likely to recur. The patient is advised not to drive, since driving puts excessive strain on the neck and back muscles. Alternate methods of relieving the pain include coolant sprays, relaxation therapy, and pressure techniques.

After the pain cycle is interrupted, treatment is directed toward restoring the normal resting muscle length through a regular program of stretching the involved muscle groups. Physical modalities including heat, cold, and correction of poor body mechanics may help accomplish this goal. Application of heat over the injected area and limbering exercises can be beneficial but are not sufficient by themselves, since many patients who develop myofascial pain are tense individuals. By habit, they tense up their muscles anytime they experience stress. Self-hypnosis relaxation therapy and biofeedback are excellent adjuncts to other modalities among such patients. Psychological intervention may be necessary if long-standing stress and tension are the underlying cause of the problem.

A long-term home modality, stretching, and aerobic conditioning program is essential in the management of patients with myofascial pain. Attention to proper body mechanics and stress reduction in daily routines significantly improves outcome.

Pain due to Facet Joint Syndrome

Pain arising from the facet joint may mimic the symptoms of radiculopathy. If objective evidence of nerve root involvement is absent, tenderness over the affected facet can usually be identified and the patient's symptoms reproduced. During the acute stage, pain may be associated with significant muscle spasm and also restricted movement of the cervical spine.

Management.   Conservative measures are the same as those outlined for the management of myofascial pain, even though some clinicians prefer manipulation of the cervical spine in order to reduce the facet displacement.

Affected patients may respond very well to a local anesthetic-steroid mixture, such as 0.5% bupivacaine with 2 mg/ml of triamcinolone, 2–4 ml of which is injected over the facet joint. This relieves acute symptoms and is useful even in alleviating chronic facet pain. More than one injection is sometimes necessary.

Good results have been reported after injection of a local anesthetic-steroid mixture into the facet joint itself. Since the facet joint space is a potential space, it is difficult to identify needle placement in the joint. Facet joint pain may also be relieved by denervating the joint or blocking the nerve that supplies it. The joint is innervated by a nerve coming from the corresponding nerve root and another branch from one level above. For example, in order to block the C5–6 facet joint, facet nerves at the C5–6 and C4–5 levels must be blocked. This is accomplished by placing a needle at the junction of the superior facet and the transverse process, the point where the nerve curves around the superior facet to innervate the joint. Here it may be stimulated to reproduce the pain. If injection of a local anesthetic relieves the symptoms, the nerve may be blocked by a local anesthetic, radiofrequency lesion, cryoprobe, or 0.5 ml of 6% phenol.

Pain due to Muscle Strain

A motor vehicle accident may initiate a sequence of events affecting the cervical spine and its joints, ligaments, nerves, blood vessels, and musculature. Abrupt hyperextension or hyperflexion of the neck are the common mechanisms of injury. The impact of a collision abruptly propels the body in a linear horizontal direction. Initially the head remains stationary, stretching ligaments and muscles in one direction, then it abruptly moves in the opposite direction. This abrupt "whiplash" movement occurs before the neck muscles can relax to permit the motion. In a rear-end impact the head moves abruptly backward, causing acute hyperextension of the cervical spine and provoking acute stretch reflex of the neck flexors. A head-on collision causes the opposite injury.

A detailed description of the accident—including direction of impact, awareness of the impending collision, and the direction in which the patient was facing at the moment of impact—is helpful in determining what tissues are affected. The physical examination and diagnostic workup are directed toward localizing the injury.

Management.   Owing to the significant variation in the type of trauma, severity of injury, and clinical presentation, the treatment program must be highly individualized. Management focuses on alleviating symptoms in the acute stage and is limited by injury to spinal cord or nerve roots and fracture dislocation of the cervical spine. Treatment in the acute stage frequently involves immobilization of the neck with a cervical orthosis, most often a soft, contoured collar that holds the neck in a comfortable neutral position. A brief course of appropriate analgesic medication is often required. Modalities that are usually beneficial in treating acute cervical pain are traction, cryotherapy, heat therapy, electrical stimulation, and massage. Traction may be positional, manual or mechanical, and static or intermittent. Proper amounts of cervical flexion may decrease pain by opening the intervertebral joint spaces and facet joints. Patients usually tolerate intermittent traction better, the weight being increased as the patient's tolerance increases. The recent literature suggests variable amounts of weight and different head positions to achieve maximal therapeutic separation of the articulating joint surfaces and musculature. As pain subsides, progressive mobilization is initiated. In the chronic stage the treatment is shifted to exercise so that the patient may undertake a more active role in controlling pain. Involved musculature must be restored to a more "normal" physiological state through a specific exercise program carried out in the patient's home, work, and recreational environment. It should be noted that when pain has reached the chronic stage, the patient has usually received extensive and multimodal treatment that may only have provided temporary relief. The goal of the exercise program is to increase the patient's functional level by increasing the activity level. Another goal is restoration of the functional range of motion and the strength of involved structures and musculature while decreasing muscle guarding.

The patient must be educated in proper body mechanics, posture, and work and sleeping habits. An exercise regimen in conjunction with supportive modalities and treatment techniques is essential for the patient to achieve maximum benefit and to return to a higher functional level.

PAIN OF REFERRED ORIGIN

Pain is a significant symptom of disorders involving the cardiovascular, gastrointestinal, and genitourinary systems. The sensory nerves from these organs traverse the posterior horn of gray matter several segments before synapsing with neurons in the dorsal horn. Sensory impulses from these organs traverse the same path to the brain as cutaneous somatic afferent fibers. The "referred pain" associated with disease processes in these organs occurs secondary to the cutaneous visceral-somatic crosstalk of afferent fibers and second-order neurons in lamina 5–7 of the spinal and medullary dorsal horns.[6] A patient with cardiac or visceral disease may experience three types of pain. Visceral pain is felt at the site of primary stimulation and is diffuse and deep. Deep somatic pain is related to parietal stimulation and is often localized and sharp. Referred pain localized to the skin is characteristically sharp. While referred pain routinely occurs in combination with visceral and somatic pain it may exist as the sole symptom.[3]

True visceral pain is the result of a diseased viscus. This pain occurs early in the disease and is usually a dull, aching pain that is poorly localized. Visceral diseases are frequently manifested by referred pain, which is often described as hyperalgesia in the dermatomes innervated by the same spinal segments that innervate the viscera. Reflex muscle contraction often occurs with visceral disease and correlates with nerve segments innervated by those supplying the viscera. The intensity of the muscle spasm is directly related to the intensity of the noxious stimuli. In addition to cutaneous hyperalgesia and reflex muscle contraction, deep tenderness and autonomic manifestations may occur.

Parietal pain is often the result of disease involving the parietal pleura or peritoneum. This pain is often intense and may be well localized and/or referred. Pain from pericarditis or disease processes near the diaphragmatic pleura is often referred to the neck, while pain from diseases involving the peritoneum may be referred to the lower chest and abdominal wall.

Chest pain may be the result of referred pain from cervical disc disease, thoracic outlet syndrome, biliary tract disease, acute pancreatitis, or many other abdominal visceral diseases. Anterior chest pain may result from myofascial disease. Costochondritis (anterior chest wall syndrome) may cause referred pain in the neck, chest, and upper extremity. Pain in the chest, shoulder, and upper arm may be the result of cardiovascular disease, including myocardial infarction, aneurysm of the aorta, pulmonary diseases, and mediastinal or thoracic tumors. Diseases of the kidney may cause a dull aching in the lower thorax or lumbar paravertebral regions that radiates to the thigh. Low back pain may be referred pain from diseases of the pelvic viscera, including prostatitis, abdominal aortic disease, and gastrointestinal disease. Shoulder and neck pain may result from abdominal visceral disorders involving the gall bladder, liver, spleen, and diaphragm. Pain may refer to the knee from diseases of the hip (such as Legg-Perthes disease), spinal stenosis, and other spinal disorders. Stimulation of the dural floor in the skull results in pain referred to various portions of the fascial anatomy. Pain of specific superficial areas of the face may be referred to a division of the trigeminal nerve with possible overflow to adjacent divisions of the nerve.[6]

Pain from deep somatic structures may be referred to other somatic regions or produce reflex changes in the viscera. For example, pain caused by degenerative joint disease may be referred to other regions of the back or radiate to the limbs. Some superficial pain is due to referred pain from a specific myofascial trigger point. In patients with referred pain, all somatic and visceral structures innervated by the segments that innervate the involved superficial cutaneous segments should be carefully examined for pathology. The optimal resolution of this type of pain derives from locating and treating the underlying disease.[3]

PAIN OF AUTONOMIC ORIGIN

Pain in the extremities may be due to overactivity of the sympathetic autonomic nervous system. Causalgia refers to partial injury of a major nerve followed by symptoms of sympathetic system overactivity. Reflex sympathetic dystrophy (RSD) refers to cases of overactivity of the sympathetic nervous system associated with minor injury or no injury. Examples include shoulder-hand syndrome, post-traumatic edema, Sudeck's atrophy, and various other syndromes in which sympathetic overactivity seems to be the primary etiologic factor.

While it is apparent that the sympathetic nervous system plays an important role in the pathogenesis of post-traumatic pain syndromes, the etiology of this phenomenon is not clear. The most common aspect of RSD is burning pain associated with hyperpathia or hypersensitivity to touch, which is relieved with an appropriate sympathetic block. The patient may show evidence of overactivity in the sympathetic nervous system, including hyperhydrosis and vasoconstriction. These symptoms result in cooling of the extremity. When accompanied by disuse, this condition may produce trophic changes, including shiny thin skin, loss of hair, and demineralization of bone. Reflex autonomic changes have been proposed as the pathological basis of this syndrome, but other factors such as alterations in central pain transmission and altered production, release, and reuptake of neurotransmitters may be involved. While many theories have been proposed, none fully explains all the findings in RSD. In fact, it is unclear whether sympathetic block produces analgesia by interruption of the sympathetic efferents or through blockage of afferent fibers traveling in the sympathetic chain.

Pain of sympathetic origin results in multiple clinical manifestations in the upper extremity, including hyperpathia and allodynia in excess of what would be expected from the original injury, vasomotor instability, edema and swelling, and dystrophic skin changes. Superficial burning pain and hyperpathia are almost universally present. Usually superimposed on these symptoms is deep pain, often of a bizarre quality described as crushing, tearing, stabbing, or throbbing. The pain is usually continuous, although its intensity can vary spontaneously. It is aggravated by any movement or stimulation of the limb or by stimuli that may evoke sympathetic responses, for example, intense auditory or visual stimuli or emotional upset. The extremity is often held away from the body and contact with clothing or bedsheets is avoided. With time, the pain may spread to previously unaffected areas. Frequently, it appears to follow arterial distribution zones rather than dermatomal patterns.[13] The time of onset for sympathetic pain is extremely variable (minutes to weeks) and depends upon the initial injury.

Trauma induces the majority of cases of reflex sympathetic dystrophy. Crush injury is a common antecedent with lacerations, fractures, sprains, and burn injuries accounting for most of the remaining cases. RSD has been reported following injury to minor peripheral nerves. Many of these cases occur after carpal tunnel decompression and palmar fasciotomy. RSD has also been reported in association with several diseases, including myocardial infarction, cerebrovascular accident, and cerebral anoxia.

Many clinicians consider the resolution of pain symptoms following sympathetic nerve block by local anesthetic to be diagnostic. Skin temperature measurements, sweat tests, and electrodiagnosis have failed to demonstrate consistent differences in response between patients diagnosed with RSD and controls.

Triple phase bone scans are considered to be essential in the diagnosis of reflex sympathetic dystrophy and have consistently revealed increased blood flow to the bone.

Establishing an absolute diagnosis for a chronic pain problem is usually difficult, as multiple pain mechanisms frequently exist. It is often possible, however, to assess the importance of sympathetic mechanisms by comparing the degree and duration of pain relief achieved by sympathetic blocks with that produced by somatic blocks and placebo injections.

Management.   The most effective treatment of a sympathetic dystrophy consists of an appropriate sympathetic nerve block using a local anesthetic agent.[32] Phenoxybenzamine has been reported effective in the treatment of causalgia.[11] If the problem originates in the head, neck, upper extremity, or upper thorax, a stellate ganglion or a cervical sympathetic block at the C6 level may be employed. If the pain is in the upper abdominal area, sympathetic denervation can be achieved using the celiac plexus block. Pain originating in the lower extremities requires a lumbar paravertebral sympathetic block at the L2 level.[29] Patients with a history of long-standing pain may receive only temporary pain relief from local anesthetic blocks. These patients may require intravenous regional guanethidine or reserpine when the nerve block ceases to provide pain relief. This technique can be applied to extremities and is useful when local anesthetic blocks are contraindicated.[13]

If the patient does not receive permanent pain relief from sympathetic blocks or from the intravenous regional technique, then permanent interruption of the sympathetic pathway may be considered. This may be accomplished by a neurolytic injection into the sympathetic trunk or by surgical sympathectomy.

In conjunction with sympathetic blockade or guanethidine injection, physical therapy must be instituted. Often the patient receives spontaneous pain relief with the sympathetic blockade, but when the extremity is moved during physical therapy the patient experiences significant pain. This pain is secondary to tight muscles, edema, or stiffness of the joint because the noxious input is carried through somatic fibers. These patients may be aided in the performance of physical therapy by somatic blocks such as brachial plexus block or epidural block. Physical therapy may be an important adjuvant to sympathetic blocks. For long-standing cases, extensive physical rehabilitation may be necessary. Active assistive range of motion exercises, muscle strengthening and conditioning, massage, and heat (whirlpool, contrast baths, paraffin, radiant heat, fluidotherapy) are particularly useful. Vigorous passive range of motion exercises and the use of heavy weights may exacerbate symptoms. Exercises are best performed during analgesic periods following sympathetic blocks.

CHRONIC PAIN MANAGEMENT

When an acute pain etiology cannot be determined or adequately treated it may lead to a persistent chronic pain state. Chronic pain may cause its sufferer to withdraw from vocation and society and thus it constitutes a major source of disability. Yet the management of chronic pain has been recognized as a major health care problem only in the last 25 years. It remains unclear why some people become chronic pain patients and others resolve their acute pain without significant difficulty.

Multidisciplinary Approach

The chronic pain problem is multifaceted. No single physician has the resources to care comprehensively for the complex psychological, social, legal, medical, and physical problems involved in chronic pain. Therefore, the multidisciplinary team approach is necessary. Using a multidisciplinary approach does not mean the patient is referred from one specialist to another, as this tends to result in conflicting and overlapping treatment and the patient's loss of confidence in treatment outcome. Ideally, the team should work together to provide a unified explanation of the illness and a comprehensive treatment program. The multidisciplinary pain service has the advantage of offering a variety of coherent treatment approaches to the patient. This type of program recognizes that a multifaceted problem requires multifaceted treatment, as well as continuity of care in which the patient is an active participant.[1]

The core group for the multidisciplinary treatment service includes a physiatrist, an anesthesiologist, and a clinical psychologist or psychiatrist. This group may vary considerably according to local needs, resources, and available expertise. However, the team must have the knowledge to manage the psychological and social problems with optimum medical and anesthetic treatments. They must also have a thorough understanding of physical treatments and the rehabilitation process.

The multidisciplinary pain approach begins with a complete clinical evaluation. Comprehensive medical and psychosocial evaluations, with particular emphasis on functional capabilities and behavioral responses to pain, are essential. All previous medical records are needed to avoid repeating appropriately performed studies and unsuccessful treatments. This comprehensive clinical evaluation also includes assessment of functional capabilities to determine impairment level. The psychosocial evaluation focuses upon the behavioral response to pain, adjustments to the physical impairment, and the degree of motivation.

The multidisciplinary team functions at several levels within the treatment process. They attempt to identify and resolve documentable organic problems when present and to improve the patient's ability to cope with the pain through medication, psychological intervention, and education. In addition, considerable effort is devoted to improving the patient's functional outcome as measured by increased activity time, improved activities of daily living, increased distance walked, and increased tolerance for specific homemaking or vocational activities. To accomplish these objectives the multidisciplinary team must use multiple skills. In many cases, the chronic pain patient is so entrenched in pain behavior that the behavior modification approach is essential. These patients are often characterized by low levels of activities of daily living, high demand for medication accompanied by physical and psychological dependency, high verbalization of pain and suffering, and the inability to work. Restoration of functional capacity to work and play often dramatically decreases the suffering that can be associated with chronic pain.

Pain Treatment Centers

The organization and operation of the multidisciplinary pain clinic have been discussed by Grabois.[12] Many behavior modification programs use the Fordyce Model.[10] This approach uses the general principles of interruption of the pain behavior reinforcement cycle, reward for healthy behavior, appropriate goals that the patient must achieve, measurement of improvement by assessment of functional ability as well as pain level, and psychosocial adjustment. Particular emphasis is placed on detoxification and medication reduction, pain reduction, increased activity, and modification of pain behavior.

If the patient is on pain medications and is determined to be physically or psychologically dependent, he or she must be detoxified. This is routinely done by establishing the equivalent dosage of other drugs for each medication type (e.g., narcotics, benzodiazepines, barbiturates, alcohol). Narcotic medications are replaced with methadone, and long-acting barbiturates are replaced with pentobarbital. Medication equivalents are placed in orange juice or given in capsulated form and are decreased at a rate of 5% to 10% per day. The medication is then given on an around-the-clock basis at fixed intervals. Gradual reduction of the pain-killing ingredients occurs without significant side effects of withdrawal. The patient is not aware of the timing of the decrease, but has been informed of the concept before starting the program. Nonsteroidal anti-inflammatory drugs and tricyclic antidepressants are routinely integrated as long-term medications. The pain management program is designed to reduce and not eliminate pain, while increasing the patient's functional capabilities.

The patient with chronic pain usually exhibits a decreased activity level, which results in a disuse syndrome. Exercise programs are based on the initial specific and general exercise that the individual can perform. The exercise regimen is progressive, with the goals rising along with the patient's ability. Rewards for accomplishing tasks are a mainstay of this program, with no reinforcement given for pain behavior. The achievable goals provide success, build confidence, and allow for frequent reinforcement when they are met. Cooperation by all staff members is essential; they must consistently ignore pain complaints and encourage improved function. Psychological intervention is used as indicated. The chronic pain behavior modification programs report good short-term success rates in medication reduction, increased activity, and more productive behavior patterns. Evaluations suggest improvements of 60% to 80% in patients with chronic pain without major psychosocial components, 30% to 50% in patients with significant psychosocial components, and approximately 20% in patients with major psychiatric components or secondary gains.[12]

Multidisciplinary chronic pain treatment is a focused, unified approach to the chronic pain syndrome. In this country, pain treatment centers differ widely in organization and emphasis. They are generally multidisciplinary centers that use some combination of anesthesiologists, clinical psychologists, dentists, neurologists, orthopedists, pharmacists, physiatrists, and psychiatrists. The goals of these centers are to diminish, if not eliminate, chronic pain; increase the patient's functional capabilities to allow for a more active life; and decrease the patient's dependence on drugs for pain control.

REFERENCES

1. Bonica JJ. Pain research and therapy: past and current status and future needs. In: Ng LKY, Bonica JJ, eds. *Pain, discomfort, and humanitarian care.* New York: Elsevier/North Holland; 1980:1–46.

2. Bonica JJ. Management of cancer pain. In: Zimmermann M, Drings P, Wagner G, eds. *Pain and the cancer patient*. Berlin: Springer-Verlag; 1984:13–27.
3. Borenstein DG, Weisel SW. *Low back pain—medical diagnosis and comprehensive treatment*. Philadelphia: WB Saunders; 1989:401–431.
4. Cleeland C. Nonpharmacological management of cancer pain. *J Pain Symptom Manage*. 1987;2:S23–S28.
5. DeJong RH. Defining pain terms. *JAMA*. 1980;244:143.
6. Donovan WH, Dimitrijevic MR, Dahm L. Neurophysiological approaches to chronic pain following spinal cord injury. *Paraplegia*. 1982;20:135–246.
7. Epstein E. Intralesional triamcinolone therapy in herpes zoster and post herpetic neuralgia. *Ear Nose Throat Mon*. 1973;52:416.
8. Farkash AE, Portenoy RK. The pharmacological management of chronic pain in the paraplegic patient. *J Am Paraplegia Soc*. 1986;9:41–50.
9. Foley KM. The treatment of cancer pain. *N Engl J Med*. 1985;313:84–95.
10. Fordyce WE. *Behavioral methods for chronic pain and illness*. St Louis: CV Mosby; 1976:41–221.
11. Ghostine SY, Comair YG, Turner DM, et al. Phenoxybenzamine in the treatment of causalgia—report of 40 cases. *J Neurosurg*. 1984;60:1263–1268.
12. Grabois M. Pain clinics—role in the rehabilitation of patients with chronic pain. *Ann Acad Med Singapore*. 1983;12:428–433.
13. Gross D. Pain in autonomic nervous system. *Adv Neurol*. 1974;4:93–104.
14. Hallett M, Tandon D, Berardelli A. Treatment of peripheral neuropathies. *J Neurol Neurosurg Psychiatry*. 1985;48:1193–1207.
15. Huber SL, Hill CS. Pharmacologic management of cancer pain. *Cancer Bull*. 1980;32:183–185.
16. Jensen TS, Krebs B, Nielsen J, Rasmussen P. Immediate and long term phantom limb pain in amputees—incidence, clinical characteristics, and relationship to preamputation limb pain. *Pain*. 1985;21:267–278.
17. Kanner RM. Pharmacological management of pain and symptom control in cancer. *J Pain Symptom Manage*. 1987;2:S19–S22.
18. Kassirer MR, Osterberger DH. Pain in chronic multiple sclerosis. *J Pain Symptom Manage*. 1987;2:95–97.
19. Kraus H. Triggerpoints. *NY State J Med*. 1973;73:1310–1314.
20. Levy MH. Pain management in advanced cancer. *Semin Oncology*. 1985;12:394–410.
21. Martin JJ. Thalamic syndromes. In: Vinken PJ, Bruyne GW, eds. *Handbook of clinical neurology; vol II: localization in clinical neurology*. Amsterdam: North Holland Publishing Company; 1962:469–496.
22. Max MB, Culnane M, Schafer SC, Gracele RH, Walther DJ, Smoller B, Dubner R. Amitriptyline relieves diabetic neuropathy pain in patients with normal or depressed mood. *Neurology*. 1987;37:589–596.
23. Merskey H, ed. Classification of chronic pain—descriptions of chronic pain syndromes and definitions of pain terms. *Pain*. 1986;3(Suppl):S1–S225.
24. O'Brien JP. Mechanisms of spinal pain. In: Wall PD, Melzack R, eds. *Textbook of pain*. New York: Churchill Livingstone; 1984:240–251.
25. Peteet J, Tay V, Cohen G, MacIntyre J. Pain characteristics and treatment in an outpatient cancer population. *Cancer*. 1986;57:1259–1265.
26. Raferty A. The management of postherpetic pain using sodium valproate and amitriptyline. *Ir Med J*. 1979;72:399–401.
27. Raj PP, Ramamurthy S. Differential nerve block studies. In: Raj PP, ed. *Practical management of pain*. Chicago: Year Book Medical Publishers; 1986:173–177.
28. Ramamurthy S, Winnie AP. Diagnostic maneuvers in painful syndromes. In: Stein JM, Warfield CA, eds. *International anesthesiology clinics, pain management*. Boston: Little, Brown; 1983:47–50.
29. Ramamurthy S, Winnie AP. Regional anesthetic techniques for pain relief. *Semin Anesthesiol*. 1985;4:237–245.
30. Ramamurthy S, Walsh NE, Schoenfeld L, Hoffman J. Evaluation of neurolytic blocks using phenol and cryogenic block in the management of chronic pain. *J Pain Symptom Manage*. 1989;4:72–75.

31. Ropper AH, Schahani BT. Pain in Guillain-Barré syndrome. *Arch Neurol.* 1984;41:511–514.
32. Rowlingson JC, Chalkley J. Common pain syndromes—diagnosis and management. *Semin Anesthesiol.* 1985;4:223–230.
33. Sherman RA, Sherman CJ. Prevalence and characteristics of chronic phantom limb pain among American veterans. *Am J Phys Med.* 1983;62:227–238.
34. Sherman RA, Sherman CJ. A comparison of phantom sensations among amputees whose amputations were of civilian and military origins. *Pain.* 1985;21:91–97.
35. Sherman RA, Sherman CJ, Parker L. Chronic phantom and stump pain among American veterans—result of a survey. *Pain.* 1984;18:83–95.
36. Swerdlow M. Anticonvulsant drugs in chronic pain. *Clin Neuropharmacol.* 1984;7:51–82.
37. Travell JG, Simons DG. *Myofascial pain and dysfunction—the trigger point manual.* Baltimore: Williams & Wilkins; 1983.
38. Twycross RG. Overview of analgesia. In: Bonica JJ, ed. *Advances in pain research and therapy, vol 2.* New York: Raven Press; 1979:3–55.
39. Waisbrod H, Panhans C, Hansen D, Gerbershagen HU. Direct nerve stimulation for painful peripheral neuropathies. *J Bone Joint Surg [Br].* 1985;67B:470–472.
40. Woolsey RM. Chronic pain following spinal cord injury. *J Am Paraplegia Soc.* 1986;9:51–53.
41. World Health Organization. *Cancer pain relief.* Geneva: WHO; 1986. 74 pp.
42. Young PA. The anatomy of the spinal cord pain paths—a review. *J Am Paraplegia Soc.* 1986;9:28–38.

Chapter 20

REHABILITATION OF PATIENTS WITH HEAD INJURY

Sheldon Berrol

Rehabilitation after brain injury is a therapeutic process designed to facilitate maximal restoration of function. Regardless of what statistics indicate about outcome possibilities, each patient must be individually assessed to determine diagnosis, associated injuries, responses, and achievable goals.

Early institution of rehabilitation principles can substantially reduce the impact of such complicating factors as bed rest, spasticity, contractures, and heterotopic ossification. The process of rehabilitation can be most effective if initiated in the phase of trauma management, so that additional levels of disability due to complications do not accumulate. Since the pathology, severity, and resultant outcome of traumatic brain injury are so highly variable, rehabilitation interventions must be individualized. Unfortunately, where medical interventions to assure survival are most acute, rehabilitation must proceed slowly.

Rehabilitation after brain injury is frequently a lengthy process that invokes many levels of intervention. Appropriate timing of these interventions, as well as availability of a knowledgeable rehabilitation team working in a coordinated effort, is required to identify and pursue reasonable goals whose achievement can be objectively assessed.

The rehabilitation team in the acute setting should involve at least the neurosurgeon, physiatrist, nurse, physical therapist, occupational therapist, speech pathologist, and social worker. This team must be involved with early discharge planning and aid in timely and appropriate placement when the patient is medically stable.

The most frequent cause of brain trauma is injury in automobile accidents. Brain injury is the leading cause of death and chronic disability among persons aged 1 to 40. It is quite common for multisystem trauma to occur, complicating the process of stabilization and rehabilitation. When multisystem injury is present, the incidence of shock and death increases dramatically. Furthermore, acute blood loss may compound the degree of brain involvement by adding an element of relative ischemia.

COMA

Coma has been defined by Jennett and Teasdale as that state in which the patient does not open the eyes, gives no comprehensible verbal response, and fails to demonstrate any motor act to command. They developed an assessment instrument, the Glasgow Coma Score (GCS), to enable numerical grading (3–15) of the various levels of coma and evolution from coma, and to assist in prognostication.[2] The numerical score allows us to avoid ill-defined terms such as deep coma, semi-coma, obtundation, etc. The lower the score, the greater the degree of brain damage and the poorer the expected outcome. A severe brain injury is defined as coma (GCS of 8 or less) persisting six hours or more. All patients who reach a 9 on this scale are considered out of coma. Moderate head injury is 9–12 and mild head injury is 13–15 on the GCS. Since eye opening, motor response, and verbal response may not be hierarchically related, it is considered best to indicate each component separately (E = , M = , V =).

Glasgow Outcome Scale.   Since the coma grading system was designed to establish an early prognosis (within the first week of injury), the Glasgow Outcome Scale was developed to categorize outcomes. It consists of five broad categories, based upon levels of independence:

1. Death.
2. Persistent vegetative state—awake but unaware.
3. Severe disability—conscious but dependent.
4. Moderate disability—independent but with obvious disability.
5. Good recovery—may have residual deficits but independent.

There is great variability in the interpretation of what "good recovery" entails. Patients who are cognitively and behaviorally severely limited but who are independent in activities of daily living (ADL) are usually considered "good recoveries."

Rancho Los Amigos Cognitive Scale.   This scale was developed to classify observed behaviors of patients who emerge from coma. It allows clinicians to adapt the interventions of all therapies so that they may be appropriately applied.[1]

I. No response—The patient is completely unresponsive to any stimuli.

II. Generalized response—The patient reacts inconsistently and nonpurposefully to stimuli in a nonspecific manner.

III. Localized response—The patient reacts specifically but inconsistently to stimuli. Responses are directly related to stimuli, such as turning the head toward a sound.

IV. Confused/agitated—The patient is in a heightened state of activity with a severely decreased ability to process information. Attempts at procedures which are uncomfortable (e.g., dynamic stretch of contractures) increase the level of agitation. A major emphasis of treatment is to decrease confusion.

V. *Confused/inappropriate nonagitated*—The patient is alert and able to respond to simple commands fairly consistently, but is unable to participate with increased complexity of command or without a high degree of structure.

VI. *Confused/appropriate*—This patient shows goal-directed behavior, but is dependent upon external input for direction. Responses to discomfort are now appropriate. He can follow simple directions consistently, and now demonstrates some recognition of staff.

VII. *Automatic/appropriate*—The patient now appears appropriate and oriented. There is increased awareness, but, as yet, little insight. There is minimal to absent confusion, some ability to learn new material. Patient is independent in self-care activities.

VIII. *Purposeful and appropriate*—The patient is now alert and oriented, able to recall and integrate past and recent events. Vocational evaluation may be considered.

EARLY REHABILITATION

The initial phase of management should be directed toward an accurate diagnosis, prognosis, and the prevention of complications. Family members should be incorporated into the process and provided with clear and accurate information so that they begin to understand the range of possible disabilities.

Areas of bony prominence such as the malleoli, knees, sacrum, occiput, and scapulae are particularly prone to decubitus ulcer formation. Initially, patients will require turning at least every two hours, day and night. Adequate padding should be provided at all points of skin contact over bone or with bed rails, foot boards, or orthotic devices, and the skin should be kept dry. As the patient emerges from coma and becomes restless, friction damage to epithelial tissue must be prevented.

Spasticity

Central nervous system injury results in increased muscle tone, characterized by hyperactive deep tendon reflexes, increased resistance to passive stretch, cocontraction, and clonus. This results in contracture formation, intertrigo, skin breakdown, positioning problems, and difficulty in maintaining hygiene. Brain-injured patients with spasticity tolerate traction poorly, so in early orthopedic management long bone fractures are best treated with internal fixation.

Noxious stimuli that could increase tone should be avoided. The side-lying hip-flexed position frequently results in temporarily diminished tone because primitive motor patterns are minimally stimulated in this position.

A vigorous range of motion exercise program should be used in physical therapy and adequate range of motion for joints should be incorporated in all routine nursing procedures to maintain maximal length of muscle fibers. As early as possible after brain swelling has abated, the patient should be evaluated for sitting in an appropriately stabilized position that minimizes tone.

Patients with widespread spasticity may benefit from drug therapy to modify muscle tone. Decisions about pharmacotherapy are based on balancing desired result against side effects. Brain-injured patients are sometimes more sensitive than normal patients to sedation: diazepam and other benzodiazepines may increase confusion. Baclofen appears to be less effective for spasticity after cerebral injury than for that of spinal origin, and may increase the risk of seizure. Dantrolene sodium is more effective for treating spasticity of cerebral origin, but can cause severe hepatic toxicity. Effective control of spasticity may require a combination of drugs in selected patients.

Physical modalities that minimize tone include sustained stretching, vibration, cryotherapy, and the use of inhibiting postures. Splints are commonly used to maintain muscle length, but to be most effective they should be individually fabricated and initiated early. Serial casting can dramatically increase muscle length and decrease spasticity. In addition, the circumferential pressure of the plaster may actually inhibit tone.

Peripheral nerve or motor-point blocks can be effective in reducing spasticity localized to an extremity or muscle group and should be considered as reasonable alternatives to systemic medications. Forty percent alcohol has been used, but 6% phenol has fewer side effects. When blocks are performed, electrical stimulation should be used to identify the myoneural junction or nerve sites for injection. Injections directly into mixed sensory-motor nerves may result in long-lasting dysesthesias. When spasticity is intense and cannot be adequately managed by the above measures, invasive orthopedic or neurosurgical measures may be indicated in the chronic phase. These might include tenotomies, muscle lengthening, releases, transposition, neurectomies (most commonly musculocutaneous and obturator), and radiofrequency rhizotomies. Procedures that are not indicated after brain injury are intrathecal phenol, simultaneous anterior and posterior rhizotomies, or chordectomies.

Contractures

Increased tone and its attendant primitive flexor or extensor reactions lead to unbalanced motor activity and loss of muscle length. Bed rest and persistent immobility contribute dramatically to the development of contractures. One major goal of early rehabilitation is mobilization and maintenance of functional muscle length.

Proper positioning of the patient in bed requires avoidance of reflex patterns that may induce spasticity, and, ultimately, contracture. Lying on the side with the hips flexed inhibits extensor tone of the lower extremities, and this position should be used, if possible. Devices to prevent shoulder adduction and internal rotation, shoulder protraction, elbow flexion, wrist flexion and pronation, finger flexion, and thumb adduction should be utilized prophylactically. Slings routinely contribute to these deforming postures. The use of arm troughs or lap trays for the wheelchair is preferred.

The lower extremities also should not be subjected to persistently deforming forces. Footboards should be avoided, since pressure over the metatarsal heads facilitates flexor spasticity, with subsequent development of a plantar flexed contracture. The patient should not be allowed to maintain the hips and knees in constant flexion. Pillows, towel rolls, and foam wedges should be placed to abduct the shoulder, limit protraction, and, in the lower extremities, partially abduct the hips. Trochanteric rolls can prevent excessive external rotation. Firm cones should be used to produce mild wrist dorsiflexion and functional positioning of the fingers. Careful attention must be directed toward maintaining the first interdigital web space. Soft rolls such as toweling may have limited utility, since their inherent elasticity places the fingers in greater extension and may reduce tone most effectively.

In the presence of severe spasticity, contracture progression may be impossible to control, even in the most aggressive program.

Sensory Stimulation

The goals of sensory stimulation are to elicit first generalized and then localized responses, to prevent "sensory deprivation" and increase environmental awareness, and, if possible, to mold responses into meaningful functions. The effort is interdisciplinary and should be incorporated into the routine daily nursing care plan.

Sensory stimulation should utilize a planned program of stimuli in the attempt to evoke normalized responses, and should use appropriate environmental stimuli as well. When intracranial hypertension is a problem, the planned stimulation program should be delayed. Noxious stimuli are to be avoided to reduce facilitation of abnormal primitive reflexes or reinforcement of spasticity. To merely elicit a startle reaction repeatedly offers no therapeutic advantage. Stimuli should be introduced singly to allow for adequate evaluation of responses and to accommodate the significant processing delay that is inevitably present. Planned stimulation with single stimuli should be provided for brief periods of time and repeated frequently; eventually, the process should be incorporated into the overall treatment program.

If radio and television are to be used for stimulation, they should be turned on only for brief intervals so that habituation to the stimulus does not occur. Patients with severe neurological deficits should be placed in rooms remote from incidental auditory stimuli. When consistent responses appear, the stimuli should be modified in order to obtain functional goals rather than provoke only response repetition.

The theoretical basis for sensory stimulation techniques as facilitators of recovery has not been established. Clearly, however, sensory stimulation requires more discrete evaluation of the patient's functional responses than standard medical assessment allows. Such serial evaluations can frequently reveal subtle neurological changes that reflect psychological contact with the environment at an early stage. Sensory stimulation also alleviates the potential negative effects of sensory deprivation (all too common in intensive care units).

Feeding

To ensure safety, it is imperative that the functioning of the oral-bulbar structures be evaluated before an oral feeding program is instituted. If doubt exists, methylene blue dye placed in a teaspoonful of food can help define when patients can safely tolerate oral feeding; blue or green color in tracheal secretions confirms unsafe swallowing. Protective mechanisms such as the gag and cough reflexes should be at least weakly present before oral feeding is initiated. Competence of the pharyngeal phase of swallowing cannot be assessed in a bedside examination, but videofluoroscopic analysis of swallowing can identify patients at risk for aspiration.

Standard nasogastric tubes are not only uncomfortable but can cause pressure ulceration, granuloma formation, stenosis, chronic blood loss, reflux, esophagitis, and aspiration. If a patient with a nasogastric tube does not make progress in oral feeding after two weeks on an oral-bulbar training program, the physician should consider inserting a gastrostomy, jejunostomy, or esophagostomy tube. Percutaneous endoscopic gastrostomy (PEG) is a safe, low-risk procedure. It can largely eliminate the problem of reflux, particularly if the feeding tube is placed in the jejunum, and it eliminates the need to suture the stomach to the anterior abdominal wall to prevent leakage.

Permanent gastrostomies generally are unnecessary, since most patients will resume oral feeding with continued training while feeding tubes are in place. Gastrostomy sites should be placed laterally in the abdominal wall to allow full movement (i.e., rolling) in the physical rehabilitation program. Esophagostomies should be avoided if a strong asymmetric tonic neck reflex or torticollis is present.

COMMUNICATION

Language comprehension usually precedes expressive language in recovery from brain injury. Thus, evaluations of linguistic parameters may be more productive than evaluation of speech in determining deficits and appropriate remediation programs. During the period of post-traumatic amnesia, a substantial number of brain-injured patients will remain mute although they still have language comprehension.

True aphasia does not appear frequently after trauma, as it does after stroke, unless focal injury to speech centers has occurred. Dysarthria is the most common expressive speech problem present after diffuse head injury. The most commonly occurring deficits are linguistic, such as dysnomia, and impaired comprehension of complex material. Attentional deficits also are characteristic of brain injury patients and limit their functional language abilities.

The initial steps in management hinge on the early development of functional communication. Since communication impairment often aggravates agitation, establishing communication will make the patient more cooperative and allow a more productive effort. Any motor act that can be repeated volitionally, such as finger movement or eye blink, can be used to develop a communication system. Consistency in response to question or command is crucial. Therefore, the entire treatment team, physician, nurse therapists, and family should be aware of and promote the development of this consistent response in the form of a previously determined motor act.

Nonoral communication systems should be simple enough to be functional. Since the patient will improve as he proceeds through rehabilitation, purchase of expensive equipment should be deferred until such time as the patient's progress has stabilized and a long-term definitive solution is needed. Simple picture or alphabet boards remain the most helpful communication devices in the early stages.

HETEROTOPIC OSSIFICATION

For many patients with central nervous system injury, ectopic calcification and ossification of soft tissue remote from sites of trauma produces major functional problems. The commonly involved joints are the hips, elbows, and shoulders, and the problem occurs with greatest frequency in the most severely brain-damaged patients. The incidence increases with prolonged coma, extremity fracture, and paralysis. Ectopic calcification may also occur secondary to direct trauma. Neurogenic heterotopic ossification (HO) may progress to total ankylosis of major joints or cause compression of nerve or vascular structures.

Early presentation signs are the sudden onset of swelling, erythema, and pain in an extremity. Clinically, the ossification may be indistinguishable from deep vein thrombosis, but venography is negative. Bone scan studies clearly define the process. Serum alkaline phosphatase elevates early (but after the process has begun) and precedes x-ray evidence of calcification. Serial alkaline phosphatase determinations are valuable in interpreting the evolution of the process.

Management includes routine, regular, full range of motion exercise; previously held beliefs that therapy might initiate the process have been discarded. In patients at high risk, it may be advisable to consider early prophylactic therapy. Diphosphonate drugs prevent crystallization of calcium into bone; these drugs are not commonly available in Latin America. Nonsteroidal anti-inflammatory agents, however, are commonly available and may be as effective in preventing ossification. They should be considered in patients who are at risk. Low-dose radiation therapy has been used prophylactically in preventing ossification around the hip joint in patients undergoing arthoplasty, and initial studies on neurogenic ossification appear encouraging.

Surgical removal of the ankylosing bony mass should be deferred until maturity of bone has occurred, usually about one and a half years post injury. In cases in which some motor function has returned, forceful manipulation of the mass under anesthesia, creating a pseudo-arthrosis, has resulted in improved extremity use.

AGITATION

Patients are disoriented and confused as they evolve from coma, owing to amnesia, the unfamiliar surroundings, and perceptual deficits. Their agitation results in impaired self-control, uncooperativeness, and, sometimes, potential danger to themselves and others. Management includes behavioral modification, environmental approaches, the use of restraints, and pharmacological interventions.

Patients should be reassured both verbally and physically as often as possible, and noxious stimuli removed or modified whenever feasible. All staff should be involved in reorienting the patient to the reality of the injury, current events, and family and friends. Staffing should be consistent, since confused patients have little tolerance for change. Daily nursing and therapy routines should be brief to prevent cognitive overload and should be performed on a consistent schedule that varies little from day to day. Activities that cause agitation should be minimized or other procedures substituted. Automatic overlearned activities such as self-care skills should be incorporated whenever possible in this early phase.

Vest restraints are reasonably well tolerated, and if necessary may be combined with soft extremity restraints. Four-point restraints should be avoided unless essential for patient safety. Even with the most agitated patient, it is important to plan periods of unrestrained extremity activity, since the restraints may contribute to confusion.

Psychotropic drugs produce sedation, alter perception, and interfere with memory and learning, and thus should be used with caution in this population. Drug therapy for agitated, disruptive behavior is indicated for safety reasons and to allow the patient to participate in rehabilitation, as long as his ability to learn is not impaired. Sedation to compensate for inadequate staffing ratios slows rehabilitation. Many of the commonly used medications, however, do impair learning and memory, may potentiate seizures, cause secondary neurological syndromes, and in theory may lead to state-dependent learning. Thus, the potential benefits of medication must be balanced against the risks. Drugs such as propranolol and carbamazepine have less effect on cognition and attention and are therefore preferable to traditional psychotropic agents.

FRACTURE MANAGEMENT

Intracranial injury and altered consciousness may obscure other injuries. As many as 10% of associated hip fractures and an equal number of occult neuropathies are undiagnosed at the time of admission to rehabilitation. The patient's insensitivity to pain and impaired level of consciousness obscure some of the usual physical signs of fracture, and abnormal postures may be mistakenly ascribed to spasticity. Persistent deformities may significantly limit the ultimate functional outcome; thus, fractures and dislocations must be recognized and corrected early during acute care. Any flaccid extremity should be evaluated for a neuropathy.

The trauma care and orthopedic intervention that are provided should assume that good neurological recovery will occur. Given that spasticity, confusion, and agitation are normally present as coma resolves, uncontrolled limb movement should be anticipated. Therefore, stable internal fixation of displaced fractures is recommended, preferably soon after injury. Joint immobilization in flexed postures and prolonged traction (skeletal and skin) should be avoided.

VISUAL SYSTEM

Injury to cranial nerves II, III, IV, and VI results in impaired acquisition of sensory information and perceptual processing. Diplopia also adds to patient confusion. An eye patch for the uninvolved eye can improve orientation and force maximal use of the involved eye. Alternate eye patching to prevent disuse amblyopia is unnecessary in the adolescent or adult. When a patient cortically suppresses the second image, the eye patch should be discontinued. Many extraocular motor palsies resolve spontaneously; pleoptic strengthening exercises may speed recovery. Once the condition has stabilized, residual dysconjugate gaze can sometimes be improved by the use of prisms. If surgical correction is indicated (generally 9 to 12 months after injury), the adjustable suture technique is preferred.

If visual field deficits are present, the patient may present with an abnormal head turn. Since this is a functional compensation strategy, no attempt should be made to correct it. The patient should be taught compensatory scanning techniques. For the patient with good cognitive function, fresnel lenses may increase functional scanning of the periphery.

Persistent convergence deficits are common after brain injury. Antiseizure drugs may also make it difficult for patients to fuse a nearby image. In some patients, eye convergence exercises may be beneficial.

NEUROPSYCHOLOGICAL RECOVERY

Physical recovery proceeds more rapidly than cognitive recovery, but the latter can continue for a much longer time.

Post-traumatic amnesia is characterized by confusion and disorientation as well as an inability to learn new information. It leads to a variety of aberrant behaviors. Most significant cognitive gains occur after the resolution of post-traumatic amnesia.

Language deficits are more common than speech problems and characteristically consist of decreased verbal fluency, dysnomias, dysgraphia, and impairment of comprehension of complex material. As language is recovered, behavior and cognitive ability usually improve as well.

Neuropsychological Testing

Neuropsychological testing that relies solely on IQ scores is inadequate for assessing the consequences of traumatic brain injury. Mental status evaluations fail to identify the functional deficits of higher-order thought processing. An adequate evaluation should determine residual areas of function, the extent and nature of the deficits, how these deficits interact with functional abilities, what and how the patient can learn, and the efficiency of memory. The patient's capacity to learn new material, including his ability to access, store, and recall information, should be established. It is only then that serial evaluations may contribute to the selection of appropriate intervention strategies.

A variety of medications, including tranquilizers, antiseizure drugs, antihistamines, and anticholinergics, may adversely affect patient performance in cognitive testing and rehabilitation. Drugs that interfere with cognitive performance should be used judiciously, if at all.

Test batteries in which the extent of impairment is represented by a single numerical value are of questionable worth for patients with diffuse brain injuries. Testing should emphasize linguistic functions rather than aphasic symptoms. Selection of specific tests on the basis of identified deficits contributes more effectively to an understanding of those deficits. Full neuropsychological testing is rarely profitable until well after post-traumatic amnesia has resolved.

Orientation Approaches

The neurotrauma unit should use environmental tools to reorient the patient. These include calendars, clocks, and signs bearing the facility name and city in the patient's room and at the nursing station. Staff should be familiar with the patient's history and know the names of significant others and of pets in order to use them in ordinary conversation. Pictures of familiar people and events should be in the room. The amount of visual information should not be overwhelming, however, in order to prevent a decay in information acquisition. Initial therapy is directed towards establishing a consistent motor act (such as finger movement or eye blinking) that can be developed into a simple communication system. It is important that physicians, nurses, therapy staff, and the family consistently use the same agreed-upon system. Prompt attention to linguistic potential may have a positive effect on patient cooperation as well as motoric recovery.

Cognitive Rehabilitation

Cognitive ability improves as a result of increased attention. Training the patient to attend to a task, to select the appropriate material for the task, and to process information from multiple sensory stimuli forms the basis of what is now sometimes called cognitive rehabilitation. This facet of rehabilitation uses techniques that have long been successful, including orientation training, behavioral modification, compensation training, and perceptual motor training. Cognitive rehabilitation now receives great emphasis in rehabilitation after brain injury. Nevertheless, it still needs better definition, more consistent application, and stronger proof of efficacy.

As patients improve after a period of rehabilitation, many may benefit from a structured learning program. Basic academic skills are the foundation on which higher order cortical functions (frontal lobe skills) can be built. Microcomputers are a valuable tool in this process, but are not a replacement for the therapist. Improved computer skills do not necessarily translate into improved cognitive or functional performance.

To benefit from cognitive retraining, the patient must have some intact abilities, the therapist must select appropriate strategies, and the patient must have the opportunity to apply the skills learned beyond the narrow confines of the therapy sessions.

LATER REHABILITATION

Brain injury can result in long-term deficits in the physical, cognitive, behavioral, and psychosocial spheres. Long-term intervention is frequently needed to maximize the process of recovery. Cost-effective intervention must rely on a supportive environment, which requires the involvement of family, friends, and the community. Although physical recovery occurs rather rapidly, years of intervention are needed to integrate the severely brain-injured survivor effectively into society.

Specialized programs for behavioral interventions and for cognitive and academic restructuring offer substantial potential for appropriate patients. Learning disability programs for brain-injured patients in educational institutions substantially lower long-term costs, while providing a peer-group setting for patients. Supportive employment also allows for ongoing vocational rehabilitation and gives the patient a chance to advance in his or her career. Adaptive physical education and recreation can improve physical skills and reduce the social isolation so common to patients after severe brain injury.

If rehabilitation is to succeed, the patient's family must be involved. Accurate information and comprehensive training throughout the patient's care can equip the family for the arduous task of reintegrating their loved one into the family and into society. We must accept the responsibility of providing and overseeing this aspect of medical service. Failure to do so can result in failure of the patient to reenter the world.

The process of rehabilitation after severe brain injury is indeed lifelong. It requires appropriate medical management, prevention of complications, aid to the patient in developing optimal relationships with family and friends, and help in achieving a productive and meaningful life within the limits of his or her nervous system injury.

REFERENCES

1. Hagen C, Malkmus D, Durham P. Levels of cognitive functioning. In: *Rehabilitation of the head-injured adult: comprehensive physical management*. Downey, California: Professional Staff Association of Rancho Los Amigos Hospital; 1979:87–88.
2. Jennett B, Teasdale G. *Management of head injuries*. Philadelphia: FA Davis; 1981. (Contemporary neurology series).

BIBLIOGRAPHY

Horn LJ, Cope DN. *Traumatic brain injury*. Philadelphia: Hanley & Belfus; 1989. (Physical medicine and rehabilitation; state of the art reviews).

Rosenthal MR, Griffith EF, Bond MR, Miller JD. *Rehabilitation of the adult and child with traumatic brain injury*. 2nd ed. Philadelphia: FA Davis; 1990.

Walsh KW. *Understanding brain damage: a primer of neuropsychological evaluation*. New York: Churchill Livingstone; 1985.

Wood RLL, Eames P. *Models of brain injury rehabilitation*. London: Chapman & Hall; 1989.

Chapter 21

ADVANCES IN ELECTROSTIMULATION IN REHABILITATION MEDICINE

W. Jerry Mysiw and Rebecca D. Jackson

INTRODUCTION

Neurostimulation is the general term that encompasses all the clinical applications of chronic electrostimulation of the peripheral or central nervous system. Although electrostimulation has been applied clinically since ancient times, proven applications did not appear until the 1950s when a functionally useful cardiac pacemaker was developed[29,41] and electrostimulation was demonstrated to cause prolonged relaxation of spastic muscles.[30] Effective application in the rehabilitation setting first occurred in 1961 with the treatment of hemiplegic foot drop by Liberson et al.[33] This event was particularly significant in that it heralded the beginning of modern functional electrical stimulation (FES), in which electricity is employed to produce useful muscle contractions in paralyzed extremities, and functional neuromuscular stimulation (FNS), which is FES restricted to the neuromuscular system.

The use of electrostimulation for rehabilitation purposes continued to expand over the next three decades with the development of better technology and the subsequent introduction of multiple therapeutic indications.[29,41] For example, the "gate theory" of pain, as described by Melzak and Wall in 1965, provided the rationale for the development of the transcutaneous electrical neurostimulator (TENS), which is perhaps the first successful application of electrostimulation for therapeutic rather than functional purposes. Other therapeutic indications for neurostimulation soon followed: the description of an implanted dorsal column stimulator in 1967; conus medullaris and sacral nerve root stimulation for the treatment of neurogenic bladder disorders in 1970 and 1977, respectively; chronic phrenic nerve stimulation in 1976; and paravertebral muscle stimulation for the treatment of scoliosis in 1977.

Acceptance of electrostimulation as an important clinical adjunct for the rehabilitation physician has been comparatively slow owing in no small part to exaggerated promises that did not withstand the test of time and to the continuing need to simplify and miniaturize the required hardware. Despite these problems, dedicated researchers have continued to develop this important tool with increasing rates of success over this last decade.

This chapter will review the status of electrostimulation as a clinical tool in the rehabilitation setting. However, because it is no longer possible to do this subject justice within the confines of a single chapter, we will limit the discussion to several selected areas of functional and therapeutic electrical stimulation with the greatest clinical implications.

Physiology

The application of electrostimulation has been advocated for disorders involving normal muscle, denervated muscle, and muscle below the level of an upper motor neuron injury. Chronic stimulation of these muscles results in a sequential biochemical, morphological, histochemical, ultrastructural, and contractile transformation.[10,34] This has been particularly well documented in an animal model in the case of chronic, low-frequency stimulation of muscle that is predominately composed of fast-twitch fibers. The transformation is, in fact, so complete that the converted fast-twitch fibers become indistinguishable from normal slow-twitch fibers. Recent evidence has documented that this transformation is related to quantitative and qualitative changes in the gene transcription of several classes of muscle protein.[11]

The ability to sustain electrostimulation as a therapeutic or functional modality is contingent on the development of a safe stimulation system. Surface electrodes remain an effective and safe strategy for therapeutic stimulation. However, the widespread acceptance of FES as a neural prosthesis is dependent upon development of an implantable system that is safe and simple and that does not require significant concentration.[1,29] Percutaneous electrodes have been utilized for research purposes, but electrode movement and breakage—to the extent that 60% of all electrodes fail within a six-month period—render this system impractical for clinical purposes.[37] The surgically implanted nerve cuff electrode remains the most popular alternative (as opposed to book, epineural, helix, or intraneural electrodes), but it too has drawbacks, such as surgical, chemical, and mechanically induced nerve injury.[1] Also, this type of system makes it difficult to selectively activate individual muscles or motor units; however, this problem may have been resolved by new methods of manipulating the electrical fields of these electrodes. Further research is required with all the above-mentioned systems before specific recommendations can be made for long-term application as part of a neuroprosthesis.

THERAPEUTIC ELECTRICAL STIMULATION

Normal Muscle

Electrostimulation of normal muscle has been advocated as an adjunct in strengthening programs, as a means of retarding atrophy around an immobilized joint, and as a means of facilitating the rehabilitation of painful musculoskeletal disorders that otherwise preclude maximum effort during voluntary muscle contraction. Unlike studies involving animal models, the studies involving humans have largely utilized isometric strengthening programs. These studies suggest that the greater the intensity of contractions, the greater the strength gains.[40] Greater intensity contractions are facilitated by larger electrodes, with a felt pad soaked in tap water serving as the transmission agent. Also, placing the electrode over the motor point increases comfort and thereby permits greater current intensity. Medium- to high-frequency stimulation rates (500–10,000 Hz) with short stimulation times followed by longer rest intervals have been advocated for strength training programs.[54] A representative regimen is the 10/50/10 design, which advocates peak amplitude stimulation (approaching 90 mA) at frequencies near 2,500 Hz (sinusoidal waveform delivered in 10 msec pulses at 30 times per second) and a pulse width of 0.45 msec. The stimulation is repeated 10 times with 50 second rest intervals. Endurance training programs typically use low-frequency electrostimulation (10–500 Hz) with contraction time and rest intervals of equal duration (4–15 sec on and off). However, the more practical consideration, and the one which ultimately determines all stimulation parameters utilized in the clinical setting, is patient tolerance. Studies have suggested that the tremendous variation in patient tolerance often precludes optimization of stimulus parameters.[40] Therefore, the clinician frequently must experiment with the two waveforms (medium frequency waveforms of 2,500 Hz or biphasic square waves) that tend to have the greatest patient tolerance. Daily training appears to be optimal, although benefit is also noted with two to three sessions per week. Finally, placing the muscle in a relatively shortened position (for example, stimulating the quadriceps with the knee at 30° of flexion) produces the greatest torque.

There appears to be a consensus that electrostimulation offers no benefit in strengthening normal muscles over voluntary isometric contraction or over electrostimulation combined with voluntary isometric contractions.[40,54] However, electrostimulation does appear to be superior to voluntary isometric strengthening programs in maintaining strength and minimizing atrophy around a joint that is immobilized secondary to trauma or surgery. In addition, electrostimulation may have a role to play in selectively strengthening muscles, such as the vastus medialis muscle in chondromalacia patella.

Denervated Muscles

During the past decade there has been little change in the literature dealing with therapeutic electrical stimulation after a peripheral nerve injury. It is known that stimulating denervated muscle attenuates the atrophy and the loss in maximum tetanic tension.[34] However, this benefit is likely to be short-lived, and electrostimulation only delays the inevitable outcome. On the other hand, evidence suggests that stimulation of denervated muscles may inhibit terminal spouting of the motor neuron or precipitate overwork weakness.[6,9] The reader is referred to other textbooks, such as *Krusen's Handbook of Physical Medicine and Rehabilitation* (fourth edition), for a review of stimulation techniques.

Electrostimulation has generally been viewed as contraindicated in myopathic disorders. However, electrostimulation two hours per day, five days per week in combination with voluntary low-resistance weight training has been shown to improve muscle strength in patients with muscular dystrophy as long as initial muscle strength was greater than 15% of normal.[38] This particular study utilized a portable unit that delivered an asymmetric, rectangular, balanced, biphasic waveform with a pulse width of 300 μsec, a 4 sec rise time, a 2 sec fall time, a 10–15 sec "cycle on" time and equal "cycle off" time, and an amplitude adjusted to tolerance. The advantage of this technique over voluntary weight training alone is not clear. Also, electrostimulation of muscle less than 10% of normal strength was not helpful.

Upper Motor Neuron Muscle

Following upper motor neuron injury, significant diffuse atrophy occurs in paralyzed muscles. The physiological consequences of such atrophy may be widespread.[27] Atrophy of the gluteus muscles is believed to contribute to the development of ischial pressure sores following spinal cord injury. Muscle atrophy of the lower extremities may decrease blood flow, leading to venous stasis and increased risk for thromboembolic diseases. Muscle weakness may also increase the risk of flexion contractures. Finally, psychological problems related to reduced self-esteem may be associated with significant muscle atrophy. All these changes can potentially be reversed by application of neuromuscular stimulation for muscle strengthening and hypertrophy.

In addition, neuromuscular stimulation plays another potentially significant role in rehabilitation medicine. Muscle strengthening is an essential prerequisite prior to application of FES technology for upper extremity neuroprostheses, cycle ergometry, standing, and gait. An example of such a strengthening approach is the isokinetic leg training used to improve quadriceps strength prior to FES ergometry and gait training. Surface electrodes are attached over the quadriceps muscle and cyclic stimulation (3–4 sec on/3–4 sec off) is given at a frequency of 20–50 Hz and with a pulse width of 300 μsec. The training protocol varies from three times weekly to daily. After successful completion of a predetermined number of leg lifts through a 45° arc, progressive resistance is added to aid in strengthening. Isokinetic leg training three times weekly results in an increase in quadriceps girth and volume (as determined by computerized axial tomography) and an increase in quadriceps muscle protein synthesis with no concomitant increase in total body protein synthesis.[45]

Cyclic use of electrical stimulation has also been shown to decrease upper extremity contractures in hemiplegic subjects.[5] Active electrodes are placed proximally on the forearm over the motor point for stimulation of the wrist and finger extensors, and the reference electrode is placed distally on the forearm. Cyclic stimulation of 7 sec on, 10 sec off is used initially for 15 minutes twice daily; treatment sessions are later increased to 30 minutes three times per day. Prospective studies have shown that flexion contractures can be prevented at the wrist, metacarpophalangeal, and proximal intraphalangeal joints in subacute hemiplegic subjects. In addition, improved range of motion in wrist extension was noted in patients with flexion contractures. Long-term studies in an outpatient setting will determine whether electrical stimulation can replace traditional range of motion activities.

Finally, a recent study suggests that FES can be employed to decrease loading on the gluteus maximus muscle by changing its shape when seated to more nearly resemble the shape of the suspended buttocks.[32] While its efficacy in preventing pressure sores is unknown, this change in tissue shape is certainly a promising and exciting new utilization of therapeutic electrical stimulation.

SPASTICITY

Spasticity is defined as an increase in muscle tone related to an increased sensitivity of stretch reflexes in upper motor neuron lesions.[24] Although spasticity can be utilized to help support a person in gait or transfers, spasticity may also result in significant functional impairment, and control of spasticity is a requirement for all modalities of FES. Three basic approaches have been used to reduce dysfunctional spasticity: pharmacological, surgical, and physical measures.[24] Baclofen, diazepam, and dantrolene sodium are the most commonly used agents in the treatment of spasticity, but pharmacological management carries the potential of significant side effects. Surgery is also useful in selected patient groups.[55] Another potential therapy, dating back to the mid-1800s, is electrical stimulation.

Both cyclic electrical stimulation (2.5 seconds on/2.5 seconds off, 0.5 seconds overlap)[52] and continuous stimulation (20 minutes duration)[4,30] have been proposed. Stimulation is supplied with a compensated monophasic pulse at 300–500 μsec duration, an amplitude of 50–100 mA, and a frequency up to 100 Hz through electrodes covered with water-soaked gauze to increase the stimulation surface. Effectiveness of therapy is determined by subjective or objective evidence of improved function or by quantitative tests such as the pendulum drop test.

Marked reduction in spasticity and improved ability to ambulate have been reported following cyclic exercises induced by peroneal nerve stimulation in a spinal cord-injured patient.[15] Decreased calf spasticity and improved voluntary control in hemiplegia have been reported following electrical stimulation for 15 minutes three times per day.[39] The use of surface electrical stimulation to muscle groups antagonistic to spastic muscle groups reduced spasticity in persons with hemiplegia,[2] and surface stimulation to the peroneal nerve decreased ankle clonus in brain-injured and multiple sclerosis patients. In spinal cord injury, sinusoidal current produced significantly greater reduction in spasticity than faradic current.[21] Other groups have used a combination of alternating and direct currents in the treatment of spasticity in spinal cord injury and have reported that up to two-thirds of patients show a decrease in spasticity and muscle spasm in the treated extremity and nearly 50% show a decrease on the contralateral side. Symptomatic relief lasted from 30 minutes to 24 hours. Quantitative objective measures have also demonstrated that spasticity responds to electrical stimulation. Stimulation of either dermatomes or muscles leads to a decrease in spasticity in approximately 50% of the subjects.

The results of repetitive long-term use of functional electrical stimulation to decrease spasticity remain somewhat controversial. Cyclic electrical stimulation consisting of a 2.5 second train at 20 Hz, with 400 μsec compensated monophasic pulses delivered in an alternating fashion, resulted in increases in spasticity after four weeks of reconditioning. This increase in spasticity was associated with gains in strength over the same interval.[53] Thus, at the present time, it appears that FES can be very effective for short-term, short-duration improvements in spasticity, but that additional studies will be required before it can be recommended for long-term treatment.

NEURAL ORTHOSIS

Since the first application of FES as a functional orthosis to improve hemiplegic gait, comparatively few advances have occurred in the use of this modality as a clinical tool. However, the application of FES as a neural orthosis has enjoyed significant development into other directions. The application of FES in the quadriplegic or even hemiplegic upper extremity is discussed elsewhere in this chapter. The balance of this section will be devoted to a discussion of the merits of FES in idiopathic scoliosis.

The Milwaukee, Boston, and Wilmington braces are all considered appropriate therapeutic options in the management of idiopathic scoliosis; their failure rates range between 8% and 16%.[41] However, since in an adolescent such extensive bracing can cause adverse psychological effects and lead to noncompliance rates of 20% to 50%,[20] electrical stimulation has been explored as an alternative treatment strategy. Protocols typically recommend placing the electrode over the paraspinal muscles on the convex side of the curve, two to three vertebral segments above and below the apex. Current intensity ranges from 0–100 mA, with pulse duration of approximately 200 μsec and firing rates of approximately 30 Hz. The on/off cycles typically involve short stimulation intervals followed by comparatively long rest intervals in an effort to prevent muscle fatigue (e.g., 5 seconds on followed by 25 seconds off). This system is utilized 8–10 hours each night during sleep. Skin irritation is the most frequent complaint, followed by rare complaints of low back pain; only 2% of patients complain of disrupted sleep. Success rates are typically identical to those for traditional bracing, although some studies suggest that electrostimulation does not alter the natural course of idiopathic scoliosis.[20,43] However, electrical stimulation is clearly psychologically superior to traditional bracing in that the subjects treated with electrical stimulation demonstrate higher self-esteem, less hostility, more advanced coping strategies, less anxiety, less depression, and better compliance.[23]

To summarize, sufficient long-term studies evaluating the efficacy of electrostimulation in the conservative management of idiopathic scoliosis have not yet been completed to unequivocally recommend this form of treatment. However, the clear psychological benefits of electrostimulation over extensive bracing and the studies reporting success rates identical to traditional bracing are compelling enough to warrant strong consideration for electrostimulation in the treatment of idiopathic scoliosis.

FES CYCLE ERGOMETRY

FES cycle ergometry as an active form of lower extremity physical therapy has been proposed for ameliorating a number of complications associated with spinal cord injury (SCI), including osteoporosis and cardiovascular deconditioning.[7,12,14,19] Within 2–12 weeks following SCI, there is a significant decline in aerobic capacity, with decrements in maximal oxygen consumption in liters per minute (VO_2 max) and minute ventilation to 40.7% and 58.3% below normal controls, respectively.[17] Traditional rehabilitation does not lead to significant recovery of this deficit.[17] After discharge from rehabilitation, the workload of paraplegics in performing ADL has been estimated at only 24% of their maximal work capacity, a percentage sufficiently less than is required to maintain cardiovascular fitness.[22] In addition, serum high-density lipoprotein cholesterol (HDL) levels are significantly decreased in SCI subjects in comparison to normal able-bodied persons,[28] and the level of HDL is much lower in sedentary SCI subjects than in SCI athletes.[8] These changes in cardiovascular risk factors may help explain why cardiovascular disease is now the leading cause of death in SCI patients.[26]

In an attempt to improve cardiopulmonary fitness after SCI, several training approaches have been investigated. Wheelchair marathoners have been shown to have significantly higher VO_2 max than sedentary SCI subjects (35.0 ± 4.8 versus 22.6 ± 5.0 ml/kg/min; $p < 0.01$),[44] but no prospective training studies have been reported. Prospective arm ergometry training protocols result in improved aerobic capacity as measured by a decrease in heart rate for a submaximal workload and an increase in VO_2 max (12.1 ± 0.54 pretraining to 23.5 ± 3.1 ml/kg/min post-training). Functionally, this improvement translated into increased endurance for wheelchair propulsion.[16]

Upper extremity training protocols may, however, be an inefficient means of aerobic training in paraplegics because arm work has been shown to be less mechanically effective than leg training, since it involves recruitment of a smaller muscle mass and results in 15–35% lower VO_2 max than similar exercise performed by the legs.[13,18,50] In addition, quadriplegic subjects may not have sufficient voluntary arm strength to pursue such training protocols. Therefore, functional electrical stimulation of the lower extremities has been suggested as an alternative training system to improve cardiopulmonary function.

FES has also been suggested as a possible therapeutic modality for preventing or reversing neurogenic osteopenia. As early as three days post-SCI, increased calcium excretion is evident, reflecting accentuated rates of bone resorption. Confirmation of bone loss below the level of the spinal cord injury is garnered from iliac crest biopsies that reveal reduced trabecular bone volume, increased resorptive surfaces, and diminished calcification rates. In addition, densitometry has shown that bone mineral content (BMC) is markedly reduced in the lower extremities in both paraplegics and quadriplegics, while BMC is maintained in the lumbar spine. The mechanism of osteopenia secondary to spinal cord injury is unclear, although the loss of active muscle contraction may be a contributing factor. Thus, FES ergometry may be useful in reversing this additional complication of paralysis.

The most frequently used technology in rehabilitation medicine for FES cycling ergometry (REGYS 1 Clinical Rehabilitation System; Therapeutic Technology, Inc., Tampa, Florida) is composed of three components: a modified Monarch lower extremity ergometer, a stimulus control unit, and a chair.[51] Six separate channels for sequential surface muscle stimulation are used. The stimulation parameters include a compensated monophasic wave form delivered at 30 Hz with a pulse width of 350 sec and an amplitude between 0–130 mA.

Three carbon-filled silastic electrodes per muscle group are used on the quadriceps, gluteal, and hamstring muscles, with the two active electrodes placed laterally and the single reference electrode medially. Muscle activation is sequential to produce a pedaling action. Pedal position sensors monitor the average velocity and instantaneous position to control the stimulus amplitude so that a cycling rate of 50 rpm is maintained.

The training protocol consists of quadriceps muscle strengthening (isokinetic leg training) followed by cycle ergometry. For knee extension, three electrodes are attached to the quadriceps, an active electrode over the distal vastus medialis and lateralis muscles and a reference electrode over the rectus femoris. Stimulation is applied to the leg, which is flexed to 90°, allowing extension to 45°. Completion of 45 leg lifts through a 45° arc of motion permits progression to extension exercises against resistive loads that do not exceed 10 lb.

Cycle ergometry begins when quadriceps strength is sufficient for more than 45 leg lifts against at least 3 lb of resistance. Initial sessions of cycle ergometry are performed at 0 kilopond (kp) resistant load for two 15-minute runs. During a session, runs are terminated at the point of fatigue, as defined by an inability to peddle at least 35 rpm, or after successful completion of 15 minutes of cycling at 35–50 rpm. Resistance is gradually increased in increments of 1/8 kp after successful completion of three consecutive 15-minute sessions of continuous cycling. All subjects are monitored for heart rate and blood pressure during training.

The medical criterion for involvement in the FES cycling program is a spinal cord injury between the level of C4–5 and T11–12 and Frankel A or B classification.[48] The upper limit of C4–5 was chosen to assure adequate ventilatory drive for aerobic conditioning. The fact that cauda equina injuries result in lower motor neuron paralysis and do not respond to functional electrical stimulation accounts for the defined lower limit. Severe spasticity interferes with the FES ergometry system by resisting cycling motions. Lower extremity x-rays should be taken prior to initiation of training to confirm the absence of degenerative joint disease or significant heterotopic bone formation. Tests of range of motion should reveal flexion to 75–90° at the knee, no mediolateral knee instability, and sufficient ankle dorsiflexion for pedaling (< 5–10° of plantar flexion).

With the training protocol described above, FES cycle ergometry has shown some evidence of an aerobic training benefit, although its effectiveness in reducing cardiovascular risk or improving endurance in ADL is uncertain. After 12 weeks of cycling, endurance for cycling is greater and a larger workload can be handled without increases in heart rate.[51] Significant increments in VO_2 max have also been noted with lower-extremity ergometry stress testing, although similar findings are not seen in the upper-extremity ergometry stress test.[51] This increase in VO_2 max seen in lower-extremity testing may be attributable to increases in peripheral oxygen consumption rather than a central cardiopulmonary training effect.

FES ergometry has also been reported to result in increased quadriceps strength and endurance.[49] It has not, however, been shown to increase bone mineral density in the lumbar spine or proximal femur in patients with long-standing spinal cord injury.[31,38,45] Finally, patients report that FES cycle ergometry improves self-image and appearance.[56] Thus, in light of the literature available at this time, FES ergometry seems to be a promising therapeutic modality, but additional studies will be needed to determine its true benefit in improving cardiopulmonary aerobic capacity and in decreasing the complications associated with long-standing inactivity secondary to paralysis.

FES IN THE CONTROL OF UPPER EXTREMITY GRASP-RELEASE FUNCTION

FES may have a role in providing prehension release in patients who have diminished or absent control of upper extremity function due to an upper motor neuron lesion.[47] Traditionally, two alternatives, tendon transfer and external orthoses, have been employed in upper extremity rehabilitation. Tendon transfers require one or two muscles of the distal upper extremity to be under voluntary control and thus cannot be used for spinal cord-injured patients with C5 or C6 quadriplegia who have voluntary control of only the shoulder or elbow. External orthoses provide only limited functional performance that often requires modification of the objects to be grasped or prior placement of the object by an attendant.[57] Over the past seven years, isolated activation of small muscles of the hand has been studied to determine its effectiveness in providing palmar and lateral prehension for both basic tasks and integrated activities.

The goal of upper extremity FES is to provide a versatile prehension-release that is graded in intensity, is repeatable, and affords adequate strength for functional activity. Stimulation can be provided by surface or implantable electrodes, although current neuroprostheses utilize indwelling intramuscular or epimysial electrodes owing to their superior performance. One such electrode is a helical coil composed of a teflon-insulated multifilament of 316 L-stainless steel wire with a deinsulated tip. Up to 10 intramuscular electrodes are placed percutaneously through the lumen of a hypodermic needle over a 4 cm area of muscle.[47] Such electrodes have a failure rate of 0.05% per month secondary to fractures. To reduce the fracture rate of electrodes, a disc containing epimysial electrodes can be surgically sutured to a muscle to reduce movement.

Stimulation parameters for upper extremity FES include a charge density of 2.0 μC per mm^2, an amplitude of up to 20 mA, and a pulse width of up to 200 $\mu secs$. The first half of each pulse wave results in a neural action potential and the second half of the pulse wave causes charge neutrality to prevent nerve injury. Control of recruitment is regulated by intensity (amplitude) or duration (width). An increased frequency results in a progressively smoother, more fused response up to 15 Hz, and increasing strength occurs with stimulations up to 50 Hz.

All subjects require an FES conditioning program before they begin to learn to control the FES upper extremity activity. Optimal stimulation parameters are not known for such conditioning programs, but a stimulation of 10 Hz for eight hours per day over a two-month period has been shown to increase the strength of contractions of hand muscles.

Coordinated movement depends upon the sequential stimulation of hand muscles to produce synergism of motion. Eight muscle groups are involved in lateral and palmar prehension-release (flexor digitorum superficialis and profundus, flexor pollicis longus and brevis, adductor pollicis, abductor pollicis brevis, extensor digitorum, and extensor pollicus longus).[25] Control of finger position, thumb, and grasp uses an open-loop myoelectric, two-axis joy stick on the contralateral shoulder coordinated through a single command source. The horizontal axis controls graded response and the vertical axis commands stimulus intensity for locking mechanisms.

The medical criteria for utilization of an upper extremity FES neuroprosthesis include C5 or C6 Frankel A or B quadriplegia with absent static two-point discrimination in the C6 dermatome. Subjects should have no evidence of muscle denervation and should have full range of motion in the shoulder, elbow, and fingers; any spasticity should be pharmacologically controlled. Patients with hemiplegia from cerebrovascular accident or with upper extremity involvement from cerebral palsy have also been amenable to such therapy.

The use of FES upper-extremity neural prostheses has shown favorable results. Patients have demonstrated the ability to pick up, hold, use, and release objects such as utensils, writing instruments, and telephones as well as to perform integrated tasks such as pouring, washing, and brushing teeth. The patient executes these activities independently, picking up an unmodified object and manipulating it without assistance, which allows for increased independence and enhancement of ADL.

FES STANDING AND AMBULATION

FES standing has a wide range of potential physiological benefits.[27] Standing may prevent disuse atrophy and the development of contractures. Weight-bearing has been shown to decrease hypercalciuria and complications of renal calculi and may prevent neurogenic osteopenia. Standing can augment blood circulation, reduce venous stasis, and lower the risk of thromboembolic disease. It has also been suggested to improve bladder and bowel function by reducing residual capacity. Finally, FES standing is a necessary prerequisite for proceeding with training for FES ambulation.

Following stimulation by surface electrodes over the quadriceps and with the use of a standing frame, T4–10 paraplegics have successfully stood,[27,46,58] supporting more than 95% of their body weight by their legs for short periods of time. Stimulation parameters for FES standing include a compensated monophasic wave with a pulse amplitude from 0–120 volts, a current intensity of 0–120 mA, a frequency of 20 Hz, and a pulse width of 400 μsec. Water-soaked sponges are used with electrodes to improve conductivity over the quadriceps. Standing is produced by a linear increase in amplitude up to 120 volts, followed by bilateral continuous stimulation of the quadriceps. The arms are utilized to augment the quadriceps power for rising and to maintain balance once a standing position is achieved.

FES standing is not successful in all subjects with thoracic SCI. Medical criteria for exclusion include the presence of joint contractures, dysesthetic pain, and spasticity. No significant complications have arisen from FES standing. At this time, FES standing is primarily a research tool, and further studies are essential to find ways to reduce fatigue of the upper-motor-neuron paralyzed muscles in order to produce the prolonged weight-bearing that is needed for potential physiological or functional improvements in patients with SCI.

FES ambulation is an active area of research worldwide and clearly beyond the scope of this chapter. Successful ambulation using surface electrodes and reciprocal walkers has been reported.[27] Recent work has focused on the use of implantable electrodes in the development of closed loop systems. Research reports to date are promising and illustrate that substantially enhanced function may be available clinically in the future by applying the techniques of functional electrical stimulation to produce walking.

TRANSCUTANEOUS ELECTRICAL NERVE STIMULATION (TENS)

Since the introduction of the TENS unit in 1966, literally hundreds of articles have been published describing the role of this modality as an adjunct in ameliorating pain. Proposed indications include virtually all forms of acute and chronic neuropathic, musculoskeletal, visceral, and arthritic pain.[42] Despite this considerable body of literature, serious methodological problems—such as failure to utilize a homogeneous patient population, the absence of controls, and the restriction of studies to subjects in whom all other forms of therapy have failed—have resulted in many unresolved issues. The mechanism of action, indications for treatment, optimal electrode placement, optimal stimulus parameters, and even efficacy of treatment are examples of important questions that have not been clearly resolved.

Two primary theories are advanced to explain the analgesic properties of TENS. The "gate theory" of pain was the first proposed mechanism, but interest has shifted to the central nervous system opioid system since its discovery. The validity of this second mechanism has been questioned after several studies demonstrated that naloxone does not always reverse the analgesia attributed to TENS stimulation.[35] However, this observation may be explained by the fact that differing stimulus parameters result in the preferential secretion of specific opioids, and naloxone is known to have variable affinities for their respective receptors.[3] For example, low-frequency FES is thought to preferentially stimulate beta-endorphin release, while high-frequency FES appears to preferentially stimulate met-enkephalin release.[56] Finally, other studies have documented that multiple neurotransmitter systems, such as serotonin and substance P, are stimulated by TENS.[3]

The stimulation parameters available for clinical use today are numerous.[36] In general, they can be characterized as either high-frequency, low-amplitude TENS or low-frequency, high-amplitude TENS. High-frequency, low-amplitude TENS (or conventional TENS) frequently involves stimulation rates of 70–100 Hz with a pulse width of up to 200 μsec and an amplitude capability between 0 and 100 mA that is adjusted to produce the minimum sensation. Low-frequency, high-amplitude TENS (or acupuncture-like TENS) usually implies stimulation rate settings of 0–10 Hz, a duration of 0–200 μsec, and sufficient amperage to produce visible muscle contractions. These TENS units can also be adjusted to produce pulse bursts separated by periods of rest.

Studies have suggested that the different stimulation systems may have specific clinical indications. For example, high-frequency, low-amplitude TENS may be more efficacious for neuropathic pain, whereas low-frequency, high-amplitude TENS may be preferable for acute pain. However, whether or not one stimulating system is more beneficial is still open to question, since the introduction of the different systems does not appear to have improved the reported rates of therapeutic success.[42]

As previously mentioned, optimal sites for electrode placement remain to be determined. Numerous approaches are advocated, but placement over the painful area remains the most common initial technique. Failure with this approach warrants experimentation with electrode placement over proximal paravertebral sites, peripheral nerves, or other acupuncture points. Considerable patience and encouragement are required during the trial phase in order to prevent premature rejection of this important modality.

In summary, the TENS unit remains an important tool for the rehabilitation physician in the treatment of pain. Despite a number of unresolved questions concerning virtually all aspects of TENS utilization, there does appear to be a therapeutic benefit directly attributable to its use. Further research is needed to identify the optimal stimulation techniques and the population of patients most likely to benefit from this expensive modality.

REFERENCES

1. Agnew WF, McCreery DB, eds. *Neural prosthesis: fundamental studies*. Englewood Cliffs, NJ: Prentice Hall; 1990:107–145.
2. Alfieri V. Electrical treatment of spasticity. *Scand J Rehabil Med.* 1982;14:177–183.
3. Almay BGL, Johansson F, von Knorring L, et al. Long-term high-frequency transcutaneous

electrical nerve stimulation (hi-TNS) in chronic pain; clinical response and effects on CSF-endorphines, monoamine metabolites, substance P-like immunoreactivity (SPLI) and pain measures. *J Psychsom Res.* 1985;29:247–257.

4. Bajd T, Gregonc M, Vodovnik L, Benko H. Electrical stimulation in treating spasticity resulting from spinal cord injury. *Arch Phys Med Rehabil.* 1985;66:515–517.

5. Baker LL, Yeh C, Wilson D, Waters RL. Electrical stimulation of wrist and fingers for hemiplegic patients. *Phys Ther.* 1979;59:1495–1499.

6. Bennett RL, Knowlton GC. Overwork weakness in partially denervated skeletal muscle. *Clin Orthop.* 1958;12:22–29.

7. Biering-Sorensen F, Bohr H, Schaadt O. Bone mineral content of the lumbar spine and lower extremities years after spinal cord lesion. *Paraplegia.* 1988;26:293–301.

8. Brenes G, Dearwater S, Shapera R, et al. HDL concentrations in physically active and sedentary spinal cord injured patients. *Arch Phys Med Rehabil.* 1986;67:445–450.

9. Brown MC, Holland RL. A central role for denervated tissues in causing nerve sprouting. *Nature.* 1979;282:724–726.

10. Brown MD, Cotter MA, Hudlicka O, et al. The effects of different patterns of muscle activity on capillary density, mechanical properties and structure of slow and fast rabbit muscles. *Pflugers Arch.* 1976;361:241.

11. Brownsom C, Isenberg H, Brown W, et al. Changes in skeletal muscle gene transcription induced by chronic stimulation. *Muscle Nerve.* 1988;11:1183–1189.

12. Chantraine A, Nusgens B, LaPiere CM. Bone remodelling during the development of osteoporosis in paraplegia. *Calcif Tissue Int.* 1986;38:323–327.

13. Crowell LL, Squires WG, Raven PB. Benefits of aerobic exercise for paraplegics: a brief review. *Med Sci Sports Exerc.* 1982;18:501–508.

14. Davis GM, Kofsley PR, Kelsey JC, Shepherd RJ. Cardiorespiratory fitness and muscular strength of wheelchair users. *Can Med Assoc J.* 1981;125:1317–1323.

15. Davis R. Spasticity following spinal cord injury. *Clin Orthop.* 1975;112:66–75.

16. DiCarlo SE. Effect of arm ergometry training on wheelchair propulsion endurance of individuals with quadriplegia. *Phys Ther.* 1988;68:40–44.

17. Ellenberg M, MacRitchie M, Franklin B, et al. Aerobic capacity in early paraplegia: implications for rehabilitation. *Paraplegia.* 1989;27:261–268.

18. Emes CG. Fitness and the physically disabled; a review. *Can J Applied Sport Sci.* 1981;6:176–178.

19. Figonl SF. Cardiac function curves for quadriplegic men during dynamic arm exercise. *Med Sci Sports Exerc.* 1986;18(Suppl):58.

20. Fisler DA, Rupp GF, Emkes M. Idiopathic scoliosis: transcutaneous muscle stimulation versus the Milwaukee Brace. *Spine.* 1987;12:987–991.

21. Gianville HJ. Electrical control of paralysis. *Proc R Soc Med.* 1972;65:133–135.

22. Hjeltnes N, Vokac Z. Circulatory strain in everyday life of paraplegics. *Scand J Rehabil Med.* 1979;11:67–73.

23. Kahanovitz, Snow B, Pinter I. The comparative results of psychologic testing in scoliosis patients treated with electrical stimulation or bracing. *Spine.* 1984;9:442–444.

24. Katz RT. Management of spasticity. *Am J Phys Med Rehabil.* 1988;67:108–116.

25. Keith MW, Peckham PH, Thorpe GB, et al. Functional neuromusclar stimulation neuroprostheses for the tetraplegic hand. *Clin Orthop.* 1988;233:25–33.

26. Kennedy EJ, ed. *Spinal cord injury: facts and figures.* Birmingham: University of Alabama Press; 1986.

27. Kralj AR, Badj T. *Functional electrical stimulation: standing and walking after spinal cord injury.* Boca Raton, FL: CRC Press; 1989.

28. LaPorte RE, Brenes G, Dearwater S, et al. HDL cholesterol across a spectrum of physical activity from quadriplegia to marathon running. *Lancet.* 1983;1:1212–1213.

29. Lazorthes Y, Upton ARM, eds. *Neurostimulation: an overview.* Mount Kisco, NY: Futura Publishing; 1985:5–10.

30. Lee WJ, McGovern JP, Duvall EN. Continuous tetanizing low voltage currents for relief of spasm. *Arch Phys Med Rehabil.* 1950;51:766–771.

31. Leeds EM, Klose J, Ganz W, et al. Bone mineral density after bicycle ergometry training. *Arch Phys Med Rehabil.* 1990;71:207–209.

32. Levine SP, Kett RL, Cederna PS, Brooks SV. Electrical muscle stimulation for pressure sore prevention: tissue shape variation. *Arch Phys Med Rehabil.* 1990;71:210–215.

33. Liberson WT, Holmquest HJ, Scot D, Dow M. Functional electrotherapy: stimulation of the peroneal nerve synchronized with the swing phase of the gait of hemiplegic patients. *Arch Phys Med Rehabil.* 1961;42:101–105.
34. Lieber RL. Comparison between animal and human studies of skeletal muscle adaptation to chronic stimulation. *Clin Orthop.* 1988;233:14–23.
35. Mannheimer C, Emanuelsson H, Waagstein F, et al. Influence of naloxone on the effects of high-frequency transcutaneous electrical nerve stimulation in angina pectoris induced by atrial pacing. *Br Heart J.* 1989;62:36–42.
36. Mannheimer JS, Lampe GN, eds. *Clinical transcutaneous electrical nerve stimulation.* Philadelphia: FA Davis; 1984.
37. Marsolais EB, Kobetic R. Development of a practical electrical stimulation system for restoring gait in the paralyzed patient. *Clin Orthop.* 1988;233:64–74.
38. Milnar-Brown HS, Miller RG. Muscle strengthening through electric stimulation combined with low resistance weights in patients with neuromuscular disorders. *Arch Phys Med Rehabil.* 1988;69:20–24.
39. Mooney V, Wileman E, McNeal DR. Stimulator reduces spastic activity. *JAMA.* 1969;207:2199–2200.
40. Morrissey MC. Electromyostimulation from a clinical perspective: a review. *Sports Med.* 1988;6:29–41.
41. Mullett K. State-of-the-art in neurostimulation. *PACE.* 1987;10:162–175.
42. Nolan MF. Selected problems in the use of transcutaneous electrical nerve stimulation for pain control—an appraisal with proposed solutions. *Phys Ther.* 1988;68:1694–1698.
43. O'Donnell CS, Brunnell WP, Betz RR, et al. Electrical stimulation in the treatment of idiopathic scoliosis. *Clin Orthop.* 1988;229:107–113.
44. Okuma H, Ogata H, Hatada K. Transition of physical fitness in wheelchair marathon competitors over several years. *Paraplegia.* 1989;27:237–243.
45. Pacy PJ, Hesp R, Halliday A, et al. Muscle and bone in paraplegic patients, and the effect of functional electrical stimulation. *Clin Sci.* 1988;75:481–487.
46. Peckham PH. Functional electrical stimulation: current status and future prospects of applications to the neuromuscular system in spinal cord injury. *Paraplegia.* 1987;25:279–288.
47. Peckham PH, Keith MW, Freehafer AA. Restoration of functional control by electrical stimulation in the upper extremity of the quadriplegic patient. *J Bone Joint Surg [Am].* 1988;70:144–148.
48. Phillips CA. Medical criteria for active physical therapy: physician guidelines for patient participation in a program of functional electrical rehabilitation. *Am J Phys Med.* 1987;66:269–286.
49. Pollack SF, Aren K, Spielholz N, et al. Aerobic training effects of electrically induced lower extremity exercises in spinal cord injured people. *Arch Phys Med Rehabil.* 1989;70:214–219.
50. Ragnarsson KT. Physiologic effects of functional electrical stimulation-induced exercises in spinal cord-injured individuals. *Clin Orthop.* 1988;233:53–63.
51. Ragnarsson KT, Pollack S, O'Daniel W, et al. Clinical evaluation of computerized functional electrical stimulation after spinal cord injury: a multicenter pilot study. *Arch Phys Med Rehabil.* 1988;69:672–677.
52. Robinson CJ, Katt NA, Bolam JM. Spasticity in spinal cord injured patients: 1, short-term effects of surface electrical stimulation. *Arch Phys Med Rehabil.* 1988;69:598–604.
53. Robinson CJ, Katt NA, Bolam JM. Spasticity in spinal cord injured patients: 2, initial measures and long-term effects of surface electrical stimulation. *Arch Phys Med Rehabil.* 1988;69:862–868.
54. Selkowitz DM. High frequency electrical stimulation in muscle strengthening: a review and discussion. *Am J Sports Med.* 1989;17:103–111.
55. Sindou M, Pregelj R, Boisson D, et al. Surgical selective lesions of nerve fibers and myelotomies for modifying muscle hypertonia. In: Eccles J, Dimitrijevic MR, eds. *Recent achievements in restorative neurology: upper motor neuron function and dysfunction.* Basel: S Karger; 1985.

56. Sipski ML, DeLisa JA, Schweer S. Functional electrical stimulation bicycle ergometry: patient perceptions. *Am J Phys Med Rehabil.* 1989;68:147–149.
57. Wise MF, Wharton G, Robinson TD. Long-term use of functional hand orthoses by quadriplegics. *Asia Bull.* 1986;4:4–5.
58. Yakony GM, Jaeger RJ, Roth E, et al. Functional neuromuscular stimulation for standing after spinal cord injury. *Arch Phys Med Rehabil.* 1990;71:201–206.

Chapter 22

REHABILITATION OF PATIENTS WITH MULTIPLE SCLEROSIS

Vinod Sahgal

The rehabilitation strategies in any disease are a function of the age of the patient, nature and course of the disease, and psychosocial determinants. These factors weigh heavily in the management of patients with multiple sclerosis (MS).

INCIDENCE AND PREVALENCE

The prevalence of MS ranges from 7 to 178 per 100,000, increasing with latitude within the range from 30° to 70°N. (The exception is Scotland, where the prevalence rate is 308 per 100,000.) Blacks have a much lower prevalence of MS than whites. In areas where it is prevalent (30°–70°N) incidence increases with age, peaking during the third and fourth decades and declining stepwise thereafter, with a deep decline to less than 5% after 40 years of age. The male to female ratio is 14:1. It has been reported that this is a disease of the socially and educationally fortunate;[3] however, studies from Minnesota, Israel, and Ireland have failed to support this. In Central and South America no good studies exist as to the prevalence, but the European experience may be applicable to the population of European extraction.

COURSE AND PROGNOSIS

The most common course of this disease is one of remissions and relapses. Of patients affected in their 20s or 30s (the peak of incidence), 90% have a relapsing course. The rest may have benign or chronic progressive courses. The probability of relapse is highest in the first few years (25–30% relapse in the first year, 50% in two years, and 75% in five years). The relapses may last from days to months. The course of the disease can change from relapsing to progressive at any time, or the patients may not have any exacerbation for 10 to 15 years. The factors that are associated with high risk of disability are: 1) progressive course (late age of onset), 2) incomplete recovery from the acute attack, and 3) frequent relapses. The benign form of the disease is characterized by optic neuritis and few cerebellar, pyramidal, brain stem, and sphincter signs. Patients recover from most of the disability caused by a relapse within one month. Krutzke[7] reports an 86% improvement rate in patients with an attack lasting one week, which drops to 36% when exacerbation lasts from two weeks to a month. The severity of the symptoms is independent of the outcome. This disease has an impact on life expectancy, which, like the above factors, affects rehabilitation planning. Actuarial life expectancy among men with MS was reduced by 9.5 years and among women by 14.4 years in the United States.

The impact of disability on the vocational profile of the patient has been examined since the 1950s. Mueller[10] reported that 40% of the patients were incapacitated for work in 5 years, 50% in 10 years, and 60% in 15 years. Kolb[6] reported that 75% of the patients gave up their work within a year and only 10% were working after 10 years. More recently, Confavreux et al.[4] calculated that 50% of cases were moderately disabled but still ambulating after six years of illness. Bauer and Firnhaber[2] further looked at the causes of inability to work. Spastic paraparesis was cited by 60% of the patients, incoordination by 39%, and sphincter disturbance by 23%. The data showed that over 60% of the patients had multiple severe deficits.

The following common signs and symptoms found among the patients have a major impact on the planning of the rehabilitative process:

Depression was the most common affective problem, as judged by Beck's depression inventory.[1,5] Intellectual deterioration has been thought to be relatively uncommon. However, in 1980 Peyser et al.[11] reported that 29 of 53 patients with MS showed evidence of intellectual deterioration. On the other hand, Marsh[9] could not correlate intellectual deficit with the extent of physical disability on Krutzke's scale.

Brain stem signs and symptoms are diplopia, ataxia, dysarthria, spasticity, atonia, facial weakness, dysphagia, ataxia, hearing problems, diminished visual acuity, and disturbed color vision. In a high percentage of cases, only spinal cord symptoms and signs may be seen. These are weakness, spasticity, sensory loss, autonomic disturbance, bowel and bladder problems (50%), and ataxia (77%). Sexual dysfunction with impotence was present in 47% of males.[13] Among females, Lundberg found an incidence of over 50% of some sexual dysfunction.[8]

In summary, multiple sclerosis would be expected to be a significant problem among the population of European descent in South America, with the highest incidence rates among people of Scottish, German, Scandinavian, and French extraction, and lower rates among persons of other backgrounds (Portuguese, indigenous, etc.).

REHABILITATION PROGRAM

The focus of the rehabilitation program will be different for the three types of clinical course: 1) remitting and relapsing, 2) benign, and 3) chronic progressive. Patients whose disease is in one of the first two categories are younger and thus in their vocationally and sexually productive years. Because those with the third variety of MS are older, work and sexuality may be less important issues, so that rehabilitation is relatively limited to maintenance of skills needed in activities of daily living (ADL).

Since the clinical course of this disease affects the patient, his family, neural control, intellect, and mentation, it is imperative that a team be assembled to address all these issues. The team should include the following: a physical therapist for strength maintenance, coordination, transfers, and ambulation; an occupational therapist for ADL and prevocational issues; a speech therapist for swallowing, articulation, and alternate communication systems; a psychologist for psychological support of the patient and family and for cognitive retraining; a physiatrist for planning the program; a social worker for providing access to community services; a vocational counselor for job placement, modification, or training; and medical consultants, including a neurologist, urologist, and internist. Meeting all the above needs demands a comprehensive Multiple Sclerosis Care Clinic, which includes representation from these disciplines and through which the physician has access to the consultants.

The classical practices of training patients for transfers, sitting and standing balance, ambulation, communication, and ADL skills are employed by the various team members. However, the following special problems have to be addressed in the rehabilitation of patients with multiple sclerosis.

Spasticity

This is a very common symptom in MS and is classified into the following categories: 1) spasticity without spasms but with intact voluntary activity of various muscles; 2) spasticity with spasms (extensor and flexor), without voluntary motor activity at the involved joint but with no fixed contracture; 3) spasticity with fixed contractures (flexor and extensor).

In dealing with symptoms of the first category, the goal is to allay spasticity and also to maintain voluntary activity and optimal muscle strength. This can be achieved by the use of various pharmacological agents. The most commonly used drugs are diazepam, baclofen, and dantrolene sodium.

Diazepam (Valium) enhances GABA-mediated presynaptic inhibition and may depress lateral reticular formation (descending) and inhibit gamma neurons. This drug is best used in patients who cannot tolerate baclofen, or as an adjunct to baclofen.

Baclofen (Lioresal) is a GABA agonist that acts at the spinal cord level on the monosynaptic extensor and polysynaptic flexor reflexes without having any effect on neuromuscular transmission or excitation-contraction coupling. Thus, patients on this medication can be kept functionally ambulatory with or without the use of appropriate ankle-foot orthoses (AFOs). These patients should also participate in a strengthening program, using progressive resistive exercises, and a program to increase endurance, using isokinetic exercises. This raises the question of the effect of fatigue on the disease. Fatigue may transiently enhance the symptoms but has not been shown to precipitate an acute attack. The dosage of baclofen should be titrated individually, starting from a small dose of 20 mg daily. The side effects generally encountered are drowsiness and nausea followed in a dose-related fashion by headache, hypotension, fatigue, insomnia, and sphincter disturbances. The dosage should be decreased if fatigue or weakness becomes profound.

Dantrolene sodium (Dantrium), because its mode of action affects calcium-dependent excitation-contraction coupling, is not a front line drug for spasticity and muscular weakness since it can exaggerate weakness.

In the second stage of spasticity the goal is to minimize spasms and maintain range of motion so that transfers and ADL skills are not compromised. This result would enable the patient to remain mobile for independent living and vocational endeavors. The drugs described for use in the first stage are also useful, in the same order, but the patient may need higher dosages (i.e., dosages higher than recommended and in combination). In our experience, dantrolene sodium, either alone or in combination, proved very useful for this condition.

If adductor spasms become a significant problem for hygiene, transfers, and other ADL functions, then obturator neurectomy or phenol nerve block should be considered, but only in patients with severe ADL limitations. Adductor tenotomy should only be used in nonambulatory patients. Achilles' tendon lengthening to permit proper positioning for fitting of orthoses should also be considered.

In the third stage of spasticity the treatment of choice is tenotomies, and the goal is to achieve proper seating and positioning for hygiene, transfers, and activities of daily living.

The various tenotomies should be strictly reserved for patients who have no voluntary function of their lower extremities and whose leg position interferes with activities of daily living. Lengthening the Achilles' tendon is a dynamic procedure to relieve plantar flexion contractures for the proper fitting of the orthotic devices needed to facilitate ambulation. If clawing of the toes poses a significant problem in skin care or the wearing of shoes, then toe flexor tenotomies are helpful. Another procedure which may be considered is the split anterior tibial transfer for relief of supination and Achilles' tendon lengthening for the equinus deformity.

The most recent development in the management of spinal spasticity is the intrathecal injection of baclofen, using a pump that delivers a continuous infusion of Lioresal (100–150 μg/day). Patients who were followed over 18 months of continuous infusion all showed a significant decrease in spasticity, which increased their ADL status significantly.

Electrical stimulation of the dorsal column of the spinal cord, though initially touted as a promising therapeutic approach, has not stood the test of time, and we do not recommend this procedure for the management of spasticity.

Tremor

In about 40% of MS patients, upper extremity tremor and lack of coordination are disabling problems affecting activities of daily living and vocational endeavors. They are also the problems most resistant to fruitful therapeutic intervention. Pharmacological, physical therapeutical, and surgical methods have been tried for the management of tremor.

Pharmacological intervention.   The most commonly tried drugs, albeit with disappointing results, have been benzodiazepines and oral choline. The rationale for supplementary dietary choline was derived from the observation of lack of acetylcholine in the brain of patients with Friedreich's ataxia. Sabra et al.[12] reported that large doses of isoniazid (approximately 1,000 mg/day) with pyridoxine reduced or abolished cerebellar tremor. The postulated mechanism is the effect on the GABA aminotransferase system.

Physical therapy.   The use of weights around the distal joints has been found helpful in limiting the excursion of the tremor by increasing inertia. The amount of weight used must be individualized, since there is a minimum amount that has no observable effect and a maximum amount that may increase the tremor.

Neurosurgical intervention.   Stereotactical thalamotomy of the venterolateral nucleus, proposed by Irving Cooper, has shown promising results; improvements in tremor of 25–80% have been reported. In all these cases tremor was the major disability. The patients had definite vocational potential, and the procedure was always performed on the most affected side.

All the above interventions are designed to complement the comprehensive therapeutic approach, that is, aggressive physical and occupational therapy with the specific goal of mobility (household, community, and vocational). They should be further augmented by an aggressive community reentry, job placement, and/or volunteer program, as well as psychological support. The comprehensive approach is extremely important, since as the patient gains mobility, the ambition for fiscal, social, and psychological independence increases. If this infrastructure is not in place, the patients can suffer significant maladjustment.

Bladder Control

The other important rehabilitative issue to deal with is the management of bladder problems. Difficulties with bladder control occur in at least 80% to 90% of all patients with MS. Over 50% of patients complain of frequency of micturition, while the rest either suffer from incontinence or retention. These symptoms have an impact on employment and hygiene. The recurrence of urinary tract infections contributes to morbidity and mortality. In recent years there has been a systematic approach to the evaluation of bladder problems of neurogenic origin. It involves the measurement of bladder and urethral pressure, electromyography of the external sphincter, measurement of flow rate, and cystometry. These techniques have helped to differentiate detrusor hyperreflexia from detrusor-sphincter dyssynergia. Having made the above statement, it must be noted that the literature reveals no one-to-one relationship between the urinary symptoms and laboratory findings.

The management can be divided into three phases: pharmacological, surgical, and physical. The pharmacological treatment is designed to decrease detrusor hyperexcitability either by peripheral or central action. The main motor supply to the bladder is parasympathetic cholinergic (muscarinic), so anticholinergic drugs that have little or no nicotinic effect (oxybutynin chloride) can be used, as can other drugs such as propantheline. Some mild cases may also respond to high dosages of imipramine. In patients with detrusor-sphincter dyssynergia, the alpha-adrenergic blocking agent phenoxybenzamine has been reported to be useful. However, in our experience it has not been very promising because of its cumulative effect, which causes postural hypotension.

The most commonly used surgical approach has been bladder neck resection or external sphincterotomy. These procedures have resulted in continence and decreased urgency in about one-third of the cases. Destructive operations on the sacral roots have not been extensively tested or performed. The most common side effect of these procedures is impotence in males.

Catheterization

Placement of an indwelling catheter is to be avoided, as it can lead to urinary tract infection. However, this method is generally preferred to the risk of bed sores. If the patient has good hands and cognitive function and can position himself or herself, intermittent catheterization is the treatment of choice. Touchless catheters are available on the market for use by either sex. This method consists of catheterization every four hours, followed by fluid restriction after 6:00 p.m. and final catheterization at bedtime.

For the male patient, an external collecting device applied to the penis has been found to be very helpful.

Sexuality

Females do not frequently cite major problems in this area. However, inability to sustain an erection is a common male complaint. If the patient experiences spontaneous nocturnal erections, then he may benefit from reassurance and psychological support. In selected cases, nocturnal electroencephalography with penile tumescence studies should be done. If spasticity makes the mechanics of sexual relations problematic, then antispasticity intervention, using the techniques described above, would be of great help.

Psychological Support

A psychologist or psychiatrist who is well versed in the course and prognosis of this disease is a valuable asset to the patient. The most common forms of psychological disturbances are apprehension and fear stemming from ignorance of future expectations. Disease course and prognosis were dealt with in detail at the beginning of this chapter, and such information should form the basis of discussion and planning. Logical planning with regard to lifestyle will almost always result in a fruitful and less fearful existence.

The most commonly used drugs in our experience have been the antidepressants. These drugs alone may not yield a significant benefit, but when combined with psychotherapy they can be very effective. Among the various modes of psychotherapy, our experience has been that sharing of experiences by family and friends in family support groups and among patients in patient groups yields the best results.

An active and aggressive vocational service is an essential component of a comprehensive MS treatment program. This program should address physical barriers in the work place, such as ramps, curbs, elevators, and inaccessibility of bathrooms; and adaptational aids, such as hand controls, dysarthria compensating techniques, optical aids, orthotic devices, special office equipment, vocational evaluation and training, and job placement to find alternative jobs compatible with the patient's disability.

Social services are also essential to address the community and legislative issues surrounding disability and to raise private and governmental awareness of the needs of the disabled.

In summary, the proper management of patients with multiple sclerosis requires a balanced medical and comprehensive rehabilitation approach which maximizes the patient's physical, sexual, social, and vocational potential and maintains his or her psychological balance to ensure optimal community involvement.

REFERENCES

1. Baretz R, Stephensen M. Emotional responses to MS. *Psychosomatics*. 1981;22:117–127.
2. Bauer H, Firnhaber W. Zur leistungs prognose multiple sklerose. *Kranker Deutscher Medizinische Wochen Schrift*. 1963;88:1357–1364.
3. Beebe G, Krutzke JF, Kurland LT, Auth TL, Nazler B. Studies in natural history of MS. *Neurology (Minneapolis)*. 1967;17:2–17.
4. Confavreux C, Airmond G, Devic M. Course and prognosis of MS assessed by the computerized data processing of 349 patients. *Brain*. 1980;103:281–300.
5. Goodstein RK, Ferrell RB. MS presenting as a depressive illness. *Dis Nerv Syst*. 1977;38:127–131.
6. Kolb LC. The social significance of MS. *Proc Assoc Res Nerv Ment Dis*. 1950;28:28–40.
7. Krutzke JF. On the evaluation of disability in multiple sclerosis. *Neurology (Minneapolis)*. 1961;11:686–692.
8. Lundberg PO. Sexual dysfunction in female patients with MS. *Int Rehabil Med*. 1981;3:32–34.
9. Marsh GG. Disability, intellectual function in MS patients. *J Nerv Ment Dis*. 1980;168:758–762.
10. Mueller R. Studies in disseminated sclerosis. *Acta Med Scand [Suppl]*. 1949;133(222):2–214.
11. Peyser JM, Edwards KR, Poser CW, Fibkov SB. Cognitive function in MS. *Arch Neurol*. 1980;37:577–579.
12. Sabra AF, Hallet M, Sudarski L, Mulloy W. Reduction of action tremor in multiple sclerosis with isoniazide. *Neurology (Minneapolis)*. 1982;32:912–913.
13. Vas CJ. Sexual impotence and some autonomic disturbances in men with MS. *Acta Neurol Scand*. 1969;45:166–183.

Chapter 23

MANAGEMENT OF THE PATIENT WITH ACQUIRED APHASIA

John E. Sarno and Martha Taylor Sarno

Physiatrists have historically concerned themselves primarily with the motor, sensory, and orthopedic ravages of disabling illnesses. In general, the disorders of speech, language, and communication confronted in the practice of rehabilitation medicine receive little attention in residency training programs. This chapter describes the management of aphasia, perhaps the most disabling sequela of acquired brain damage. Current concepts and practices in the management of dysarthria have been expertly discussed in the recently published fourth edition of *Krusen's Handbook of Physical Medicine and Rehabilitation* (F.J. Kottke and J.F. Lehmann, eds., 1990),[4] to which the reader is referred. Such entities as functional articulation disorders, voice disorders, stuttering, cleft palate, and laryngectomy are generally managed by medical and paramedical specialists other than those in rehabilitation medicine.

APHASIA

The term aphasia refers to a language disorder resulting from acquired disease of the brain, such as cerebral infarct, infectious processes, neoplasia, or trauma, and not from genetic causes or perinatal trauma. The distinction is important because patients in the former category have normal language function prior to the onset of disease.

The neuropathology of aphasia results in a disturbance in the ability to transmit and receive verbal messages in either the spoken or written form. The ability to formulate and comprehend messages in verbal form is referred to as language. The term speech is not synonymous with language; it refers to the motor act of orally transmitting verbal messages.

The preparation of this chapter was supported in part by the National Institute on Deafness and Other Communication Disorders (NIDCD), Grant # R01 NS25367-01A1, of which one of the authors is Principal Investigator, and the National Institute of Disability and Rehabilitation Research (NIDRR), Grant #G008300000.

Patients with aphasia have trouble formulating verbal messages, comprehending them, or both. This applies to both spoken and written language. Their difficulties may be in finding or using the correct words or in using the proper grammatical construction. Ordinarily, there is a predominance of deficit in either the production of language or its comprehension, but many patients have some degree of trouble with both. The problems of people who are deaf or who have lost their voices are not to be confused with aphasia. Deaf individuals can transmit and receive language if it is in an appropriate sensory mode, for example finger spelling or sign language. The individual with absent phonation is able to formulate and present written messages and comprehends what is said if hearing is intact.

The group of disorders known as dysarthria must also be distinguished from aphasia, since these patients suffer damage to some part of the speech motor system and have difficulty with such mechanical parameters of speech as phonation, resonance, and articulation. The pathology of dysarthria may be in the brain, brain stem, or cerebellum and affects the function of one or more parts of the speech motor system, including the vocal cords, respiratory apparatus, larynx, pharynx, and tongue. The pathology of aphasia involves only the brain.

MANIFESTATIONS OF APHASIA

The following is a brief review of some of the common signs of aphasia.

Abnormal Fluency

An important characteristic of aphasic speech is its abnormal fluency relative to normal speech. Spontaneous speech is said to be fluent if it approaches normal with respect to its relative speed, length, and melody. In some cases, aphasic speech is more prolific than normal speech. It may be so full of errors, however, that it is almost impossible to understand. Nonfluent speech may be slow or halting, or may consist of single words or short phrases that adversely affect normal melody. It is basically agrammatical. Table 1 indicates where the locus of pathology generally is in fluent and nonfluent aphasia.

Naming Difficulties

Each of us has a kind of dictionary (lexicon) in our brains, from which we select the right words when attempting to transmit a thought. The person with aphasia may not be able to find the desired word at all (usually referred to as a naming disturbance) or may use the wrong word (called a paraphasia). Paraphasic errors take many forms. The patient may say *table* when he means *chair*, or *label* instead of *table*; he may make up an entirely new

Table 1. Aphasia syndromes.

	Broca's aphasia	Wernicke's aphasia	Global aphasia	Conduction aphasia	Anomic aphasia	Transcortical motor aphasia
Locus of lesion	Third frontal convolution	Posterior portion of superior temporal gyrus	Third frontal convolution and posterior portion of superior temporal gyrus	Parietal operculum or posterior temporal gyrus	Angular gyrus	Supplementary motor area
Speech fluency	Nonfluent	Fluent	Nonfluent	Fluent or nonfluent	Fluent	Nonfluent
Auditory comprehension	Good	Impaired	Impaired	Good	Good	Good
Repetition	Poor (but may be better than spontaneous speech)	Impaired	Impaired	Very good	Good	Normal
Naming	Poor (but may be better than spontaneous speech)	Impaired	Impaired	Impaired	Very poor	Impaired
Reading comprehension	Good	Impaired	Impaired	Variable	Variable	Good
Writing	Impaired	Impaired	Impaired	Impaired	Variable	Impaired

word, like *cabrew*. When there are many paraphasias in a sentence the speech is called jargon, and if the words are all new ones (like *cabrew*), it is called neologistic jargon.

Repetition Deficit

Another sign of aphasia is impairment in the ability to repeat words, phrases, or sentences. It is a fairly common manifestation and is found in many different types of aphasia. A repetition deficit is the most important sign in conduction aphasia and is consistently associated with an anatomical lesion in the perisylvian area of the dominant hemisphere (Table 1).

Auditory Comprehension Impairment

Comprehension of the spoken word is frequently impaired in aphasia. The deficit varies considerably in severity, with some patients being able to follow the general idea of a conversation and others understanding very little. Special testing will often reveal deficits not apparent in casual conversation. Aphasic patients with lesions in the parietotemporal region usually have comprehension deficits.

Reading and Writing Deficits

One may refer to reading and writing as the visual mode of language, while oral communication and auditory comprehension are the oral-aural mode. Both require the formulation, transmission, and understanding of language. Therefore, it is appropriate to include disturbances in reading and writing as part of aphasia when they are found in conjunction with other evidences of aphasia. Occasionally, a patient may have an impairment in reading but no difficulty in writing or auditory comprehension. In the majority of cases, however, all communication modes are impaired to varying degrees.

Grammatical Disturbances

Difficulty with grammar is a common sign of aphasia. Patients may use the wrong type of word (e.g., a noun instead of a verb) or use the wrong verb ending (e.g., "tomorrow I walked"). Words may be used in the wrong sequence. It was once thought that these difficulties were seen only in patients with anterior lesions, those with so-called Broca's aphasia, but it is now recognized that such deficits may occur in the other large category of aphasics, those patients with lesions in the parietotemporal area (Wernicke's aphasia).

Verbal Apraxia

This is a special type of motor disorder associated with nonfluent aphasia. It often accompanies other manifestations of aphasia but rarely occurs in isolation. Apraxia is best described as dysfunction in the ability to execute learned motor patterns when there is no evidence of weakness, incoordination, or sensory loss. The disorder may involve limb function; it is not uncommon to see a patient with aphasia who cannot use his/her hand for fine motor activities, although there is no loss of strength or sensory function. Verbal apraxia is characterized by an obvious motor struggle to produce speech.

MAJOR TYPES OF APHASIA

The clinical syndrome called aphasia has been studied for over 100 years. A number of systems of classification have been suggested, generally reflecting either a clinical or research emphasis. In keeping with the purpose of this textbook, the classification presented here will be clinically oriented.

A rational classification is possible because the signs of aphasia tend to cluster with great consistency. They do so because damage to certain neural structures tends to result in particular and consistent signs of dysfunction. Variations within categories are a function of differences in size and location of the lesion, in vascular and neural anatomy, and in other more subtle neuroanatomical and neuropsychological factors. The types of aphasia are summarized in Table 1.

Broca's Aphasia

Broca's aphasia has also been called expressive or motor aphasia. It is characterized by nonfluent, hesitant, telegraphic speech; reduced vocabulary; short sentences; and many pauses in the course of speaking. The preserved vocabulary usually consists of substantive, high-information words such as nouns, verbs, and adverbs. There tend to be many grammatical errors. In addition, the melody of speech is impaired and the patient may struggle to find words. This difficulty in production is to be differentiated from the struggle of the person with verbal apraxia, who knows the words but has a difficult time enunciating them. Auditory comprehension in these patients tends to be grossly preserved but is not completely normal in many cases. Repetition of words, phrases, and sentences is not normal.

The lesion in Broca's aphasia involves the third frontal convolution of the dominant hemisphere. There is invariably a right hemiparesis, more severe in the arm than in the leg (Table 1).

Patients with Broca's aphasia tend to be aware of their deficits and are depressed. They also often exhibit uncontrollable rage or aggression and may cry or be uncooperative. As we shall see, depression is not limited to this group of patients.

Wernicke's Aphasia

In these patients speech is fluent, contains many paraphasic errors, and is generally well articulated. They make grammatical mistakes, but not with the same frequency or of the same type as Broca's patients. Those with Wernicke's aphasia tend to omit substantive words (e.g., nouns and verbs) so that speech often sounds "empty." Auditory comprehension is impaired, as are reading and writing, and these patients have trouble with repetition. Based on the latter features, this type of aphasia is often called receptive aphasia, although there are clearly significant disturbances in language output as well.

The posterior part of the superior temporal gyrus is the locus of the lesion (Table 1). Wernicke's aphasia patients tend not to have motor, sensory, or visual field deficits. In view of the absence of these other neurological sequelae and the confusing nature of their communication disorder, they may be mistaken for psychiatric patients. This possibility is enhanced by the fact that some are paranoid. They may be anxious and depressed, are often inappropriate in their behavior, and present a confusing pattern of loss and recovery of awareness and control. Even though a Wernicke's aphasia patient may appear psychotic, the clinician should exercise a conservative approach and insist that a careful language evaluation be administered by someone who is sophisticated and experienced in the aphasias. If a language disorder is of sudden onset in a middle-aged or elderly person, it is highly unlikely that the individual is psychotic.

Global Aphasia

When patients with aphasia are profoundly impaired in all language modalities (i.e., speech, understanding, reading, and writing), resulting in an almost total loss of the ability to produce and comprehend language, the condition is referred to as global aphasia. Those with global aphasia tend to have a hemimotor defect as in Broca's aphasia, and react emotionally much like those patients. Broca's, Wernicke's, and global are the most common varieties of aphasia.

Conduction Aphasia

The major deficit in patients with conduction aphasia is the inability to repeat. Spontaneous speech is quite fluent and the patient may manifest only minor problems with auditory comprehension. Repetition, however, is characterized by great difficulty with function words (e.g., prepositions) and a tendency to omit or substitute words or, most frequently, to make paraphasic errors. The locus of the lesion is thought to be the parietal operculum or posterior temporal gyrus (Table 1).

Transcortical Motor Aphasia

Patients with transcortical motor aphasia can usually repeat accurately, which distinguishes them from conduction and Wernicke's aphasics. Their major problems are lack of fluency, the loss of connective words, and a marked tendency to make paraphasic errors and to perseverate. They comprehend well enough to follow simple conversation, but demonstrate deficits in formal testing. (See Table 1 for locus of lesion.)

Anomic Aphasia

Pure anomic aphasia, also referred to as amnesic aphasia, is an uncommon type of aphasia in which the major problem is word finding; speech is fluent and grammatically correct. Historically, the lesion has been thought to involve the angular gyrus, but its location is still under study.

DIAGNOSTIC MEASURES IN THE EVALUATION OF APHASIA

Over the past 25 years a number of excellent measures have been developed to assess aphasic disorders. Historically, diagnostic tests of aphasia have identified losses and deviations from normal language function, measured according to the general concepts employed in intelligence and educational tests. In recent years these tests have been standardized and thoroughly studied, so that the classical syndromes of aphasia can be consistently identified. Most of these tests were designed for speakers of English. Therefore, they are of no value in Spanish- or Portuguese-speaking countries since, unfortunately, one cannot simply translate test items from one language to another. Knowledge of test construction and neurolinguistics is necessary for the adaptation of an aphasia test into another language. An aphasia test that has been standardized in Spanish is described below.

The best known of the linguistic performance tests for aphasia are the Boston Diagnostic Aphasia Examination (BDAE), the Western Aphasia Battery (WAB), and the Neurosensory Center Comprehensive Examination for Aphasia (NCCEA). The NCCEA has been modified for use in Spanish and Portuguese (as well as Chinese, French, German, and Italian) and is known as the Multilingual Aphasia Examination (MAE).[1] The manual for this test is available from a source in the United States.*

---

*The Multilingual Aphasia Examination/Spanish may be obtained from: AJA Associates, Inc., P.O. Box 8740, Iowa City, Iowa 52240-8740, USA.

The MAE consists of seven subtests: Visual Naming; Sentence Repetition; Controlled Oral Word Association (i.e., word fluency); Spelling; a version of the Token Test (a subtest of the NCCEA that tests auditory comprehension); Aural Comprehension of Words and Phrases; and Reading Comprehension of Words and Phrases. Two rating scales are included: the first rates speech articulation, based on the patient's verbal performance throughout the test session; the second, writing praxis, is scored on the basis of the patient's performance on a task such as writing to dictation. Material from the MAE spelling subtest can be used for this task.

Increasingly, professionals engaged in the rehabilitation of patients with aphasia have been impressed with the importance of assessing the functional usefulness of language ability in the everyday life of the patient. An important dimension of aphasia assessment consists of the evaluation of functional communication, which involves considerably more than a person's linguistic performance, the attribute measured by traditional aphasia tests. Functional communication refers to a combination of all the verbal and nonverbal (gestural, pantomime, etc.) behaviors used to transmit thoughts, ideas, and feelings. Effective functional communication need not correlate with linguistic performance. A person may have very little verbal ability but be extremely effective in making himself understood through gestures, facial expression, and signs, for example.

Since communication is essentially a social behavior, a functional assessment must take into account the person's family setting, living situation, personality, and personal lifestyle. Additional extralinguistic factors include alertness, level of awareness, level of initiation of activity, reliability of the yes-no response system, and the ability to use gestures and pantomime. The setting in which the assessment takes place makes a difference for some individuals with aphasia. There are those who do less well in a test situation than when engaged in social conversation, and vice versa. It has been commonly reported that some patients speak better on the telephone than face to face. These are some of the many factors to be taken into account in a functional communication assessment.

The primary purpose of aphasia rehabilitation (speech therapy) is to improve functional communication effectiveness to the patient's maximum potential. This is accomplished by the patient developing compensatory verbal and nonverbal strategies.

Because the field of rehabilitation medicine is primarily concerned with teaching people to function in the face of disability, it is not surprising that the first functional communication assessment scale was developed in a rehabilitation medicine setting. It is known as the Functional Communication Profile (FCP).[7,9] Subsequently, two other functional measures have become available, the Communicative Abilities in Daily Living (CADL)[3] and the Communicative Effectiveness Index (CETI).[5]

Regrettably, none of the functional assessment measures are available in

Spanish or Portuguese. Nevertheless, clinicians will want to keep functional language factors in mind when clinically evaluating the patient with aphasia.

RECOVERY AND REHABILITATION

The rehabilitation management of patients with aphasia is particularly difficult because of the complexity and crucial importance to human beings of the ability to communicate. More than any other behavior, the faculty of speech identifies us as human. Of even greater importance, speech behavior is highly individual and unique for each of us. As a consequence, the loss or impairment of the power of speech is a mortal blow to self-esteem and to that important sense of identity. A language disorder affects every aspect of a person's life: occupation, social relationships, community status, and, perhaps most crucial, his/her role in the immediate family. A man who is paraplegic and in a wheelchair may still function as the "head of the house" and command the respect and attention of his family members. But a man with a significant aphasia, although he may have no other physical disability, usually loses his accustomed place in the family constellation.

It is to be expected, therefore, that patients with aphasia usually have severe psychological reactions. They are usually depressed, and when they are sufficiently aware of the nature of their aphasia, as are patients with Broca's aphasia, they may become angry and even agitated to the point of violence.

Planning for the management and rehabilitation of these patients must consider not only linguistic deficits but also the psychological and social sequelae of having aphasia. In addition, the expected course of recovery must be understood in order to plan effectively. For example, it was generally believed that recovery from aphasia ceased after three to six months, but recent research has provided strong support for the idea that functional (compensatory) improvement may continue for many more months and sometimes years. In one documented case, a poststroke aphasic patient showed gradual improvement for 10 years after onset.

Another commonly held idea is that younger aphasics do better than middle-aged and elderly patients. Current research is challenging this opinion by demonstrating that the severity of the lesion, psychological status of the patient, availability of support and treatment, the family situation, and other social factors are more important than age in determining outcome. A patient who is highly motivated, who can make adjustments, and who can use compensatory strategies tends to have a better outcome regardless of age.

In their eagerness for recovery, patients and their families often try to arrange for speech therapy more frequently than is appropriate or necessary. A program of one-hour sessions three to four times a week seems adequate. The intensity and frequency do not necessarily correlate with improvement.

Too much treatment may be negative by inducing unrealistic expectations of recovery, which lead to disappointment, frustration, and depression in both patient and family.

It is often thought that people who are highly intelligent or had high-level jobs prior to their illness will do better, but this is not necessarily so. Once more, the social and psychological factors mentioned above, plus the severity and type of the aphasia, are more important in determining outcome than a patient's premorbid level of intelligence and/or achievement.

The patient's premorbid personality is one of the most important factors in recovery. Those who tended to be anxious or depressed before becoming aphasic will invariably have a more difficult time. Patients who are perfectionists or always had a strong need to be in control will be angry and frustrated at their inability to function exactly as they did before. Passive individuals may become even more passive when confronted with the daunting reality of having aphasia. These common examples of the effect of personality on adjustment to life with aphasia suggest that talking to family members in order to learn about a patient's premorbid personality is desirable for sound rehabilitation planning.

The recovery timetable, though still poorly understood, seems to correlate with type and severity of aphasia. Spontaneous recovery is believed to take place up to three to six months after onset. One recent study that followed treated aphasic patients for the first year poststroke determined that all aphasic patients improved during that period, that fluent aphasic patients improved most in the first six months after onset, and that global aphasic patients improved most in the second six months. The study results suggest that in severe aphasia a longer period of time is required to develop compensatory communication strategies. Furthermore, severe patients who do not appear to be good candidates for treatment during the initial postacute stage should be reevaluated at later points to determine candidacy for treatment. Also, several recent studies found that chronic, severe patients who were provided speech therapy for several years showed notable improvements in communication function and decreased depression.

An ideal aphasia rehabilitation program is based on sound neurolinguistic and psychological principles and is composed of many parts. Various formats for speech therapy are currently in use and serve different purposes. In addition to the traditional one-to-one treatment format, which utilizes specific, direct language remediation techniques, group therapy is now being employed with greater frequency. Groups are generally designed to provide an opportunity for socialization, stimulation, facilitation, or practice in a specific modality (e.g., visual language skills). The group format is also used for patient or family education, which is an essential component of a comprehensive aphasia rehabilitation program. It is important for both patient and family to know something about aphasia; mystery and lack of knowledge breed fear and anxiety. The family is better able to deal with the patient and with their own feelings if they understand the nature of the disorder. By the same token, the patient needs to acquire certain basic information if he/she is to address some of his/her reactions and expectations.

In the ideal program, the services of a social worker are of great value. A recent national survey conducted by the National Aphasia Association[6] reported that over 92% of respondents considered personal and social isolation to be their principal problem. Friends tend not to maintain contact because of difficulties in communication, and communities are not prepared to integrate individuals with communication problems. An associated motor deficit, of course, makes matters worse. Social workers are skilled in identifying and helping to address some of these difficult realities and the feelings they evoke. In some cases the social worker will suggest services, programs, clubs, or other community activities that might be appropriate.

In the case of a patient with mild to moderate aphasia, it is often possible and appropriate to arrange for consultation with a psychologist or psychiatrist. Though traditional psychotherapy may be difficult because of language impairment, the therapist may still be able to find ways of working with an aphasic person, employing the help of the speech pathologist if necessary. In addition, psychiatric referral is sometimes needed for prescription and monitoring of a psychoactive drug, as when the patient is particularly anxious or depressed. Drug therapy can be a useful adjunct to other treatment modalities.

Speech therapy administered by a trained speech pathologist should be started early and continued as long as possible. The obvious impediments to long-term treatment are lack of availability of such treatment and financial constraints.

A number of theories have been promulgated regarding approaches to aphasia rehabilitation. It is generally agreed that one does not "teach" language to the patient and that language is not "lost" but that it is inaccessible. Recovery from aphasia is not the same as learning a language. It is the therapist's task to stimulate and facilitate the use of whatever language is still available to patients and to help them compensate by using other ways or means of transmitting their thoughts and feelings. The therapist must walk a narrow line between encouraging patients to try to develop compensatory strategies and at the same time helping them to adjust to limitations. Throughout this process patients must be allowed to experience denial and depression about the aphasia and to mourn the loss of normality. Patients appreciate commiseration, the knowledge that someone knows how badly they feel. They don't like being told to "cheer up."

In addition, the effective therapist knows how to select tasks that will be within the patient's capacity, for it is imperative that the patient avoid failure during treatment sessions, since treatment must endeavor to stimulate self-confidence. The enlightened, competent aphasia therapist develops a partnership with the patient, becomes the patient's advocate, and tries to help in the long and arduous task of adjusting to life with a communication disorder. Excellent results have been obtained in difficult cases when a speech pathologist and psychologist have worked together with the patient.

Considerable research in recent years has focused on designing and testing new treatment methods. It is beyond the scope of this chapter to describe them in any detail. Those readers interested in pursuing the specifics of the treatment of aphasia are referred to a volume by Roberta Chapey.[2] For the most current literature review and state-of-the-art information concerning classification, localization, assessment, neurolinguistics, cognition, and emotional factors in aphasia, readers are referred to the second edition of the book *Acquired Aphasia*, edited by M.T. Sarno.[8]

A new area of study with potential application to aphasia rehabilitation is the field of "alternative and augmentative communication systems," which is based on recent technological advances. The development of synthetic speech, advances in microcomputers, and new knowledge in artificial intelligence and electronics have contributed to the knowledge base in this new area. To date, none of these methods can be said to have resulted in significant improvement in functional communication across broad categories of aphasic patients. However, some of the experiments with severe global aphasic patients have been promising. The usual approach has been to develop methods of communication that are alternatives to the oral mode, such as sign languages of different kinds, gestures, or systems of symbols. Application of the latter has made use of computer technology, with some experimental success. The availability of synthetic speech and microcomputers has stimulated interest in trying to employ these technologies in aphasia rehabilitation.

The success of rehabilitation can be measured only by the degree to which the disabled person can resume a reasonably comfortable, meaningful life. This goal represents a formidable challenge in the patient who has sustained a stroke and has both physical and aphasic deficits. The field of rehabilitation medicine has accepted that challenge, and the doctors, speech pathologists, physical and occupational therapists, psychologists, and social workers have made substantial progress toward that goal in the years since this medical specialty came into being. We are confident that the dedicated, compassionate professionals trained in the techniques and philosophy of rehabilitation medicine will continue to explore the frontiers of knowledge in behalf of the severely disabled.

REFERENCES

1. Benton AL, Hamsher K de S. *Multilingual aphasia examination/Spanish.* 2nd ed. Iowa City: AJA Associates, Inc; 1989.
2. Chapey R. *Language intervention strategies in adult aphasia.* 2nd ed. Baltimore: Williams and Wilkins; 1986.
3. Holland AL. *Communicative abilities in daily living.* Baltimore: University Park Press; 1980.

4. Kottke FJ, Lehmann JF. *Krusen's Handbook of Physical Medicine and Rehabilitation*. 4th ed. Philadelphia: WB Saunders; 1990.
5. Lomas J et al. The communicative effectiveness index: development and psychometric evaluation of a functional communication measure for adult aphasia. *J Speech Hear Disord*. 1989;54:113–124.
6. National Aphasia Association. *Questionnaire survey*. New York: National Aphasia Association; 1987.
7. Sarno MT. *The functional communication profile: manual of directions*. New York: Rusk Institute of Rehabilitation Medicine, New York University Medical Center; 1969.
8. Sarno MT (ed). *Acquired aphasia*. 2nd ed. New York: Academic Press; 1991.
9. Taylor ML. A measurement of functional communication in aphasia. *Arch Phys Med Rehabil*. 1965;46:101–107.